Child Maltreatment

Contemporary Issues in Research and Policy

Volume 13

Series Editors

Jill E. Korbin, 3089 Warrington Road, Shaker Heights, Ohio 44120 USA, Cleveland, OH, USA

Richard D. Krugman, University of Colorado School of Medicine, Aurora, CO, USA

This series provides a high-quality, cutting edge, and comprehensive source offering the current best knowledge on child maltreatment from multidisciplinary and multicultural perspectives. It consists of a core handbook that is followed by two or three edited volumes of original contributions per year. The core handbook will present a comprehensive view of the field. Each chapter will summarize current knowledge and suggest future directions in a specific area. It will also highlight controversial and contested issues in that area, thus moving the field forward. The handbook will be updated every five years. The edited volumes will focus on critical issues in the field from basic biology and neuroscience to practice and policy. Both the handbook and edited volumes will involve creative thinking about moving the field forward and will not be a recitation of past research. Both will also take multidisciplinary, multicultural and mixed methods approaches.

More information about this series at http://www.springer.com/series/8863

Bernard Gerbaka • Sami Richa • Roland Tomb

Child Sexual Abuse, Exploitation and Trafficking in the Arab Region

Springer

Bernard Gerbaka
Chair of Pediatric Department
Saint Joseph University
Beirut, Lebanon

Sami Richa
Chair of Department of Psychiatry
Saint Joseph University
Beirut, Lebanon

Roland Tomb
Dean of Faculty of Medicine
Saint Joseph University
Beirut, Lebanon

ISSN 2211-9701 ISSN 2211-971X (electronic)
Child Maltreatment
ISBN 978-3-030-66506-7 ISBN 978-3-030-66507-4 (eBook)
https://doi.org/10.1007/978-3-030-66507-4

This Springer imprint is published by the registered company Springer Nature Switzerland AG.
The registered company address is: Gewerbestrasse 11, 6330 Cham, Switzerland

Acknowledgments

The Arab Professional Society for the Prevention of Violence on Children, the Lebanese Institute for Child Rights, the Kempe Foundation for the Prevention and Treatment of Child Abuse and Neglect, the Kempe Center for the Prevention and Treatment of Child Abuse and Neglect, Child Helpline International, Save the Children, the Oak Foundation, ECPAT, Susan Bissel, Anthony Lake, Marta Santos-Pais, Henrietta Fore, Kathleen Cravero, Howard Taylor, Etienne Krug, Hans Zollner, Asa Regner, Anila Ahmed, Elisabeth Dahlin, Sarah Stevenson, Alex Butchart, Sabine Rakotomala, Sergio Paulo Pinheiro, Raymond Sayegh, Charaf AbouCharaf, Awais Raoof, Cesar Bassim, Ziad Khoury, Ghassan Khoury, Antoine Maalouf, Nagib Geahchan, Joseph Otayek, Pierre Yared, Jean-Claude Lahoud, Roland Tomb, Shanti Raman, Zulficar Buttha, Fadlo Khoury, Selim Daccache, Fady Yarak, Violette Safadi, Amal Farhat-Bassil, Marie-Claude Fadous-Khalife, Myriam Amm-Abi Ghosn, Nidal Barakat-Hage, Habib Hage, Elie Attieh, Angy Fenianos, Gisele Daccache-Dagher, Miguel Abboud, Zaki Ghorayeb, Gaia Gerbaka, Nour-Estelle Gerbaka, Joe Gerbaka, Marianne Naami-Majdalani, Bassem AbouMerhi, Maha AbouAlfa, Mona-Lisa Alame, Maroun Mattar, Mhamad Mahdi, Michel Khoury, Gaby Fallakha, Abdallah Bissar, Ghaiss Makhoul, Elie Aramouni, Mhamad Itani, Leila Akoury-Dirani, Claire Ghafari-Zablit, Rima Mawad, Lena Ghannage, P. Marek Cieslick, Nabil Diab, Georges Beyrouthy, Hadi Fakih, Ghassan Baassiri, Diala Hamdane, Catherine Daubrege, Zeina Hobeiche, Nagi Souaiby, Elie Mikhael, Hani Jahshan, Majid El Eissa, Jamila Bia, Aida Gorbel, Adib Essali, Afra ElBasti, Hassan Kassim, Abdelouadoud Kharbouch, Fadheela Al-Mahroos, Randa Yousef, Mona Saadoon, Mona Khawari, Aisha Midfa, Essam Ali, Faouzi Bendridi, Fatma Eissa, Mohamad Sheikh, Suad Marzooqi, Richard Roylance, Jenny Gray, Joan Van Niekerk, Martin Finkel, Howard Dubowitz, Irene Cheah, Kevin Lalor, Myriam Caranzano-Maitre, Randall Alexander, Isabel Cuadros, Sue Foley, Toshihiko Yanagawa, Florence Bruce, Michael Dougherty, John Myers JD, Judge Carlos Rozanski, Arnon Bentovim, Donald Bross, Barbara Bonner, Danya Glaser, Marcellina Mian, R. Kim Oates, Irene Intebi, Tufail Muhammad, Rajeev Seth, Richard Krugman, Jill Korbin, Desmond Runyan, Henry Plum, Patricia Peterson,

Itamar Batista Goncalves, Marianne Bentovim, Alessandra Guedes, Benedito Rodrigues dos Santos, Yumiko Kirino, Carlos Rozanski, Janet Saul, Julia Sloth-Nielsen, Katrina Legarda, Marielle Dekker, Brenda Mirabal, Jill-Ellyn Straus, Reinhard Fitchl, Suzanne Tiapula, Viola Vaughn-Eden, John E. B. Myers, and Chris Newlin.

Countries' reports to the CRC. 1997–2003. Concluding Observations of the Committee Algeria, Iraq, Kuwait, Yemen, Jordan, Saudi Arabia, Egypt, Oman, Qatar, Bahrain, Emirates, Israel, Lebanon, Tunisia, Libya, Morocco, Sudan, and Syria.

Abstract

Child sexual abuse and exploitation (CSAE) is a violation of child rights. The diverse manifestations of CSAE and child trafficking (CT) are associated with significant adverse consequences throughout the child's life.[1]

Extensive research on adverse childhood events (ACE), over the past few decades, indicates that children who are victims of sexual abuse are significantly more likely to suffer emotional problems throughout their lives; such problems include anxiety, anger, PTSD, low self-esteem, impaired self-concept, depression, and suicidal thoughts and behaviors; they are also more at risk to run away from home, to use illegal drugs, to bear substance abuse, including legal products (alcohol, tobacco, marijuana—where applicable—etc.), and to engage in risky sexual behavior.[2]

Obviously, much of this knowledge is based on data from North America; however, diverse findings across Europe and the Arab region overall corroborate similar consequences of child sexual abuse on child health, in terms of morbidity and survival.[3]

In light of the recent growing and spreading armed conflicts and social events in the MENA and Gulf region, Arab states increasingly face new challenges in child protection from CSAE and CT. Many other types and contexts of violence expose the child to the added burden of abuse: on one hand, abduction and kidnapping, early marriage and rape, armed conflicts and riots, refugee and displaced children, child labor and exploitation, etc., and on the other hand, institutions often shut down or become virtual; child-related observatories are either politicized or hardly listened to; and even professionals find this political turmoil hard to cope with, in terms of delivery of expertise and services.

[1]English, D.J. The extent and consequences of child maltreatment. The Future of Children, Protecting Children from Abuse & Neglect 1988; 8: 1: 39–53 13.

[2]Berlinger and Elliott (2002).

[3]May-Chahal and Herczog (2003).

In such contexts, the prevention of child abuse and neglect (CAN) and violence against children (VAC) is at stake, in terms of social programs, child rights implementation, and national processes, mainly in the fields of CSAE and CT.

The 2010 OIC recommendations, the 2016 Global Partnership to #endviolence against children, the INSPIRE WHO strategy, and Agenda 2020 offer a new hope for children in the Arab region.[4]

End Violence Against Children
THE GLOBAL PARTNERSHIP

[4] Cairo Declaration on the Convention (CRC) and Islamic Jurisprudence. Cairo. November 23 and 24, 2009.

Contents

Abbreviations

#endviolence	The Global Partnership to End Violence against Children
ACCD	Arab Council for Childhood and Development
ACHR	Arab Charter on Human Rights
ACRWC	African Charter on the Rights and Welfare of the Child
AGFUND	Arab Gulf Program for United Nations Development Organizations
AIHR	Arab Institute for Human Rights
ALESCO	Arab League Educational, Cultural and Scientific Organization
APSPVAC	The Arab Professional Society for Prevention of Violence against Children
ARC	Arab Resource Collective
AU	African Union
CAN	Child abuse and neglect
CHI	Child Helpline International
CPI	Child Protection Initiative
CRC	Convention on the Rights of the Child
CSO/CSOs	Civil society organization/Civil society organizations
CSA	Child sexual abuse
CSE	Child sexual exploitation
CSAE	Child sexual abuse and exploitation
CPS	Child Protection Services
CRC	Convention on the Rights of the Child
CT	Child trafficking
ECM/EFCM	Early child marriage/forced child marriage
ECPAT	End Child Prostitution and Trafficking
ERW	Landmines and explosive remnants of war
EU	European Union
FGM/FGC	Female genital mutilation/cutting
GC13	the 13th comment of the CRC articles, currently Article 19, on the protection of children from violence

GCC	Gulf Cooperation Council (also known as the CCASG: Cooperation Council for the Arab States of the Gulf)
HIV/AIDS	Human immunodeficiency virus/acquired immunodeficiency syndrome
HRC	Human Rights Commission
HRW	Human Rights Watch
IBCR	International Bureau for Children's Rights
I-CAST	The International Child Abuse Screening Tool
ICRC	International Committee of the Red Cross
I-CRC	International Committee on the Rights of the Child
ILO	International Labour Organization
INSPIRE	WHO Strategy to #endviolence
INTRAC	International NGO and Training Centre
ISESCO	Islamic, Educational, Scientific and Cultural Organization
ISPCAN	The International Society for the Prevention of Child Abuse and Neglect
KPH	Killing for the purpose of Honor (Honor crimes)
LAS	League of Arab States
MENA	Middle East and North Africa
National body	the high-level structure in charge of the strategy in Arab States
NCCI	NGO Coordination Committee in Iraq
NGO/NGOs	Non-Governmental Organization/Non-Governmental Organizations
NPA	National Plan of Action
OAU	Organisation of African Unity
OIC	Organization of the Islamic Conference
OMCT	World Organisation against Torture/Organisation Mondiale Contre la Torture
OPT/oPt	Occupied Palestinian Territories
SCS	Save the Children – Sweden
SCUK	Save the Children – United Kingdom
SCUS	Save the Children – United States
SIDA	Swedish International Development Cooperation Agency
STD	Sexually transmitted disease
UAE	United Arab Emirates
UN	United Nations
UNCRC	United Nations Convention on the Rights of the Child
UNDP	United Nations Development Programme
UNESCO	United Nations Educational, Social and Cultural Organization
UNHCR	UN Refugee Agency/Office of the UN High Commissioner for Refugees
UNODC	United Nations Office on Drugs and Crimes
UNICEF	United Nations Children's Fund
UNOHCR	Office of the United Nations High Commissioner for Human Rights

UNRWA	United Nations Relief and Works Agency for Palestine Refugees in the Near East
UNVAC	The United Nations Secretary-General's Study on Violence against Children
VAC	Violence against children

About the Author

Bernard Gerbaka is Professor of Pediatrics at St Joseph University in Beirut, Chair of the Pediatric Department, Chair of the Mother-and-Child Pole, and member of the Faculty of Medicine Council. He is Chairperson of the Pediatric Division, Director of the Child Protection Unit, and coordinator of Pediatric Emergencies in Hotel-Dieu University Hospital.

He works in the fields of child health, child abuse, violence against children, and child injuries prevention and safety promotion; he developed child safety and protection programs with MoH, MoSA, MoE, MoJ, UNICEF, and WHO, as well as health, social, education, and law schools and professionals.

He is a former member of the City Council of Beirut, and has founded the first Child safety committee in the LOP in 1998, the first Child and Youth Commission in Beirut Municipal Council[5] in 2004 and the child protection committee[6] in the Higher Council for Childhood in 2004,[7] and the first hospital-based child protection unit in Lebanon in 2009, leading to introduction of child abuse and neglect into the health curriculum.

He also works on research on child protection with the United Nations and the League of Arab States and the I-CAST instrument. He participated in the setting of the UNVAC in 2004,[8]the Lebanese report on the Situation of Children in 2004,[9] the

[5]Deeb M, Gerbaka B, Ajouz-Sidani R, Kheir-El-Kadi M,: The vulnerable and disadvantaged children in Arab cities. Child and the City Conference, Amman, 2004.

[6]BUILDING A MULTISECTORAL TASKFORCE IN LEBANON FOR THE PREVENTION OF CHILD ABUSE AND NEGLECT; Public Health Approaches to Child Maltreatment: Prevention as a Priority; Bernard GERBAKA, TOWN AND COUNTRY RESORT & CONVENTION CENTER, SAN DIEGO, CA; JANUARY 23, 2006

[7]Ministère de la justice http:www.justice.gov.lb/alahdath

[8]The MENA Regional Consultation on Violence against Children, Cairo, June 2005.

[9]The MENA Regional Consultation on Violence against Children, Cairo, June 2005.

Lebanese delegation to the 2006 Geneva ICRC meeting,[10] and the Lebanese response to the UNVAC in 2007.[11]

He is the President of the Lebanese Institute for Child Rights www.ChildOfLebanon.org, former President of the Lebanese Union for Child Protection www.UPEL-lb.net, and Vice-President of the University Child and Youth Observatory in Lebanon Oeil@usj.edu.lb

He has published on child health, child injuries, child safety, child abuse, violence against children, and child protection.[12,13]

Within the child protection network in the Arab region, Prof. GERBAKA founded, with colleagues from the Arab region, the Arab professional network for the prevention of CAN (2004) and the Arab professional society for the prevention of violence against children (2012) and was elected within the board of the International society for the prevention of CAN (2008–2014 and 2014–2020) where he chaired the TCER (Training, Consultation and External Relations), and was recently elected President of ISPCAN for the period 2016–2018, www.ISPCAN.org. He also worked in the data collection working group (WGDCCM, ISPCAN) and the RAP committee of Child Helpline International www.ChildHelplineInternational.org

Bernard Gerbaka also created 3 websites dedicated to child protection www.ChildOfLebanon.org, to vaccine preventable diseases www.infovac-lb.org, and to community education on child heath www.ChildHealthRight.org.

Bernard Gerbaka has published on child health, child injuries, child safety, child abuse and neglect, violence against children, and child protection; he presently works on study and promotion of adolescent health, strengthening breast-feeding and cocoon vaccination, data collection on VPDs, training of health professionals on vaccinations, pediatric emergencies, and child protection, as well as on CM and child sexual abuse, bullying and cyberbullying, VAC in the Arab region, child deaths, corporal punishment, and positive parenting; university courses on immunization and emergency pediatrics; VPD awareness campaigns (HPV, flu, PCV, adolescent and cocoon vaccination); and advocacy for the universal rights for protection from VPDs, as an integrated component of the CRC. Bernard GERBAKA is also a member of the INSPIRE WHO board on Violence and Injuries Prevention and contributes to the global strategy and the parenting program; he is also a member of the board of the UN Global Partnership to End Violence against Children.[14]

---

[10]The reply of the Lebanese state on the UN questionnaire on VAC, Bernard GERBAKA, Sana' AWADA, Elie MIKHAEL, 2004.

[11]The National Report of Lebanese Associations and NGO's. Narrative Report (Supplement). Presented to the Committee on the Rights of the Child, Geneva, November 1995.

[12]The reply of the Lebanese state on the UN questionnaire on VAC, Bernard GERBAKA, Sana' AWADA, Elie MIKHAEL, 2004.

[13]The prevention of child abuse and neglect [CAN] is a long-standing teamwork, relies on a regional expertise and needs an international cooperation; Bernard GERBAKA, TOWN AND COUNTRY RESORT & CONVENTION CENTER, SAN DIEGO, CA. January 26, 2006.

[14]Toward an Efficient Child Protective Strategy in Lebanon: A Call for Pediatricians' True Child Advocacy. G. Hage, B.Gerbaka, Pediatrica 2007.

Sami Richa Chair of Department of Psychiatry, Saint Joseph University, Beirut, Lebanon.

Roland Tomb Dean of Faculty of Medicine, Saint Joseph University, Beirut, Lebanon.

Part I
Perspectives and Purpose

Chapter 1
Objectives of the Present Book

This book collates and brings together the available information on CSA in the Arab region, as well as efforts to address the multiple types of CSAET and respond to the expanding burden of its diverse presentations. The purpose of the book is to show the quality of the work already done and the terrible plight of CSAET on children.

More specifically, this book will:

- Present a background for the situation of Rights of the Child in the Arab region, in terms of child protection from CSAE and CT.
- Build the knowledge base on CSAE and CT.
- Reflect the extent of challenges and achievements to the recommendations of the UNVAC.
- Assess the Arab efforts to stop sexual violence against children during the past years.
- Contribute in the monitoring of sexual violence against children and to identify specific problems and priorities.
- Highlight the implementation of the Arab countries to the UNVAC concerning CSAE.
- Propose mechanisms of implementation for child protection within Arab countries
- Share a road map on an Arab vision of the future steps of children protection from CSAE and CT
- Help setting an action plan to combat sexual violence against children, including:
  - Developing policies and programs.
  - Identifying agencies responsible for coordination of implementation.
  - Stressing on the needs in terms of funds and human resources.
  - Developing indicators to evaluate performance and follow-up implementation.
- Advocate for peaceful, safe , healthy and happy environments for children and their families

B. Gerbaka et al., *Child Sexual Abuse, Exploitation and Trafficking in the Arab Region*, Child Maltreatment 13, https://doi.org/10.1007/978-3-030-66507-4_1

Chapter 2
Introduction

The definition of the child is contained in article 1 of the Convention: "every human being below the age of 18 years unless, under the law applicable to the child, the majority is attained earlier". The present definition is adopted by most countries in the Middle East and North Africa regions (MENA).[1]

Violence is defined as presented in the WHO World Report on Violence and Health: "the intentional use of physical force or power, threatened or actual, against oneself, another person, or against a group or community that either results in or has a high likelihood of resulting in injury, death, psychological harm, mal development or deprivation".

Violence against children is a global problem. Children experience violence in schools, in institutions, on the streets, in the workplace, in prisons, as well as in their own homes. Violence can affect children's physical and mental health, impair their ability to learn and socialize and undermine their development as functional adults and good parents later in life. In the most severe cases, violence against children leads to death.[2,3]

Violence against children, including sexual violence, is a violation of children's rights. Article 19 of the Convention on the Rights of the Child (1989) calls all countries for legislative, administrative, social and educational actions to protect children from all forms of violence and abuse.[4]

Child sexual abuse or child molestation is a form of child abuse in which an adult or older adolescent uses a child for sexual stimulation. Forms of child sexual abuse

---

[1] *Child Sexual Abuse in the Middle East and North Africa: A Review.*

[2] Finkelhor, D , Hotaling, G., Lewis, L.A., Smith C. Sexual abuse in a national survey of adult men and women: Prevalence, characteristics, and risk factors. Child Abuse & Neglect 1990;14/1:19–28.

[3] Schwendinger, J. and Schwendinger, H. A Review of the Rape Literature. Crime and Social Justice. 1976; (Fall-Winter):79–85.

[4] Scher, C., Forde, D., McQuaid, J. and Stein, M. Prevalence and demographic correlates of childhood maltreatment in an adult community sample. Child Abuse & Neglect. 2004; 28: 167–180.

B. Gerbaka et al., *Child Sexual Abuse, Exploitation and Trafficking in the Arab Region*, Child Maltreatment 13, https://doi.org/10.1007/978-3-030-66507-4_2

include engaging in sexual activities with a child (whether by asking or pressuring, or by other means), indecent exposure (of the genitals, female nipples, etc.), child grooming, or using a child to produce child pornography.

Child sexual abuse can occur in a variety of settings, including home, school, or work (in places where child labor is common). Child marriage is one of the main forms of child sexual abuse; UNICEF has stated that child marriage "represents perhaps the most prevalent form of sexual abuse and exploitation of girls". The effects of child sexual abuse can include depression, post-traumatic stress disorder, anxiety, complex post-traumatic stress disorder, propensity to further victimization in adulthood, and physical injury to the child, among other problems. Sexual abuse by a family member is a form of incest and can result in more serious and long-term psychological trauma, especially in the case of parental incest.

The global prevalence of child sexual abuse has been estimated at 19.7% for females and 7.9% for males. Most sexual abuse offenders are acquainted with their victims; approximately 30% are relatives of the child, most often brothers, fathers, uncles, or cousins; around 60% are other acquaintances, such as "friends" of the family, babysitters, or neighbors; strangers are the offenders in approximately 10% of child sexual abuse cases. Most child sexual abuse is committed by men; studies on female child molesters show that women commit 14% to 40% of offenses reported against boys and 6% of offenses reported against girls.

The word pedophile is commonly applied indiscriminately to anyone who sexually abuses a child, but child sexual offenders are not pedophiles unless they have a strong sexual interest in prepubescent children. Under the law, *child sexual abuse* is often used as an umbrella term describing criminal and civil offenses in which an adult engages in sexual activity with a minor or exploits a minor for the purpose of sexual gratification. The American Psychological Association states that "children cannot consent to sexual activity with adults", and condemns any such action by an adult: "An adult who engages in sexual activity with a child is performing a criminal and immoral act which never can be considered normal or socially acceptable behavior."

The UN study on violence against children examined violence in the Middle East, North Africa and the Gulf Region, its different forms, its causes, and its impact on children, thus identifying the necessary measures for eradicating this phenomenon and the responsible actors, including children themselves, in protecting themselves from exposure to violence [recommendation of the UN General Assembly in its resolution no. 57/190].

The Committee on the Rights of the Child (CRC) also recommended that this study should lead to the development of intervention strategies that aim at protecting children from all forms of violence, with a view to effectively providing the needed protection and prevention [A/56/488].

The regional 2005 UNVAC consultation in Cairo was the first step in the development of regional interaction, followed by the meeting of national teams with the I-CRC in Geneva in 2006 and again the Cairo conference in 2007. Those important landmarks allowed stakeholders in a growing number of Arab countries to enhance interaction between international organizations and national representatives, while increasing the networking with Councils for Childhood, National Committees for the prevention of violence, Women and children ministries, as well as other official bodies within governmental structures.

The purpose of this process is to combat CAN and reduce VAC in the Arab region, while installing appropriation structures for efficient programs that would be accepted and developed by diverse cultures in the region.

Chapter 3
The Rationale

3.1 Abstract

Child sexual abuse and exploitation (CSAE) is not a new phenomenon—it is documented in the written and verbal histories from all cultures.[1]

Child sexual abuse and exploitation remains an issue for all peoples of all nations—regardless of race, culture or religion.

Children are sexually abused and exploited in all their livehoods and environments:

- homes;
- extended kinship and friendship networks;
- 'physical' neighborhoods;
- 'virtual' neighborhoods;
- 'formal' institutions (e.g. schools and churches); and
- 'informal' institutions (e.g. sports and recreational clubs).

3.2 CSA Occurs in All Settings and Cultures[2]

Specific definitions of child sexual abuse vary between disciplines, nations and cultural groups; such definitions and norms have further evolved within those groups over time. This is not dissimilar to other areas of human interaction where significant change has occurred in the globalization of standards of what constitutes acceptable human behavior (i.e. abolishment of slavery, establishment of guidelines for

[1]Yazdi, S. 2000. On Prevalence of Physical Child Abuse among Admitted Cases in Selected Pediatric Clinics and Emergency Wards in Tehran.

[2]Finkelhor, D. and associates. A Sourcebook on Child Sexual Abuse. Beverly Hills: Sage, 1986.

B. Gerbaka et al., *Child Sexual Abuse, Exploitation and Trafficking in the Arab Region*, Child Maltreatment 13, https://doi.org/10.1007/978-3-030-66507-4_3

management of physical violence at the national (i.e. armed conflict), community (i.e. neighborhood violence) or family (i.e. inter-personal) level.

Despite variation in some aspects of definitions, there is universal acceptance across national, cultural and religious groups that there are aspects of sexual interaction (including some which are acceptable in sexually and developmentally mature humans—i.e. 'adults') for which children are developmentally unprepared; and that these sexual interactions are predominately harmful to children.[3] Such child sexual abuse and exploitation has been universally declared as unacceptable and harmful by all national, cultural, and religious sects.

Child sexual abuse commonly does not exist in isolation from the other forms of child abuse and neglect (i.e. child physical abuse, child emotional abuse, child neglect), and shares many of the same risk factors. In different settings and cultures, interventions aimed at the prevention and treatment of child sexual abuse and exploitation must be designed with this complex social and professional interaction in mind.

3.3 CSA in the Global Perspective

Global changes in communication technologies are associated with changes in the 'type' and 'degree of risk' for sexual abuse and exploitation to which children may be exposed (e.g. electronic media; electronic social networks; digital imagining; etc.)—through entrapment and by exposure to developmentally inappropriate 'sexualized' material. This risk may transcend local community, national, cultural or religious boundaries. The 'globalization' of world economies and increased ease of travel have led to an increased vulnerability for children to sex trafficking, sex tourism, internet sex and bullying as examples of child trafficking.

As child sexual abuse and child sexual exploitation of are not issues which fall solely within the family environment, nor solely outside of it—the responsibility for the prevention and treatment of child sexual abuse and child sexual exploitation must be shared between parents/guardians, the State, and the international community more broadly (Article 19 of the UN CRC).

[3]This statement needs to be used appropriately. What makes a sexual interaction problematic can be the age difference, degree of force involved or just how sexual (i.e. intrusive) the behavior is). Children of about the same age involved in non-coercive exploitation would not necessarily result in harm.

3.4 CSA Is a National and Multidisciplinary Problem in All Countries

The development of a global, trans-national, trans-cultural, trans-ethnic and trans-religious approach to the prevention, identification, and treatment of child abuse and neglect is an important goal.

The prevention of child abuse and neglect (CAN) and violence against children [VAC) is based on a human rights vision, involving universal child rights and national processes. The consequences of CSAE are damaging on many aspects of the child's present and future life. In fact, several studies reported on the consequences of CSAE. For example, Hay-Yahia and Tamish (2001: 1318–1319) found that child sexual abuse was related to numerous measures of mental health problems 'including psychoticism, hostility, anxiety, somatization, phobic anxiety, paranoid ideation, depression, obsessive-compulsiveness, and psychological distress.'[4]

The research on women in Morocco and on college men in Jordan likewise found a strong relationship between CSA and poorer mental health later in life as an adult (Jumaian 2001; Alami and Kadri 2004). In Egypt, Afifi et al. (2003) found that CSAR significantly increased the odds of the victim subsequently perpetrating physical and sexual abuse as a teen.[5]

These results for the Middle East and North Africa are consistent in finding that child sexual abuse has serious adverse consequences. In turn, these findings are consistent with the prior research in North America, Europe and elsewhere on the adverse effects of child abuse.

Given the neurobiological research that has demonstrated the changes in the child's brain and central nervous system as a result of child maltreatment, it is not surprising that arrays of adverse consequences of CSA throughout the victims' life are found globally (Perry 1997; Anda et al. 2006). Among many others, those are reasons to justify tackling CSAE and taking corrective measures at State and community levels, as well as in family and individual lifestyles.

3.5 CSA Is a National and Multidisciplinary Problem in the Arab Region

Since the meeting with the UN special representative for the study on violence in 2003, the Arab region was involved in the UNSV (UN Study of Violence) in many tracks

[4]Haj-Yahia, M., et. al. 2002. "The Incidence of Adolescent Maltreatment in Arab Society and Some of Its Psychological Effects." In Journal of Family Issues, 23/8.

[5]Afifi, Z.E. M., El-Lawindi, M., Ahmed, S. and Basily, W. Adolescent abuse in a community sample in Beni Suef, Egypt: prevalence and risk factors. Eastern Mediterranean Health Journal 2003; 9: 5/6.

- Research, through studies, questionnaires and qualitative data - involving academic sectors and NGOs,
- Advocacy, with the involvement of multiple agencies in the UNSV, including governmental structures and civil societies,
- Training of professionals, with multidisciplinary tools, some of them developed with the WHO and UNICEF, as frameworks and guidelines for intersectoral approach to the prevention of child abuse,
- Capacity building, by setting or developing multidisciplinary teams within national structures
- Tools for child protection, culturally adapted by national teams, in order to set strategies for the prevention of VAC
- Evaluation, integrated within program implementation, with the purpose of enhancing transparency, sustainability and efficiency.

3.6 Multi-dimensional Issues

Child sexual abuse and exploitation can be considered from a number of different (but independently legitimately) perspectives. Examples of such perspectives are to consider child sexual abuse as a:

3.6.1 Criminal Justice

Child sexual abuse and exploitation are universally recognized as criminal acts that require some type of legal and correctional response. The role of punishment as a means to prevent future child sexual abuse, and as a response to the harm suffered by the victim is a corner stone of the legal response. In some systems, a therapeutic response is also attached to the criminal response. Restorative justice may also play a part in this process. Legal and investigative services need to keep the rights of the child—in addition to the right of the accused in mind. Specific developmental issues in regard to children (cognitive, linguistic and social) need to be accommodated by legal and criminal systems to allow children equal rights and opportunities within these systems. However, ad hoc criminalization and isolated punishment have shown to provide a limited and incomplete mechanism to prevent, treat and protect children from child sexual abuse and exploitation; more social and individual interventions are often needed in order to provide optimal resilience and reintegration of victims, as well as rehabilitation of perpetrators.

3.6.2 Child Rights

Child sexual abuse and exploitation is a child rights violation because children have the right to be safe from sexual abuse and exploitation—which may also be associated with other forms of abuse and maltreatment. International meetings and programs have expressed an aspirational consensus regarding the well-being of children that encompasses the problem of child sexual abuse. These include:

- the UN Convention on the Rights of the Child (CRC) and optional protocols;
- the role of national government policy and resource allocation to ensure that efforts are made to ensure the creation of a world fit for children;
- the Millennium Development Goals;
- the United Nations Secretary-General's Study on Violence against Children (2006).

3.6.3 Child Health and Well-Being

Child sexual abuse and exploitation are a child health and well-being issue because child sexual abuse poses serious physical health and mental health risks for children across their lifespan. In order to improve well-being, people adversely affected by child sexual abuse need effective assessment, treatment, and intervention. These include medical, mental health, reparative developmental care, non-offending caregiver support and reunification consulting.

3.6.4 Family and Community Well-Being Concepts

Child sexual abuse and exploitation are well-being issues for families and communities because child sexual abuse erodes trust, reinforces abuse of power, and adversely impacts family relationships.

3.6.5 Public Health Perspective

Child sexual abuse and exploitation is a public health issue because of its pervasive nature; the adverse effects upon the health and well-being of individuals, their families and the broader community; and because effective identification, treatment and prevention requires interventions at all levels of the community. An opportunity for sexual offenders and community members affected by child sexual abuse to access effective interventions is an essential part of the public health approach.

3.6.6 Risk Management

Child sexual abuse and exploitation are risk management issues for families, organizations, and the broader community. System measures need to be established to protect children; and to manage risks of potential future harm after incidents of sexual abuse have occurred (e.g. screening of possible offenders) in order to ensure the safety of children in organizations, schools and other institutions.

3.6.7 Related Services

Child sexual abuse and exploitation are related services issues because child sexual abuse victims are overly represented in healthcare and mental health services, and overly represented in juvenile services and criminal institutions. Therefore culturally appropriate and effective intervention and prevention strategies need to be developed—capable of effectively bridging historical organizational divides.

3.6.8 Employment and Essential Education

Child sexual abuse and exploitation are employment and education issues because child sexual abuse adversely affects children in terms of their education and employment options—the effects potentially extending throughout the adult life-cycle, and extending into the next generation.

3.6.9 Professional Education

Child sexual abuse and exploitation are professional education issues because all professional and ancillary staff involved with children, adults and families require specialized training to maximize effective identification, prevention and intervention capacities.

3.6.10 International Issues

Child sexual abuse and child sexual exploitation are international issues because modern changes in transport, information technology and migration require an international approach for the implementation of effective interventions.

Child sexual abuse and exploitation is an important issue for:

- Governments;
- Law Makers, Law Enforcement & Courts;
- Policy Makers;
- Communities & Societies—regardless of their specific linguistic, cultural, ethnic, geographical or political characteristics;
- Organizations & Institutions: esp. schools, religious and recreational organizations;
- Prisons & Treatment Facilities for offenders;
- Cultural & Religious Groups;
- Practitioners—working with children and their families;
- Families;
- Individual adults;
- Individual children;
- Media Organizations;
- Organizations with roles in promoting health, well-being, education and justice.

3.7 The Situation of CSA in the Arab Region

Despite initiatives at the level of countries as well as regional bodies on working for the welfare of children through strengthening existing instruments or producing new ones the situation of the rights of children in the MENA region is still in need to be improved in a number of areas.[6] There is a sense that the system is not totally independent of the powers of the religious communities and senior community members. The functioning of the statutory child protection mechanism is influenced by its relationship with the religious courts—to an extent, it was suggested, that the government judges work in the shadow of the religious courts. This pattern stands in stark contrast to the pattern for the sexual abuse of girls which can be seen within the larger societal context of oppression of women. The more patriarchal a society is, the greater the discrimination against females, the more unequal access to resources and power, including the power to protect oneself from violence, and the greater the violence against women and girls including rape, incest, child sexual abuse of girls, sexual harassment and exploitation.[7] Understood within this context, the similarities between rape and child sexual abuse/incest are more clear including the fact that for both the majority of victims are females, the majority of perpetrators are males and more often family members (for incest/CSA, fathers, uncles, mother's boyfriend, older brothers or cousins, etc.; for rape, husbands, boyfriends, dates). As Heise (1994) states, *while men and women are victims of violence, men tend to be attacked and killed by strangers or casual acquaintances, whereas women are most at risk at*

---

[6]Shalhoub-Kevorkian, N. The politics of disclosing female sexual abuse: A case study of Palestinian society. Child Abuse & Neglect 1999;23:1275–1293.

[7]Russell (1984), Schwendinger and Schwendinger (1976).

home from men whom they trust . . . . Violence against women is grounded in power imbalances between men and women and is caused and perpetuated by factors different than violence against men. As such, it must be analyzed and addressed differently. Likewise, at least for the US, research suggests that sexual abuse of girls and boys may have a different etiology (i.e., male perpetrators of sexual violence against girls and women more likely to have been physically abused as a child, while perpetrators of sexual abuse of boys more likely to have been sexually abused themselves as a child). If so, prevention of CSA of boys and girls would require at least some differences in policies to address each.

All the states in the Middle East and North Africa (MENA) region have ratified the United Nations Convention on the Rights of the Child (CRC). Following the ratification of the CRC, MENA countries have enacted or propose to enact laws to protect children from violence, abuse, neglect or exploitation. A number of countries have put in place comprehensive Child Laws that bring together legal provisions for the protection of the child.[8] In countries where no comprehensive child law has been introduced, specific laws have been adopted or amended to better promote child protection.

The Committee on the Rights of the Child has welcomed these legislative reforms, but consistently recommended MENA countries to expedite the adoption and enforcement of proposed laws, to strengthen efforts to provide better legal protection for children, and to ensure that relevant domestic laws are in full conformity with the principles and provisions of the CRC, through enacting new legislations and or amending existing ones.

[8]Marrakech Declaration, 2010, Fourth Arab High Level Conference on the Rights of the Child, Marrakech, 19–21 December 2010, adopted by the 23th Session of the Council of the League of Arab States at the Summit level in Baghdad, 2012: http://www.childsrights.org/html/site_fr/cnews/userfiles/file/Marrakech_Declaration%20English%20final%20version.pdf

Chapter 4
Background of the Book

4.1 Abstract

4.1.1 The Recognition

Within the sphere of international development, the move towards developing a more comprehensive approach to child welfare has been gathering pace in recent years.[1] There is increasing global recognition that a more integrated and systems-based approach is required at the national level to prevent and protect children from all forms of violence, abuse, neglect and exploitation.

4.1.2 The Global Debate

Within the global debate, emphasis is increasingly shifting towards a more holistic approach, encompassing proactive and preventive child and family welfare services rather than simply reactive interventions after violence or abuse has occurred. Exclusive focus on the child victim is gradually moving towards interventions directed at the whole family, aiming to improve parents' capacities to provide appropriate care and protection or to provide alternative family based care for children who cannot live with their own family. Although a systems approach has long been a feature of countries with more developed social welfare provisions, the traditional model of service provision in developing countries has generally focused on 'categories' of children: orphans, trafficked children, street children, working children.

[1]Finkelhor, D. The international epidemiology of child sexual abuse, Child Abuse & Neglect 1994; 18: 5: 409–417.

B. Gerbaka et al., *Child Sexual Abuse, Exploitation and Trafficking in the Arab Region*, Child Maltreatment 13, https://doi.org/10.1007/978-3-030-66507-4_4

4.1.3 Challenges

In countries experiencing multiple and complex child protection challenges in a context of limited resources, this 'one-off' issue-based approach reduces potential for synergy between direct services provided. Similarly, the often uniform categorization used is problematic and rarely based on actual needs of individual children. Without a holistic perspective of the lives of children and families, critical interconnected aspects of the situations and problems confronting them may be missed.[2]

Understanding the influence of politics, religion and cultural or traditional systems is another essential aspect of advocating social and behavioral change in the way children are perceived and treated. Sensitivity is clearly required when violent, exploitive or abusive practices are linked to prevailing traditions or cultural beliefs.[3]

4.1.4 Shifting the Paradigm

In such cases, a paradigm shift may be needed; one that approaches the proposed programs and services in an integrated manner and with a systematic frame of reference. Another feature of the system-building approach is the emphasis placed upon early intervention and family support. Priority is given to prevention measures and long-term care rather than reactive crisis intervention for individual child protection cases.

There is increasing recognition that to ensure this more holistic approach, it is essential to develop a strong local-level infrastructure for child welfare and justice, including organized and regulated continuum of care and protection services.

4.2 The Cassandra Data on Boys and Girls

Given these serious consequences, data on the prevalence of child sexual abuse (CSA) are even more disturbing. Estimates from national epidemiological as well as regional samples of adults over 18 in the US using similar measures of CSA have been remarkably consistent since the mid-1980s.[4] On average, roughly 16% of males and 27% of females report experiencing at least one episode of CSA, either

[2]Heise, L., Ellsberg, M. and Gottemoeller, M. Ending Violence against Women. Population Reports, Series L, No. 11. Baltimore: Johns Hopkins University School of Public Health, Population Information Program, 1999.

[3]Ashoori, M. et al. 2002. The Study of the Situation of Child Abuse in Iran. UNICEF. Iran.

[4]Russell (1986), Finkelhor et al. (1990, 1997), Dong et al. (2003), Briere and Elliott (2003), Scher et al. (2004).

non-contact (e.g., exhibition) and/or contact (fondling and/or penetration) abuse, before the age of 18. The best estimates for contact sexual abuse including both fondling and rape are 6%–9% for males and 23%–30% for females; for contact abuse-fondling, 8% for males and 22% for females; for contact abuse—intercourse or any penetration, 6% for males and 12% for females.

Boys and girls are victims of sexual abuse. In part this reflects the powerlessness of children in societies or what has been referred to as adultism.[5] Children as a group are more vulnerable to violent victimization as they are denied access to societal resources including protection from violence, and are to varying degrees seen as the property of parents. It is also clear from research to date that girls are much more likely to be victimized than boys, with gender differences even more pronounced at the more severe levels of sexual abuse—i.e., both categories of contact abuse. In addition, while girls are the majority of victims of CSA, males are the majority of perpetrators who sexually abuse boys (80%) and girls (95%) both for reported cases of abuse and general population surveys.[6] Girls are much more likely than boys to be sexually abused by family members; in contrast boys are more likely to be older when victimized, abused by non-family members, and by men who are known to have sexually abused other children.[7] The latter point fits with discussions who found evidence that males who abuse boys were themselves more likely to have been sexually abused as a child by a male,[8] and that these men were not 'homosexuals' as their attraction was to older boys not men.[9]

4.3 The Timing of This Book: More Than 15 Years After the Arab Regional Consultation on Violence Against Children

This work comes in the framework of the follow-up and implementation of the study of the Secretary General of the United Nations "on combating violence against children". In order to achieve the objectives for the plan, the second Arab Children's Fund on the protection of children invested in careful management of the family and children, with the purpose of following up the Arab region efforts as well as the international achievements to stop VAC, including the regional consultation of the UNVAC (2006).

---

[5]Lombardo and Polonko (2010), Freeman (1997).

[6]Finkelhor et al. (1986: 126).

[7]Berlinger and Elliott (2002: 57).

[8]Russell (1984: 197) and Finkelhor et al. (1986: 102–103) of the early classic studies by Gebhard, Groth and others.

[9]Berliner, L. and Elliott, D. 'Sexual Abuse of Children.' In: Myers, J., Berliner, L., Briere J., Hendrix, C., Jenny, C., and Reid, T., editors. The APSAC Handbook on Child Maltreatment, second Edition. Thousand Oaks, CA: Sage Publications, 2002. Pp. 55–78.

The UNVAC mechanism developed this regional consultation,[10] which reviewed national efforts, presented during the special session of the General Assembly of the United Nations in 2006. Based on the recommendations of the UNVAC, the Arab Children Commission included the issue of violence against children as a permanent item on the agenda of the twelfth meeting,[11] in order to coordinate the Arab position that reflects the concern of Arab governments to provide protection for children. The Department of Family and Children circulated the Final Report and Recommendations, a comparative draft on the implementation of Arab States to stop violence against children. New data was received from seventeen countries, namely: Jordan, United Arab Emirates, Bahrain, Tunisia, Algeria, Sudan, Saudi Arabia, Syria, Iraq, Oman, Qatar, Kuwait, Lebanon, Libya, Egypt, Morocco, and Yemen. It is clear that the report did not include any information on five countries: Djibouti, Somalia, Comoros, Palestine and Mauritania. As part of its on-going commitment to understanding, studying and strengthening child protection in the Middle East and North Africa (MENA) region, the UNICEF Regional Office developed a strategic framework to guide future actions—the Regional Child Protection Implementation Framework (2010–2013). This framework is underpinned and guided by the overall Regional Office Management Plan (2010–2011).

4.4 The Information Gap on Violence Against Children

Little information has been gathered to date on child protection systems in countries in the Middle East and North Africa. Although a number of evaluations have been undertaken, they tend to be limited to individual projects or programs or have been thematic in nature. There appears to be a paucity of research on national systems of protection, local definitions of child protection and, critically, on positive cultural practices and protective mechanisms. This information gap has important implications for mapping and analyzing systems in the MENA region as well as for creating a platform to support the development of national child protection systems.

[10]Cairo (2005, 2006, 2007).

[11]Damascus (2006).

Part II
SWOT Analysis of CSA in an Arab Country: LEBANON

The National Framework for Child Protection in Lebanon

Abstract
In Lebanon, based upon the actual perceived number of cases, it becomes evident that an undefined number of child sexual abuse protection cases, even more serious cases, may not be systematically referred to the existing formal mechanism. Three basic child protection response pathways are identified:

1. The cultural and religious mechanisms and practices used by families, communities and sectoral political leadership to deal with child protection issues;
2. The non-statutory child welfare services provided by NGOs and government agencies, but not mandated under Law 422; and
3. The statutory child protection mechanism, mandated under Law 422, with the Union for Child Protection in Lebanon and other NGOs.

Gerbaka, B., S. Awada, E. Mikhael. The reply of the Lebanese State on the UN Questionnaire on VAC. 2004.

Chapter 5
The Settings Within Lebanon

5.1 Social Settings

In the sectoral frame of family and personal religious jurisdiction, each pathway impacts and has important ramifications for the other and is therefore representing a duality within the child protection system; it is therefore not possible to develop an accurate picture of the national child protection system by analyzing any of these pathways in isolation. In order to genuinely strengthen the national child protection system in Lebanon, it is necessary to understand and identify the positive aspects of each of these pathways and develop strategies to build upon, coordinate and strengthen existing mechanisms in a way that is practical, coherent and acceptable to the general population, within the essential and consensual CRC and the Lebanese obligations towards the convention and its optional protocols.

5.2 Limitations

Repeatedly, discussions with community leaders and case-management with families reveal a core set of cultural values and beliefs that help to provide a contextual explanation behind the child protection responses that exist in Lebanon, more than in other Arab countries where the leading jurisdiction in the Islamic rule. At the center of these values is a fundamental belief in the sanctity of the family unit and its inherent right and responsibility to manage its affairs in an autonomous way.

Many cases of child sexual abuse and exploitation seem to be occasionally disclosed directly to service providers. It appears that the primary responsibility for finding solutions is often maintained within the circle of extended family, engaging identified respected individuals to help find solutions. In this way, family members work together to appeal to the reason of the perpetrator and encourage more positive patterns of behavior. Professional opinions agree that cases of children

B. Gerbaka et al., *Child Sexual Abuse, Exploitation and Trafficking in the Arab Region*, Child Maltreatment 13, https://doi.org/10.1007/978-3-030-66507-4_5

at high levels of risk, including sexual abuse, should be reported to statutory protection services, but in reality these same people signaled their personal reluctance to become involved in judicial processes themselves, for a number of reasons, including personal security and professional safety.

In Lebanon, a wide array of government and civil society organizations provide essential assistance to children and families at risk of CSA. These organizations are considered to provide appropriate, practical support to families in difficulty and children at risk. Such organizations are often bred and based in communities and, with a clearer delineation of their responsibilities, could potentially play a much greater role in the identification of children at risk of CSA. These diverse organizations may have no legal mandate under Law 422 to provide child protection services and may therefore be required but not mandated to report identified cases of CSA to the statutory authorities. Such hazy operating conditions imply a certain degree autonomy but also uncertainty about the child safety and best interests. A number of ideological and professional factors appear to influence the decisions made by service providers when faced with child protection concerns: a trust in family cohesion and resilience; a fear of breaking up families; a lack of trust in statutory services; the preference for flexible, voluntary interventions; and the potential harm to their own organization.

Although UPEL is a statutory agency mandated within the whole Lebanese territory, some other agencies state that, without a clearer legal mandate and algorithm, CBOs may feel powerless to intervene to protect children unless the beneficiary consents or to persuade alleged perpetrators to seek help. However, it is also clear that mandatory reporting for NGOs and professional bodies should promote the nature of trusting relationships with families. Service providers may offer children and families, rather than an alternative to the formal legal system, a more enabling relationship of trust to promote resolution of problems.

At conceptual levels, the statutory measures under Law 422 have come to define the national child protection system. However, the measures in reality are designed as a response system for the most egregious cases of sexual abuse, violence, neglect and exploitation, and have not been revised in the last 16 years, whereas additional types of CSA and exploitation have emerged, like within virtual reality and armed conflicts, just to name a few. In many ways, current legal frame is investigatory and closely aligned to criminal procedures: when children are referred, they immediately enter a judicial system comprised of judges, forensic doctors and statutory social workers, which means that the resilience and rehabilitation track is somewhat neglected, in spite of specific attention given to those dimensions by—young—judges who are more aware of the possibilities of combining child safety, perpetrator treatment and family reunification.

5.3 Resources

The human resources—especially judges and social workers—are extremely limited for application of Law 422; the current financial situation in Lebanon suggests that there is little potential for scaling up at this point in time, in light of the overwhelming burden of child refugees and population displacement, complicated by conflicting trans-territorial jurisdictions. Unless those complications are controlled and child protection situation changes, the statutory child protection system will continue to function with limitations, as a measure of last resort only. However, at professional levels, there is a considerable effort to develop a more proactive, dynamic and preventive role, starting with a position statement on Violence against children, that the Lebanese Order of Physicians and some Medical schools in Lebanon have endorsed; such a strategy would certainly require consequent funding for implementation. On a more operational level, a number of factors still impede the functioning of the statutory child protection mechanism at regional and local levels, especially in areas where the concentration of child refugees is critical. Basic field professionals operating under Law 422 have received limited specialized skills-based training for applying the law's provisions and the government system of rotation was cited as a real challenge for the consistency and sustainability of social and justice sector services. Again, professional bodies need to address those gaps and coordinate their strategies in order to respond positively to those needs.

The poor dissemination of standard operational procedures, in implementing the child protective provisions of the law, represents a significant obstacle. Within a limited series of supplementary protocols and guidance, those professionals that are responsible for applying the sectoral or general procedures of Law 422 often do so based upon personal intuition and professional experience rather than by inter-professional codes. By addressing many of these factors, the professional bodies may overcome the challenges of poor clarity in some of the provisions of Law 422 and would consequently facilitate the application of more effective and efficient algorithms. However, it is important to stress that these operational solutions need to address more fundamental reasons why a limited number of children at risk are referred to statutory authorities.

The deeper questions of cultural and religious factors that influence the functioning of the statutory child protection mechanism should not be under-estimated, whether in regions or within sects; the consequences and interfaces of these limitations have been addressed in 2 studies in the health sector, about child protection sectoral response and case management on one side, and multidisciplinary preparedness and institutional support on the other. It appears that when communities and service providers are identified as poorly capable to resolve complex or serious cases, there is a fundamental reluctance to seek a starting point or to apply the end-point provisions of Law 422 for child victims of abuse, violence, neglect and exploitation. The family in Lebanon is considered in most communities as the recognized primary unit of protection, which means that initial efforts are driven to focus on resolving the problem in the home and in cooperation with the family.

There appears to be a strong motivation to preserve the perceived dignity of family and the social integrity of the child and the family. Thus, even in the most egregious cases, concealment of sexual abuse from law enforcement and welfare agencies seems to be common, even when such scenarios involve worst forms of child labor.

5.4 Legal Frame in Lebanon

Law 422/2002 is the legal framework for child protection in Lebanon; cases of CSA are managed within this law; perpetrators are judged in separate courts and respond to other provisions of laws in terms of punishment and imprisonment, depending on severity of aggression; decisions of judges may vary from placement in correctional facilities in cases of minors (under 18) perpetrating CSA to death penalties in cases of CSA with aggravated abuse leading to death of child. Children are generally offered health management, rehabilitation, placement in culturally sensitive foster family or placement in institution, by civil court decision, potentially overruling religious family courts.

5.4.1 The Law 422

Since 2000, a number of legislative measures relating to child welfare have been introduced, most importantly Law 422 of 6 June 2002, on 'Protection of Minors in Conflict with the Law or At Risk'.

This law represents the first and most significant effort to create a legal framework for the delivery of protective services. Essentially, the law establishes judicial processes for dealing with serious abuse, violence, neglect and exploitation perpetrated against children. For the first time it establishes the powers of children's judges and social workers to make protective orders for children at risk. However, Law 422 has a number of important limitations, including age and emergence. It is important to perceive the law as an essentially reactive juvenile justice law, not a comprehensive protective and preventive child protection law; it is therefore infrequently applied or applicable for child victims. Furthermore, the law does not provide a series of welfare service measures, but creates a 'last resort' response mechanism for children already in crisis. The debate continues as to whether it is possible to rewrite Law 422 to ensure more rigorous child protection measures or whether a new specialized law should be encouraged. It also appears to be more accessible to include emergent definitions about types of CSA and explore the availability of requested services to victims and families, often involved in interpersonal and family violence.

The SWOT represents a promising milestone for the inter-sectoral approach in Lebanon. The pathfinding program offers a draft for a National Action Plan for the Prevention of child abuse and neglect as well as a Protection frame for Children from

Violence; the pioneering program that Lebanon failed to engage in 2018 should be reactivated in order to establish a more structured framework of programs and activities for promoting the welfare of children and families. Even in the absence of a timeframe for a national plan or an allocated provisional budget, a common platform should identify the diverse sectoral roles and engage the different professional agencies, then lead the movement of child protection, within the position statement against violence and a consequent implementation plan; a broader policy paper would clarify the existing foundations of the child protection system and highlight its guiding values, principles and purpose, following an already triggered effort.[1] Such a policy would help to establish clear guiding values, principles and responsibilities upon which the action plan should be based.

The different studies performed in Lebanon highlight the priorities of different health, education and social sector agencies, as per their individual plans of action. Despite the solid efforts of the Higher Council for Childhood to harmonize strategic planning, underpinned in its recent reports, the child protection responsibilities of all sectors involved in child protection need be articulated with clear interfaces. While the Higher Council for Childhood will continue to lead the recommendation in terms of child protection, different Ministries must be involved in implementation, including the Ministry of Social Affairs, of Health, of Labor, of Justice, as well as the Ministry of Interior and Municipalities, in order to clarify the sectoral role and responsibilities, within a broad strategic role for ensuring the welfare and protection of children and families, and avoid the conflicts of "disinterest" in their practical roles at national and local levels. Although there is an abundance of commitment and enthusiasm for a child protection system that meets different international standards and respond to the ICRC comments on the Lebanese national strategy, current ambitions should dependent upon stable road map and growing budgetary allocation.[2] However, as a percentage of total government expenditure, social sector expenditure has continued to be reduced in recent years. Although there are positive government initiatives—such as Social Development Centers—it is clear that the private sector (including welfare, education and healthcare providers) will increasingly assume the responsibility to provide and operate basic social services. While the MOJ and MOSA provide some funding to child protection non-governmental organizations, these agencies nonetheless are required to secure their own external funding for their work. It is therefore essential that the Government increases the number of contracts with such semi-governmental service providers like orders and syndicates, as well as academic resources to provide skills' building about specialized services to children at risk and/or in conflict with the law. When more agencies are contracted and mandated under Law 422, there will be stronger coordination in interventions and better stability of UPEL to provide social services to those at most

[1]WHO. Lebanon, 2005. Global Student-Based Student Health Survey. WHO: Geneva, Switzerland, 2007. http://www.who.int/chp/gshs/2007_Lebanon_GSHS_Country_Report.pdf 16

[2]Usta, J., Mahfoud, Z., Chahine, G. and Anani, G. Child sexual abuse: The situation in Lebanon. KAFA (enough) Violence & Exploitation. Save the Children: Sweden, 2008. 15

risk. There is am consensual recognition that current funding for the optimal functioning of services under Law 422 remains fragile and scattered.

While Government financing of the child protection system has traditionally prioritized residential care for children, the CPS in Lebanon should de-institutionalize child protection. Indeed, both out-of-home care and statutory based responses under Law 422 are expensive and detract financing for other essential services. The current approach leaves little opportunity to fund either:

- Essential preventive family strengthening services like home visitation or
- Appropriate welfare and rehabilitation services for child victims for the purpose of resilience.

Beyond the judicial processing of cases, there is a gap in budgeting for services that work with families in crisis with the specific aim of restoring the wellbeing of the child victim.

5.4.1.1 Comments on Law 422/2002

In 2002, the Lebanese Parliament overhauled the juvenile justice system by enacting a self-contained law titled "Protection of Children in Violation of the Law or Exposed to Danger" to deal with juvenile courts emphasizing educational and rehabilitative measures rather than punishment.

The issued Law no. 422/2002 related to the protection of juveniles in conflict with the sanctions law or at risk, is a milestone for ensuring the legal protection of children. This Law has taken into consideration in many of its articles the general principles of the Convention on the Rights of the child. Whereby it has set educational non-restraining measures that are in line with the non-retributive approach and gave authority to social workers in charge of pursuing juveniles matters from the beginning of investigation till the issuing of a court decision and subsequently, and to suggest the proper and adequate measure that is convenient for the juvenile, preceded by an extensive social investigation and after hearing the juvenile's point of view on the matter in question. This Law has defined the "juvenile at risk" and ensured for him the proper protection in order to secure his/her rehabilitation and reintegration into society.

However, this Law has some matters in stake that are controversial and ought to be revised per se, it has set the legal age for legal criminal responsibility at the age of seven years which is contradictory to the best interest of the child, in addition to the participation of the juvenile in the court hearing procedures with adults in the case where partnership in crime. This surely denies the juvenile's right to privacy in all procedures of the court hearings in relation to public hearings, and this constitutes an obstacle to the juvenile's freedom of expression of views, and the presence of specified people that are authorized by the court to attend court hearings. In addition to other loop holes which are today the main concern of the civil society that actively advocate for amending the Law in accordance with the Convention on the Rights of the Child

Article 2 declares the supreme importance of the interests of juvenile offenders and the need for an autonomous procedure to deal with them where alternative forms of sentencing and rehabilitation are the norm.

The law requires compliance with the following principles in its implementation:

1. The juvenile is in need of special help that enables him or her to play a role in society;
2. Under all circumstances, the interest of the child shall be taken into consideration to protect it against delinquency;
3. A juvenile who violates the law should benefit from humane and fair treatment; the manner by which he or she is prosecuted, investigated, and tried shall be subject to special procedures that save him or her, to the extent possible, from normal criminal procedures through adopting amicable settlements and solutions, away from liberty depriving measures. The juvenile judge shall have the most discretion in this regard with the authority to amend or rescind whatever measures ordered, based on the results of its implementation on the child.
4. The juvenile court is the authority in charge of juveniles and the application of the law and the competent ministries provide all necessary means needed to this implementation

Measures and punishment that may be imposed upon juveniles are:

1. Public blame;
2. Placement under probation;
3. Protection;
4. Supervised freedom;
5. To provide labor to the benefit of the public or to compensate the victim.

- Those measures may be modified by the judge during the course of their application.
- Alternative sentences have reduced the number of juveniles in prison.
- Although the Law reduced sentences in exceptional cases for offenders aged 15–18 who had committed serious crimes, such sentences were counterbalanced by the power given to judges to suspend execution of sentences or to replace them with rehabilitation measures where the offender was not deprived of his or her freedom.
- Although the Law retained the possibility of preventive detention, it restricted its application to certain crimes and under precise conditions.
- In addition, the Law provided for exhaustive protective arrangements for juvenile offenders in particular danger of recidivism. Such measures can either be decided by the judge or at the request of the young offender himself. Increases in the number of homeless minors, often engaged in begging and vagrancy, justified such measures.
- The presence of the social worker throughout the proceedings, from the preliminary inquiries to the reintegration phase, is required by law.

- In order to ensure effective application of the Law, the importance of the Department for Minors of the Ministry of Justice has been underlined, in particular its function as coordinating office between the different services and the organizations concerned.

Under this Lebanese law, juveniles between the ages of 12 and 18 can be sentenced to prison. There were 1121 in this age bracket accused of crimes in 2007, according to statistics from the Ministry of Justice. Any law-breakers under the age of 12 (15 were accused in 2007) are either released to their parents or to an NGO that can care for and rehabilitate them. The juveniles in Roumieh share a building with adults and come into contact with and are even supervised at night by them. This contact is in direct contradiction to part of Article 37 of the UN convention, which says that any child (defined as any person under the age of 18) arrested, detained or imprisoned "shall be separated from adults," except in rare cases.

5.4.1.2 Article 25 of Law No. 422/2002

The juvenile is considered threatened in the following cases:

1. If he was found in an environment exposing him to exploitation, threatening his health, safety, ethics or conditions of raising him.
2. If he was exposed to sexual abuse or physical violence exceeding the limits of what is allowed by custom as a manner of harmless disciplining.
3. If he was found begging or homeless.

He is considered homeless if he left his house to live on the streets and on public places or if he did not have a house.

5.4.1.3 Article 26 of Law No. 422/2002

Any person knowing that the juvenile is exposed to ill-treatment:

- Persons dealing with children: physicians, teachers, and social workers...
- Parents or the custodian of the minor
- The minor himself

....Should report this case to adequate authority.

5.4.1.4 Article 26 of Law No. 422/2002

Any notification to the adequate authority, aware by its status or its profession of the situation of the child exposed to danger, is not considered disclosure of a professional secret and is not subject to the penal code provisions in the cases specified in article 25 of this law.

5.4.2 *Legal Settings*

Legal (nonspecific but specialized child judges, child lawyers, including child advocacy services within Lebanese Orders [Physicians, Lawyers], Academic institutions and NGOs, within the officially mandated body, the Union for Child Protection in Lebanon [www.UPEL.net-lb and use of www.UPEL.org]; Health (physicians, mental health, midwives, nurses, emerging hospital child protection units); Social (social workers within formal settings and NGOs); Educative (rehabilitation for perpetrator if minor within correctional facility or in civil service, education for child in placement in institution).

5.4.3 *Constitutional Rights*

Main problems are related to: situation of child and family in constitution; situation of vulnerable children (refugees, street children); civil unrest and conflicts in relation with community issues.

Chapter 6
Services to Children and Families in Lebanon

6.1 Abstract

Many services to children are available in Lebanon; however, there is a need to review the role of government welfare structures, specifically in the spectrum of protection services. This review should consider:

(a) the types of services that could be integrated for families and children in crisis and disasters,
(b) the qualities of obligations and mandates that staff have to intervene when protection cases are disclosed or suspected and
(c) Standardized procedures and regulations for addressing child protection cases. This does not necessarily imply mandatory reporting but rather some form of unified procedures to ensure quality of service.

As part of the continuum of care, a range of positive Government support initiatives that help families to care for their children at home is lacking. These might include financial and material assistance and family mediation services, as well as further developing the fostering and the peculiar "kafala" systems to strengthen and building upon positive community practices already in place that contribute to the protection of children.

6.2 Government Contracted Services

- Beyond the eleven child protection agencies already contracted by the Government, identify and contract specialist protection agencies in all regions.
- Identify and contract agencies in all regions that are specialized in family support and assistance. Align these agencies so that they form the foundation of preventive services.

B. Gerbaka et al., *Child Sexual Abuse, Exploitation and Trafficking in the Arab Region*, Child Maltreatment 13, https://doi.org/10.1007/978-3-030-66507-4_6

- Review the nature of the contracts that these agencies sign with the Government. Under these contracts, all child protection agencies should be subject to standard regulation and compliance, including standards of care.
- As is already prescribed in Law 422, review further the potential to increase -beyond UPEL, the number of semi- and non-governmental agencies with powers of protective intervention.

6.3 Non-Governmental Agencies[1]

- Review the types of INGOs and NGO services that are currently being provided to help children and families; and identify those that potentially represent a balance of different types of services within the continuum of care, including universal, targeted and individual services.
- Review the current policy of financing residential institutions in favor of moving towards support for family-based interventions aimed at keeping families united.
- Conduct a national assessment of community based welfare organizations to identify services that aim to strengthen families, whether by addressing factors such as unemployment and livelihoods, or by more targeted prevention programs that address child abuse and neglect.

6.4 Regulation of Services

- Establish a comprehensive central registry of all approved child welfare and protection providers, outlining their core mandates and services.
- Establish standards, independent monitoring processes, and accountability mechanisms for all agencies working in child care and protection.[2]

Establish rigorous standards for all residential care institutions. These should include rigorous gate-keeping procedures, care planning processes, and staff capacity.

[1]Save the Children Sweden, MENA Regional Office. Child Rights Situational Analysis for the Middle East and North Africa (MENA) Region, 2008. http://mena.savethechildren.se/Middle_East_and_North_Africa/Resources/Child-Rights-Programming

[2]Salem-Pickarta, J. 2005. Violence in Schools in the Middle East and North Africa: Features, Causes, Intervention, and Prevention. UNICEF MENARO.

6.5 Long Term Reform

The above short-term measures will undoubtedly increase the range and improve the quality of social services for families and children. However, there are several longer term strategic challenges to address in order for the service paradigm to be holistic and function in an optimal way.

Challenges to be considered in the future include:

- A comprehensive review of budget allocations in line with national child welfare and protection priorities. Important decisions need to be made regarding the very significant investment in residential and day-care facilities every year. While the amount per child per day is relatively not substantial, it is suggested that this investment could be better spent on promoting strong families. This would represent not only a financial shift, but also an ideological one.
- The future need for the Government to assume a greater role in the regulation of the child protection system, based on the Lebanese State obligations to the CRC and the recommendations of the Global partnership to end violence against children. As per the SDGs, semi- and NGOs should assume a greater service provision role and more sectoral leadership in the future, in coordination with CPS. Therefore, it is recommended that a broad, sustainable government regulatory function be delineated and specific agency roles be defined, as per the pathfinding strategy. This regulatory function will need to be costed so that financial investment can be sought and allocated from the central level.
- Included with the development of a stronger regulatory framework, it is recommended that there be a deeper reflection about the relatively autonomous nature of the private sector. This is not limited to social welfare NGOs, but includes other sectors. At the current time, there is a pioneering initiative about the operational autonomy of private education and health facilities, under the leadership of the LOP, in particular for ensuring that private and academic institutions operate by agreed protection codes and guidelines.

6.6 Obstacles Are

6.6.1 Legal

Child protection is managed by civil courts while family matters are managed by religious courts; there are no dedicated and exclusive child judges; there is still no child police; in response, settlement of mixed cases is made through informal conjunction and discussion between courts.

6.6.2 Health

Health coverage is not universal; mental rehabilitation is not mandatory or systematically implemented for perpetrator; in response child protection units are emerging tools in hospitals.

6.6.3 Social

Mandated social workers may face challenging situations in terms of security and their safety is often in risky positions; even representatives of law may face threats in some areas where weapons are present; in response, child protection issues are discussed with cultural resources and child protection policies are managed within the Higher Council for Childhood, as an inter-ministerial body anchored to the Ministry of Social Affairs.

Social Response
This question should specify what types and levels of evidence are at task; On the contrary, home visitation and visitation of minors in conflict with law by family is helpful, as well as civil service by minor perpetrators.

6.7 Potential Strategies

"Children come first" would be the slogan of the strategy at the beginning; as for the environment, creating a mandatory space for children, in Constitution then within policies, would enforce the natural and socially compatible implementation of child friendly processes, including development plans.

6.8 Short Term Actions

6.8.1 Policy Framework

The existing system is defined by a series of strategies and action plans, but requires a more defined vision. Based upon the documented opinions of policy makers, service providers, community leaders and service beneficiaries, the process of developing a comprehensive national child protection system policy should begin. This policy should outline the contours of the system and its functioning at the local level, and reflect the unique situation and context of Lebanon. The policy should outline, for example:

- The values and principles that underpin the national child protection system: e.g. the way in which international standards will be promoted within a national system that is based upon respect for the norms and autonomy of the religious communities.
- The roles and mandates of different service providers: e.g. the responsibility of different government and non-government agencies within the child protection system.
- The specific functions of the education and health sectors for protecting children.
- The duties and powers of religious communities, and their leaders, for the protection of children.
- The typology of service paradigm: e.g. the balance of prevention and response services and the framework for intervention.
- The structures that will make the system operational: e.g. the structures to be bolstered or established at national, regional and community level for the protection of children.

6.8.2 Legal Framework

Ideally, the policy framework above would be approved before any changes to Law 422 are finalized. However, at the time of writing, revisions to the existing Law 422 are already being debated and are expected to be agreed by mid-2012. These measures would significantly enhance the legal framework for protecting children. Essential features of a revised law would include:

1. Establish the scope of legal mandates and powers of different government and non-government agencies and individual actors within the system.
2. Establish a range of protective mechanisms, including early intervention, rather than the limited responses available now.
3. Establish procedures and protocols for decision-making about children's cases.
4. Reallocate funds to ensure that the application of Law 422 is viable. In order to recruit more social workers and other professionals, the structure requires significant investment. To this end it is recommended that the proposed system be fully costed to ensure that it is feasible and sustainable.
5. Provide training to ensure that professionals working with children and families understand the extent and potentials of Law 422.

6.8.3 Implementing Protocols

Whether Law 422 is revised or whether a new child protection law is created, a series of standard operational procedures are required for applying the legal provisions. These include:

- Standardized reporting and referral protocols, and guidance for professionals.
- Case management procedures and standards.
- Gatekeeping procedures for residential care institutions.

6.8.4 Training of Professionals

- Compulsory professional training for all professionals (at a minimum of sectoral tasks) with responsibilities to apply the provisions of Law 422.
- Training of para-professionals at community level in child welfare and protection, ensuring that they understand some basic procedures for identifying and launching a response to children at risk.

6.9 Long Term Measures

The measures given above are designed to ensure that the local level child protection mechanism is strengthened, allowing it to function optimally in the short term. However, it is strongly recommended that comprehensive reform of the legislative framework will be required in the longer term.

Simply amending Law 422 will probably be found inadequate. Thus, when there is the political and social 'space' for major legal reform, it is recommended that a comprehensive new law on child protection is created, moulded to the Lebanese context and designed in a way that, where possible, works in coordination rather than conflict with traditional and religious authorities and decision-making processes.

Religious leaders and people of influence, including lawyers, from each of the confessionals should be invited to participate in the development of child welfare and protection policy and legislation. The effective application and functioning of a new nationwide law will depend upon the balance of authority and responsibility that is achieved between civil and religious law and the establishment of a mutually agreed conceptual framework for child protection.

6.10 Short Term Actions

- Identify and promote cultural practices and values that have a positive impact upon the wellbeing and welfare of children and families. Consider ways to integrate these practices within the wider child protection framework.
- Identify and collaborate with 'champions' from the different religious communities. Study the positive ways in which the communities protect children and support families in crisis, using a partnership approach to build upon good community protection strategies.

- Target campaigns and initiatives designed to change the attitudes and behaviours of men, especially fathers, in relation to domestic violence and physical punishment of children.
- Target campaigns towards the rights and protection of children and women, especially mothers, and in accordance with the priorities of any potential Domestic Violence Law in the future.
- Promote greater equity in the distribution of and access to information for all citizens about the child protection law and available social assistance and services, especially in the remote areas.

6.11 Long Term Reform

All the recommendations suggested above will contribute to evolution of social norms and practices on child welfare and protection. These types of interventions should be initiated as soon as possible within the framework of a targeted prevention strategy. However, in order to affect longer term, nationwide change, some macro issues need to be addressed.

- The traditional authority of the religious communities to regulate and respond to child welfare and protection issues will need to be defined more clearly. Continuing debate will be required to determine the powers of the communities in family matters: a balance needs to be struck between autonomy and compliance with national standards in relation to child protection.
- National strategies will need to be developed to build upon the positive aspects of child protection practices within families and communities. At the same time, given the reported prevalence of different forms of abuse and violence, strategies to challenge negative attitudes and behaviours towards children will be required.

Part III
SWOT of CSA in the Arab Region

The Present Situation in Arab Countries v/s UNVAC

Abstract
In 2008 Jordan drafted a Child Rights Act, later withdrawn from the National Assembly. Another draft was prepared in cooperation with all organizations concerned with children's rights and UNICEF. Article 62 of the penal code was amended with the stipulation that no harm should be caused by parents disciplining their children, in addition to social norms. Amendments of the penal code also included an increase in punishments for crimes against family, women and children. The age of protection for sexual offences and crimes against public ethics and morals has also been raised to 18 years of age for the girl child in accordance with international conventions, and punishments for perpetrators have been intensified. The United Arab Emirates completed its Child Rights Act prepared by the Ministry of Social Affairs and the Ministry of Interior. Many countries in the region followed the child protection track, while some others failed, in the context of social riots and armed conflicts.

Chapter 7
The Value of Research

7.1 Prior Reviews of International Research on CSA

7.1.1 *Abstract*

Attempts to examine patterns of child sexual abuse internationally has been limited for many reasons. Outside of the US, Canada and England, few countries have research on child sexual abuse published in scholarly-refereed venues, and regardless of source, comparability is difficult with respect to methods and measurement. This reflects in part the lesser status of children and females as well as a resistance in societies globally (even those who have conducted research) to acknowledge the problem of child sexual abuse, instead relying on myths to continue denial such as "child sexual abuse doesn't happen here" or "only disturbed strangers do that." This is unfortunate, as information on child sexual abuse allows for the possibility of acknowledging the problem in society which in turn is necessary if victims are to be assisted and child sexual abuse to be prevented in the future.[1]

7.1.2 *The Data*

There are increasing reviews of research on CSA internationally published in refereed scholarly journals. Published in 1994 and 2009, both were based primarily on a literature search of relevant databases focusing on published academic sources on child abuse, including data from national probability samples to college classes. Finkelhor (1994) found data on CSA from 21 countries—sixty percent from Europe and at least one country from North America, Central America, sub-Saharan Africa

[1]Finkelhor, D., Moore, D., Hamby, S. and Straus, M. Sexually Abused Children in a National Survey of Parents: Methodological Issues. Child Abuse & Neglect 1997; 21:1–9.

B. Gerbaka et al., *Child Sexual Abuse, Exploitation and Trafficking in the Arab Region*, Child Maltreatment 13, https://doi.org/10.1007/978-3-030-66507-4_7

and Oceania, but not one from 5 the Middle East or North Africa. Pereda et al. (2009) secured data for 21 countries (12 countries overlapped with the first study but with updated data), 40% in Europe, and at least one in North America, Central America, Asia, sub-Saharan Africa, Oceania and North Africa and the Middle East.[2,3]

In analyzing these data, Finkelhor (1994: 411) found: *'The international studies are generally consistent with the North American literature in the profile of the sexual abuse problem…'* For almost all of the 21 countries, CSA was higher for girls than boys.

Regarding prevalence, over 70% of the rates of CSA of boys were under 10%; while 80% of the rates of CSA of girls were over 10% and 50% were approximately 20% or higher. Results mostly showed 'rates for females to be 1.5 to 3 times that of males'; 'intrafamily abuse to be consistently more common for girls than boys, constituting about one-third to one-half of girls' experiences'; and 'offenders against girls to be disproportionately male (above 90%), while boys were abused by males in proportions that varied' (Finkelhor 1994: 411). He concluded that:

Studies from a variety of countries suggest that sexual abuse is indeed an international problem. In every locale where it has been sought, researchers have demonstrated its existence at levels high enough to be detected through surveys of a few hundred adults in the general population. These rates are far higher than anything suggested by the level of reported cases in these countries. As such epidemiological findings are available for more and more countries, the responsibility of proof shifts to anyone who would argue that sexual abuse is rare or nonexistent in their locale.

Almost 15 years later, the findings by Pereda et al. (2009: 337) yielded remarkably similar conclusions with respect to a pattern of higher prevalence of childhood sexual abuse among women than men and prevalence rates internationally that remained fairly constant over time and continued to be deeply concerning—indicating that '. . .child sexual abuse remains an international problem.' The consistency in pattern and prevalence of CSA across countries and time points in large part to how deeply entrenched adultarchy and patriarchy remain.

7.1.3 Prevalence

Based on self-disclosure data, Pereda performed in 2011 a meta-analysis of 217 studies, which estimated a global prevalence of 12.7%–18% for girls and 7.6% for boys. The rates of self-disclosed abuse for specific continents were as follows:

---

[2]Frederick, J. Sexual Abuse and Exploitation of Boys in South Asia. Innocenti Working Paper, Florence, UNICEF Innocenti Research Centre 2010. Freeman, M. The Moral Status of Children: Essays on the Rights of the Child. The Netherlands: Martinus Nijhoff Publishers, 1997.

[3]Pereda, N., Guilera, G., Forns, M., and Gómez-Benito, J. The international epidemiology of child sexual abuse: A continuation of Finkelhor (1994). Child Abuse & Neglect 2009; 33:6:331–342.

Region	Girls	Boys
Africa	20.2%	19.3%
Asia	11.3%	4.1%
Australia	21.5%	7.5%
Europe	13.5%	5.6%
South America	13.4%	13.8%
USA/Canada	20.1%	8%

Previously, a 2009 meta-analysis of 65 studies from 22 countries found a global prevalence of 19.7% for females and 7.9% for males. In that analysis, Africa had the highest prevalence rate of child sexual abuse (34.4%), primarily because of high rates in South Africa; Europe showed the lowest prevalence rate (9.2%); and America and Asia had prevalence rates between 10.1% and 23.9%.[4]

7.1.3.1 Africa[5,6]

A ten-country school-based study in southern Africa in 2007 found 19.6% of female students and 21.1% of male students aged 11–16 years reported they had experienced forced or coerced sex. Rates among 16-year-olds were 28.8% in females and 25.4% in males. Comparing the same schools in eight countries between 2003 and 2007, age-standardized on the 2007 Botswana male sample, there was no significant decrease between 2003 and 2007 among females in any country and inconsistent changes among males.[7]

The prevalence of child sexual abuse in Africa is compounded by the virgin cleansing myth that sexual intercourse with a virgin will cure a man of HIV or AIDS. The myth is prevalent in South Africa, Zimbabwe, Zambia and Nigeria and is being blamed for the high rate of sexual abuse against young children. Indeed, Child rape is on the rise in the war ravaged eastern Democratic Republic of the Congo. Aid workers blame combatants on all sides, who operate with much impunity, for a culture of sexual violence. South Africa has some of the highest incidences of child

---

[4]Pereda, N.; Guilera, G.; Forns, M. & Gómez-Benito, J. (2009). "The prevalence of child sexual abuse in community and student samples: A meta-analysis". *Clinical Psychology Review*. 29 (4): 328–338. doi:https://doi.org/10.1016/j.cpr.2009.02.007

[5]Madu, S. and Peltzer, K. Prevalence and patterns of child sexual abuse and victim-perpetrator relationship among secondary school students in the Northern Province (South Africa). Achieves of Sexual Behavior 2001; 30: 311–321.

[6]Lalor, K. Child sexual abuse in sub-Saharan Africa: a literature review. Child Abuse & Neglect 2004, 28 (4): 439–460.

[7]Andersson, N.; Paredes-Solís, S.; Milne, D.; Omer, K.; Marokoane, N.; Laetsang, D.; Cockcroft, A. (2012). "Prevalence and risk factors for forced or coerced sex among school-going youth: National cross-sectional studies in 10 southern African countries in 2003 and 2007". *BMJ Open*. 2 (2): e000754. doi:https://doi.org/10.1136/bmjopen-2011-000754. PMC 3293138.

rape (including the rape of babies) in the world.[8] A number of high-profile baby rapes appeared since 2001 (including the fact that they required extensive reconstructive surgery to rebuild urinary, genital, abdominal, or tracheal systems). In 2001, a 9-month-old was raped and likely lost consciousness as the pain was too much to bear. In February 2002, an 8-month-old infant was reportedly gang raped by four men. One has been charged. The infant has required extensive reconstructive surgery. The 8-month-old infant's injuries were so extensive, increased attention on prosecution has occurred.[9]

Gang rape is also prevalent: CIET found in a survey that around 11% of boys and 4% of girls admitted to forcing someone else to have sex with them. In a related survey conducted among 1500 schoolchildren, a quarter of all the boys interviewed said that "jackrolling", a term for gang rape, was fun. More than 67,000 cases of rape and sexual assaults against children were reported in 2000 in South Africa, compared to 37,500 in 1998. Child welfare groups believe that the number of unreported incidents could be up to 10 times that number. The largest increase in attacks was against children under seven. The virgin cleansing myth is especially common in South Africa, which has the highest number of HIV-positive citizens in the world; Child abusers are often relatives of their victims—even their fathers and providers."

7.1.3.2 Asia

Nineteen percent of the world's children live in India, which constitutes 42% of India's total population. In 2007, the Ministry of Women and Child Development published the "Study on Child Abuse: India 2007." It looked at different forms of child abuse, including sexual abuse and girl child neglect in five evidence groups, namely, children in a family environment, children in school, children at work, children on the street and children in institutions. The study's main findings included: 53.22% of children reported having faced sexual abuse. Among them 52.94% were boys and 47.06% girls. Andhra Pradesh, Assam, Bihar and Delhi reported the highest percentage of sexual abuse among both boys and girls, as well as the highest incidence of sexual assaults. 21.90% of child respondents faced severe forms of sexual abuse, 5.69% had been sexually assaulted and 50.76% reported other forms of sexual abuse. Children on the street, at work and in institutional care reported the highest incidence of sexual assault. The study also reported that 50% of abusers are known to the child or are in a position of trust and responsibility and most children had not reported the matter to anyone. Despite years of lack of any specific child sexual abuse laws in India, which treated them separately from adults in case of sexual offense, the 'Protection of Children Against Sexual Offences Bill,

[8]"Oprah Scandal Rocks South Africa". *TIME.com*. 5 November 2007.

[9]*"Child rape in South Africa". Medscape. Retrieved 2010-12-31.*

2011' was passed the Indian parliament on May 22, 2012, which came into force from 14 November 2012.[10]

In Bangladesh, child prostitutes are known to take the drug Oradexon, an over-the-counter steroid, usually used by farmers to fatten cattle, to make child prostitutes look larger and older. Charities say that 90% of prostitutes in the country's legalized brothels use the drug. According to social activists, the steroid can cause diabetes, high blood pressure and is highly addictive. In one survey, 2.5% of Taiwanese adolescents report having experienced childhood sexual abuse. UK Ambassador Craig Murray has written that the government of Uzbekistan, under president Islam Karimov, used child rape to force false confessions from prisoners.

7.1.3.3 Pacific

Almost half of reported rape victims in Papua New Guinea are under 15 years of age and 13% are under 7 years of age [UNICEF] while a report by ChildFund Australia citing former Parliamentarian Dame Carol Kidu stated 50% of those seeking medical help after rape are under 16, 25% are under 10 and 10% are under 8.[11]

Additionally, a study found that men with a history of victimization, especially having been raped or otherwise sexually coerced themselves, were more likely than otherwise to have participated in both single perpetrator and multiple perpetrator non-partner rape. 57·5% (587/1022) of men who raped a non-partner committed their first rape as teenagers.

7.1.3.4 United States and Europe

Child sexual abuse occurs frequently in Western society. The rate of prevalence can be difficult to determine. Research in North America has concluded that approximately 15% to 25% of women and 5% to 15% of men were sexually abused when they were children. In the UK, a 2010 study estimated prevalence at about 5% for boys and 18% for girls (not dissimilar to a 1985 study that estimated about 8% for boys and 12% for girls). More than 23,000 incidents were recorded by the UK police between 2009 and 2010. Girls were six times more likely to be assaulted than boys with 86% of attacks taking place against them. Barnardo's charity estimates that two thirds of victims in the United Kingdom are girls and 1 third boys. Barnardo's is concerned that boy victims may be overlooked.

In the United States, estimates vary widely. A literature review of 23 studies found rates of 3% to 37% for males and 8% to 71% for females, which produced an average of 17% for boys and 28% for girls, while a statistical analysis based on

[10] *Parliament passes bill to protect children from sexual abuse". NDTV. May 22, 2012.*

[11] *Davidson, Helen (26 November 2013). "Papua New Guinea takes first steps to combat 'epidemic' of abuse". Guardian News and Media Limited. Retrieved 9 March 2014.*

16 cross-sectional studies estimated the rate to be 7.2% for males and 14.5% for females.[12] The US Department of Health and Human Services reported 83,600 substantiated reports of sexually abused children in 2005. Including incidents which were not reported would make the total number even larger. According to Emily M. Douglas and David Finkelhor, "Several national studies have found that black and white children experienced near-equal levels of sexual abuse. Other studies, however, have found that both blacks and Latinos have an increased risk for sexual victimization".[13]

Surveys have shown that one fifth to one third of all women reported some sort of childhood sexual experience with a male adult. A 1992 survey studying father-daughter incest in Finland reported that of the 9000 15-year-old high school girls who filled out the questionnaires, of the girls living with their biological fathers, 0.2% reported father-daughter incest experiences; of the girls living with a stepfather, 3.7% reported sexual experiences with him. The reported counts included only father-daughter incest and did not include prevalence of other forms of child sexual abuse. The survey summary stated, "the feelings of the girls about their incestual experiences are overwhelmingly negative." Others argue that prevalence rates are much higher, and that many cases of child abuse are never reported. One study found that professionals failed to report approximately 40% of the child sexual abuse cases they encountered. Lawson & Chaffin indicated that many children who were sexually abused were "identified solely by a physical complaint that was later diagnosed as a venereal disease...Only 43% of the children who were diagnosed with venereal disease made a verbal disclosure of sexual abuse during the initial interview." It has been found in the epidemiological literature on CSA that there is no identifiable demographic or family characteristic of a child that can be used to bar the prospect that a child has been sexually abused.[14]

In US schools, "nearly 9.6% of students are targets of educator sexual misconduct sometime during their school career." In studies of student sex abuse by male and female educators, male students were reported as targets in ranges from 23% to 44%. In U.S. school settings same-sex (female and male) sexual misconduct against students by educators "ranges from 18% to 28% of reported cases, depending on the study"[15] Significant underreporting of sexual abuse of boys by both women and men is believed to occur due to sex stereotyping, social denial, the minimization of male victimization, and the relative lack of research on sexual abuse of boys. Sexual victimization of boys by their mothers or other female relatives is especially rarely researched or reported. Sexual abuse of girls by their mothers, and other related

[12]*Gorey KM, Leslie DR (April 1997). "The prevalence of child sexual abuse: integrative review adjustment for potential response and measurement biases". Child Abuse & Neglect.*

[13]Child Sexual Abuse Fact Sheet. (PDF). Emily M. Douglas and David Finkelhor.

[14]*Finkelhor D (1993). "Epidemiological factors in the clinical identification of child sexual abuse". Child Abuse & Neglect. 17 (1): 67–70. doi:*https://doi.org/10.1016/0145-2134(93)90009-T. *PMID 8435788.*

[15]Shakeshaft, C, "Educator Sexual Misconduct: A Synthesis of the Literature", U.S. Department of Education, 2004.

and/or unrelated adult females is beginning to be researched and reported despite the highly taboo nature of female–female child sex abuse. In studies where students are asked about sex offenses, they report higher levels of female sex offenders than found in adult reports.[16] This underreporting has been attributed to cultural denial of female-perpetrated child sex abuse, because "males have been socialized to believe they should be flattered or appreciative of sexual interest from a female."[17] Journalist Cathy Young writes that under-reporting is contributed to by the difficulty of people, including jurors, in seeing a male as a "true victim".[18]

7.2 Forms and Prevalence of CSEC in the Region[19]

Although statistics on CSEC inevitably understate the extent of the problem, which is largely hidden and therefore impossible to measure, there are some reliable figures on cases of CSEC that have been reported to law enforcement entities. As far in time as1999:

- Algeria recorded 1180 cases of sexual mistreatment;
- Jordan recorded 17 cases of rape, 3 of attempted rape and 202 indecent assaults;
- Lebanon recorded 40 cases of sexual abuse, 65 of homosexuality (illegal in Lebanese law); 56 cases of rape and prostitution;
- Morocco recorded 17 cases of rape, 63 indecent assaults, 19 cases of prostitution, and 3 unspecified related crimes.

Two-thirds of these recorded cases involved girls. Since the loss of virginity of a girl victim of sexual abuse or exploitation is considered to dishonor the family, there are often serious repercussions for the child. She may be rejected, sent away, locked up, forced to marry the aggressor or imprisoned. In some countries she may be subject to 'crimes of honor' (considered as the worst form of domestic violence) and, for her own protection, might be taken into preventive custody. Jordan is one of the few countries in the region where the concept of 'crimes of honor' is a subject of public debate: 25 girls and women are victims of such crimes each year in that country.

Should the girl become pregnant, then family and society rejection is even more serious: both girl and baby might be rejected, abandoned, stigmatized or victimized. Of 38 sexually abused girls who were the subject of a study in the Palestinian

[16]Watkins, B.; Bentovim, A. (1992). "The sexual abuse of male children and adolescents: a review of current research". *Journal of Clinical Psychology & Psychiatry*. 33 (10): 197–248. doi:https://doi.org/10.1111/j.1469-7610.1992.tb00862.x. PMID 1737828.

[17]Educator Sexual Misconduct: A Synthesis of the Literature", U.S. Department of Education, 2004, p25, Shakeshaft, C.

[18]*Cathy Young (2002).* "Double Standard". *The Boston Globe.*

[19]Jumaian, A. Prevalence and long-term impact of child sexual abuse among a sample of male college students in Jordan. Eastern Mediterranean Health Journal 2001; 7:3: 435–440.

Autonomous Areas of Gaza and the West Bank, only three girls were accepted back into their communities.

Crimes registered between 2002 and 2006 revealed that perpetrators and victims of non-domestic violence among adults are generally men. In the last five years 6186 persons have been victims of these criminal acts; 924 (15%) women compared to 5258 (85%) men and 4 cases of unspecified sex. Perpetrators of these crimes also tend to be mostly men, out of 9227 criminals 95% of non-domestic crime perpetrators are men, compared to 5% women perpetrators. Generally, this corroborates the male aspect of violence in Lebanon.

The same observations regarding non-domestic violence among adults applies to minors. The number of minors that are perpetrators of non-domestic crimes between 2002 and 2006 reached 806 minors: 26 (3%) girls and 780 (97%) boys. Minors committed acts of crime against 609 victims, 514 (84%) male and 95 (16%) female.

Furthermore, perpetrators and victims of domestic violence among adults are generally men. The number of victims registered between 2002 and 2006 was 1501 victims, 734 (49%) women, (51%) 765 men, and 2 unspecified. Perpetrators of domestic violence among adults were 2034 criminals, 1714 (84%) men and 318 (16%) women. In two cases, the sex of the perpetrator was not specified. The majority of juvenile perpetrators of domestic violence are also male. 111 minors were perpetrators of domestic-crimes of who 86 (77%) were boys and 25 (23%) girls. However, the number of female-minors that were victims of this violence exceeded that of males: out of 83 minors that were victims of domestic violence, 52 (63%) were girls compared to 31 (37%) boys.

The abovementioned forms of violence are related to sexuality, while only the two latter forms are sexual activities as such. Still, we categorize all three forms as sexual violence. Furthermore, since we are analyzing these forms of sexual violence from a gender perspective, we can conclude that this violence is gender-based. Although boys are also victims in honor- cultures, in the sense that they somehow are forced to "guard" and commit acts of violence against their sisters, we believe that the victims are primarily girls. We are concerned that girls are the most marginalized group in the region because they often face discrimination as females and as children. To focus too much on boys and other victims in honor cultures such as homosexuals, we believe would be another betrayal against the girls in the region.

It should be stated that sexual violence against children exists in all societies around the world and is not a particular problem restricted to the MENA region.[20] However, each society has its particular cultural-logic and mechanisms in the field of sexuality that have to be discerned and acknowledged. Some trends are general and almost universal, such as patriarchalism, as well as the shame and trauma associated to the victim of sexual abuse. Polonko study emphasizes analyzing in-depth

[20]Karen A. PolonkoNicholas Adams, Nazia Naeem and Ava Adinolfi; Department of Sociology and Criminal Justice; Old Dominion University;Norfolk, VA USA; Paper presented at the fourth Annual International Conference on Sociology Athens, Greece on 10–13 May 2010. Forthcoming chapter in edited book by ATINER.

gender-based sexual-abuse in the MENA region, rather than comparing the different problems between various cultures regarding this issue. Sexuality is often a controversial and charged topic touching the inner and existential aspects of our identity. Therefore, sensitivity of the subjects include gender roles, family building, religious morality, identity and kinship relations. Since this is a thorough analysis some of these aspects are criticized in the way that they are exploited for legitimizing sexual abuse, for instance, Islam might be used to legitimize honor violence.

By acknowledging this we do not say that Islam or other religions accept honor-violence. Close kinship relations might be used as a method of psychological pressure on girls to marry early. Discussing this is not a criticism of kinship societies but only on some aspects of its practice.

7.3 Research and Reviews in the Middle-East

7.3.1 Abstract

As expected, an extensive review of the prior research in 21 countries in the Middle East and North Africa, published in refereed academic outlets and/or NGO documents, yielded few studies with prevalence data on CSA. Information on the studies is presented in Appendix A and prevalence rates of CSA by gender and country are presented in Table 7.1. What is striking is the absence of prevalence data available, even just from a small convenience sample of a class of college students, for all countries in the Middle East and North Africa except Israel—Bedouin Arabs, Jordan, Occupied Palestinian Territory, Lebanon, Egypt and Morocco.

Given the few studies available and how little we know about CSA in MENA, as much information as can be gleaned from these studies will be presented and discussed within the framework of global trends.

7.3.2 Prevalence

The first and most important point to note about the results is that child sexual abuse of boys and girls does indeed exist in the Middle East and North Africa as it does in the rest of the world. Regardless of the country, region, sample size (from 100 to over 3000), age group (secondary school, college, adults over 20) or gender studied or measure used, results showed that child sexual abuse is a problem.[21]

[21]Briere, J. and Elliot, D. Prevalence and psychological sequelae of self-reported childhood physical and sexual abuse in a general population sample of men and women Child Abuse & Neglect 2003; 27: 1205–1222.

Table 7.1 Prevalence Rates of child sexual abuse prevalence studies

Middle East North Africa	All CSA combined Non Contact and Contact & Hugs		Non-Contact Only		Contact only Fondling & Rape		Contact Only Fondling		Contact Only Rape-Penetration	
Country Author	Male ALL Non-Cont & hug	Female All Non-C &Cont &hug	MaLe Non-Cont Only	Female Non-Cont Only	Male Conta Only F&R	Female Contac only Fondle & Rape	Male Contac Fondle	Female Contac Fondle	Male Rape	Female Rape
Middle East										
Israel Bedouin Arab Elbedour et al	31%		16%+		17%+		13%+		4%+	
Jordan Jumaian					27%					
OPT Al-Rafi Palestinians Haj-Yahia&Tam	46% for M&F	20%+	13%+	25%	22%	15%+	8%+	12%+	5%+	
Lebanon Usta et al WHO			18% 20%				15% 15%			
North Africa										
Egypt Afifi et al						8% for M&F Males Higher				
Morocco Alami&Kadri						9% (13%)				

Although scarce, these studies add some insights on CSAE, with comparable potential, in terms of measures and results. Several studies used variations of the Finkelhor scale/questions, covered many aspects, and secured information on non-contact and contact CSA for girls and/or boys, and consequently ensured some results in terms of actual prevalence and maximum comparability to prior research internationally. The problem is that these authors either did not present the data for both males and females for all items (Usta el al. 2008)[22] or more importantly, did not present results for males or females on the categories of any contact CSA (e.g., yes to any question on touch, fondling, etc.) and any non-contact (e.g., yes to any question on proposition, exhibition, etc.) in addition to an overall category of any contact or non-contact combined item (Usta et al. 2008; Elbedour et al. 2006[23]; Hay-Yahia and Tamish 2003).[24] In spite of the variation and limits to comparability, one can discern several patterns. As expected, percentages decrease as severity of contact CSA increases from fondling to penetration. In addition, the prevalence of the overall rates of combined contact and non-contact CSA appear to be higher for Bedouins and Palestinians than those in Lebanon and Morocco. (Regarding the study on Morocco by Alami and Kadri,[25] one-third of the respondents ended the interview when questions on child sexual abuse were asked. These respondents should have been treated as 'missing data' and deleted from the prevalence rate instead of counting them as 'no child sexual abuse.' These "missing" cases yield a rate of 13%, which is much closer to the prevalence, for the same category for females, in both Lebanese studies. For the three categories of contact CSA, comparable findings are found for North America and Europe; it also appears that a much higher percent of boys are victims of CSA, while a similar or lower percent of girls (particularly lower on the category of penetration) are victims in the Middle East. For example, for the category of contact CSA (all contact items combined), rates for males in the US range from 6% to 9% in contrast to 25% to 27% in Jordan and OPT. Corresponding rates for females in the US are 23% to 30% compared to 17% to 22% among Arab Bedouins in Israel and Palestinians. In addition since the estimates for males and females in the contact categories are the lower estimates based on one item, it could be possible that these differences are even higher for boys and less (more similar) for girls.

---

[22]Usta, J., Mahfoud, Z., Chahine, G. and Anani, G. Child Sexual Abuse: The situation in Lebanon. KAFA (enough) Violence & Exploitation. Save the Children: Sweden, 2008. 15.

[23]Elbedour, S., Abu-Bader, S., Onwuegbuzie, A., Abu-Rabia, A. and El-Aassam, S. The scope of sexual, physical, and psychological abuse in a Bedouin-Arab community of female adolescents: The interplay of racism, urbanization, polygamy, family honor, and the social marginalization of women. Child Abuse & Neglect, 2006; 30: 215–229.

[24]Haj-Yahia, M. and Tamish, S. The rates of child sexual abuse and its psychological consequences as revealed by a study among Palestinian university students. Child Abuse & Neglect 2001; 25: 1303–1327.

[25]Alami, K. and Kadri, N. Moroccan women with a history of child sexual abuse and its long-term repercussions: A population-based epidemiological study. Archives of Women's Mental Health 2004; 7: 237–242.

7.3.3 Analysis

Rates of CSA of boys in the Middle East are not only higher than that for boys in western cultures but also higher than rates of CSA of girls in the Middle East. This is opposite to findings in North America and Europe and authors in the studies reviewed commented on this. For example, in observing that male students were significantly more likely than female students to be victims of CSA (recall 20% v. 15%), WHO (2007, 47) concludes: 'Contrary to expectation, males are more likely to report sexual harassment than females.' Hay-Yahia and Tamish (2003) found a similar pattern of differences by gender, on average, across a multiplicity of indicators, although not significant. They conclude '... in contrast to those contexts—mainly North America and Western Europe ...where females reported higher rates of sexual abuse than males, the current research findings indicate that the rates of the problem are similar among female and male Palestinian students' (Child Abuse & Neglect 2001; 25: 1303–1327; p. 1320). Afifi et al. (2003) found that gender was not related to the risk of child physical or emotional abuse, but it was for child sexual abuse as results from multivariate analyses showed boys were significantly more likely to be victims of CSA than girls. The authors conclude: 'The sex of the child was an important risk factor only for sexual abuse as males were more exposed than females. This contradicts studies from the United States and might be attributed to the relative freedom male children in Egyptian society enjoy ...compared with their female counterparts.... Another possibility is that females are less likely to disclose abuse, especially sexual abuse.' In reference to that point, several authors including Elbedour et al. (2006), Haj-Yahia and Tamish (2001), Ouis and Myhrman (2007)[26] frame child sexual abuse within the larger context of gender-based violence and the extremes of patriarchy and sex segregation in many countries in the Middle East and North Africa. Related factors include seclusion and segregation of women from the public domain, imposition of veiling, hindrance to access to education and other resources, female genital mutilation, early marriages of girls and crimes of 'honor' where female victims of sexual violence can be forced to marry the rapist or even killed to restore family honor (Shalhoub-Kavorkian 1999: 1278[27]; Elbedour et al. 2006). This would provide theoretical support for the hypothesis that rates for females are lower because of strong fears of disclosing the actual abuse.

---

[26]Ouis, P. and Myhrman, T., editors. Gender-Based Sexual Violence against Teenage Girls in the Middle East: A Comparative Situation Analysis of Honour Violence, Early Marriages and Sexual Abuse in Lebanon, the Occupied Palestinian Territories and Yemen. Save the Children Sweden, Regional Office for the Middle East and North Africa, 2007.

[27]Shalhoub-Kevorkian, N. The politics of disclosing female sexual abuse: A case study of Palestinian society. Child Abuse & Neglect 1999;23:1275–1293.

7.3.4 Comments

It is not clear why prevalence rates of boys are higher than girls in the Middle East and North Africa and there are two separate issues that must be addressed in future research. Regarding girls, their lower rates than boys could reflect underreporting due to females fear that disclosing CSA may lead to substantial costs they could suffer. It could also reflect lower rates due to less access of girls to non-family members hence reducing the portion that extrafamilial sexual abuse contributes to the prevalence of CSA. In other words, the rates of CSA of girls would reflect more exclusively the CSA due to incest or intrafamilial abuse as the portion of extrafamilial CSA could be less. It could be due to a pattern reflecting other aspects of Middle Eastern and North Africa culture. It is certainly clear that the extremes of patriarchy and sex segregation do not prevent the sexual abuse of girls.

Regarding boys, having more freedom than girls would not necessarily lead to expecting higher rates of CSA of boys per se, particularly since in the US boys also have freedom and rates for CSA of boys are lower. Also, recall that evidence suggests a different etiology for the CSA of boys v. girls in North America. The pattern seems to be one where boys are abused by men who tend to be asexual with adults as they tend to be exclusively drawn to boys. Girls are more likely to be sexually abused by heterosexual men who also commit violence against adult women.

There is nothing conceptually thus far that would help understand why lower rates of CSA of girls in a region would lead to higher rates of sexual abuse of boys. More research is needed to explore the many aspects of MENA cultures in this regard.

7.4 The Importance of Measurement and Analysis

The regular collection of accurate demographic data about child sexual abuse in affluent cultures induced a sometimes forceful change in how people in those cultures perceived and responded to the issue of child sexual abuse. This process of collection and meaningful analysis should be entrenched as part of recognized child sexual abuse prevention and treatment systems within all countries and social settings, for the purpose of child protection systems in the Arab region; it may also be extended globally.

When data are poorly collected, low 'reported numbers' cannot be taken to reflect a 'real' low incidence or low prevalence of the problem. The collection of data alone is insufficient, if that data are of poor quality.

The regular collection of demographic (e.g. incidence and prevalence data) data about child sexual abuse is fundamental to any purposeful analysis, and any strategy to positively effect change.

In order to respond appropriately to the needs of their children, their families and their communities, and the decision makers within all countries, cultures, ethnic groups and religions need to know the incidence of the different types of CSA, as well as adverse consequences of child sexual abuse on their children, their families and their society.

The confident identification of child sexual abuse is not always possible:

- *Objective 'physical' markers* of child sexual abuse are present in only a small minority of cases of child sexual abuse. Those markers, if present, may only persist for a short time period (measured in hours and days). The absence of 'physical' markers of child sexual abuse cannot be the basis for dismissing concerns about the possibility that child sexual abuse has occurred. Those signs may include the presence of sexually transmitted infections, pregnancy, etc.
- *Subjective 'behavioral' markers or physical consequences* of child sexual abuse may include drug-use disorders, subsequent behavioral and/or mental disorders in accordance with self-report, other report of CSA or the findings of legal or child protection action, as well as "founded" cases, reported cases, or some combination.

7.5 Research and Evaluation

Research into the etiology, prevention, identification and treatment of child sexual abuse is essential to provide effective interventions.[28]

The development of evidence-based approaches to the prevention, identification and treatment of child sexual abuse that are universally applicable is an important strategy. The present literature is predominately generated from affluent countries, and published in English. Although there is reason to believe that much of this research is globally relevant—significant further investment is required to confirm this possibility, and therefore encouraging publications through regional offices of UN agencies and regional resource centers of ISPCAN.

Specifically, there is a need to demonstrate effective interventions in Arab languages that are culturally attractive, practically implementable (both financially and in regard to available expertise), and politically acceptable, especially in circumstances of limited financial resources, social conflicts and specific regulations.

There are substantial difficulties in researching child sexual abuse, including the challenges:

- to identify the actual prevalence of child sexual abuse versus incidence reports;
- in definition, which relate to both diagnosis and to the development of descriptive data on child sexual abuse;

[28]Russell, D. The incidence and prevalence of intrafamilial and extrafamilial sexual abuse of female children. Child Abuse & Neglect, 1983; 7:133–146.

- to avoid additional harm to victims while respecting their rights;
- to engage offenders while protecting their rights;
- to tackle the cost of conducting the research and disseminating research outcomes;
- to meet scientific requirements for reliability, validity and generalizability of research findings across cultures; and
- related to intra-familiar versus extra-familial child sexual abuse.[29]

There is a need to better understand (both qualitatively and quantitatively) the developmental trajectory of 'normal' childhood sexuality (and expected 'normal but atypical variants') to better understand how we can prevent its exploitation.

When child sexual abuse incidence and prevalence figures are based on surveys, and other indicators (such as crime records, sexually transmitted diseases—STDs—, pregnancies), then researchers can better define what it is being counted, and also describe what they believe the results represent or fail to represent. Research indicates that it is likely that one in five ten, or even more children experience child sexual abuse and exploitation.[30] When incidence and prevalence studies are based on mandatory reporting laws, the data rely on definitions prescribed by law in the jurisdictions mandating reporting. Such data systems are not common yet, but do provide some advantages in terms of management and research.

7.6 The Need for Knowledge on CSA in the Middle East and North Africa

Data on CSA from many new countries continue to add to our knowledge, most impressively, a wealth of data from countries in sub-Saharan Africa (Lalor 2004) and South Asia (Frederick 2010). However, data on CSA from countries in the Middle East and North Africa are still most notably lacking. In discussing the consistency of findings on prevalence and higher rates for girls across countries, Finkelhor (1994: 412) long ago noted that regions of the world such as Africa and the Middle East that lack data on child abuse and have cultures different from 'the predominantly Caucasion, western and Christian countries' that have been most studied, could yield differences in patterns of CSA. In this direction, it is interesting to note that in the Pereda et al. study, atypically high rates for child sexual abuse of boys were found for South Africa, Turkey and Jordan, although South Africa showed similarly high rates of CSA for girls as well. The lack of data on child abuse in general in the

[29]Al-Rafai, A. Political Instability and Nation-Building: Sexual Violence against Female Teenagers in the Occupied Palestinian Territories, Chap. 3 In: Ouis, P. and Myhrman, T., editors. Gender-Based Sexual Violence against Teenage Girls in the Middle East. Save the Children Sweden, 2007.

[30]Most estimates actually indicate higher levels of CSA. The number of cases can vary by the definition and the methodology used. (e.g. the more behaviorally specific questions asked the higher the hit rate of CSA cases.

Middle East and North Africa has been noted by diverse sources, in part reflecting the impact of the near universal ratification of the UN Convention on the Rights of the Child (CRC).[31]

For example, the Child Rights Situational Analysis for the Middle East and North Africa (MENA) Region (2008: 8) states: '. . .despite progress in the legislative and programmatic fronts—with many of the governments of MENA countries working with civil society groups, international NGOs, regional bodies, donors and United Nations agencies to better protect children—child protection remains a serious issue every country of the region. The nature and extent of child protection issues varies country to country, and includes issues such as violence against children—whether at homes, schools or institutional settings—harmful practices, particularly female genital mutilation and early marriage, juvenile justice, exploitative child labor and birth registration' (emphasis added). In the summary of the "Commercial sexual exploitation of children: the situation in the Middle East/North Africa region" (2001), it is acknowledged that all 21 countries covered have ratified the UN CRC, but also that in all the countries of the region, there is cultural resistance to addressing the problem (of child abuse) because the subject is largely taboo.'[32]

It is critical that government and non-government officials in the Middle East and North Africa acknowledge a serious problem in child protection, similar to the rest of the global community. However, without data on CSA in this region, children in this area suffer disproportionately. Without research, there is little chance to overcome societal resistance to acknowledging the problem, there is little understanding of the prevalence, causes and consequences, and therefore less chance to help children who are victims of sexual abuse now and prevention of future victims. The research on child sexual abuse in the Middle East and North Africa contributes to understand CSA in the region and in turn to our understanding of CSA globally. Every research maximizes comparability to Finkelhor and Pereda et al. regarding definition, sources, prevalence and distribution by gender.

Although most Middle Eastern and North African States have endorsed the CRC, few included in their country reports replies to the comments made by the UN regarding the rights of the child. Finally, the voices of children is almost absent from replies to the questionnaire with the exception of one or two countries, reflecting the absence of children's participation in defining the problem or possible solutions.

Furthermore, although the participation of civil society organizations is mentioned in almost all reports, yet the voice of civil society remains virtual in reports, as the critical voice of NGOs is represented in discussing the impact of protective

[31]Alami, K. and Kadri, N. Moroccan women with a history of child sexual abuse and its long-term repercussions: A population-based epidemiological study. Archives of Women's Mental Health 2004; 7: 237–242.

[32]Elbedour, S., Abu-Bader, S., Onwuegbuzie, A., Abu-Rabia, A. and El-Aassam, S. The scope of sexual, physical, and psychological abuse in a Bedouin-Arab community of female adolescents: The interplay of racism, urbanization, polygamy, family honor, and the social marginalization of women. Child Abuse & Neglect, 2006; 30: 215–229.

measures for children. In that report, the views of both the executive bodies and those of civil society are however highlighted.

A review of the available studies clearly shows that there is a great similarity between countries of the Middle East and North Africa region concerning the causes behind the high prevalence of violence against children in the different areas, including its most common forms. Discrepancies between countries exist regarding certain types of violence such as FGM (female genital mutilation) or "honor killings" and the size of other phenomena such as street children and child labor. Risk factors may be classified as follows:

- Economic factors: increased rates of poverty and unemployment, which will increase with global economic crisis.
- Social factors: dysfunctional families in multicultural contexts, marital disputes of parents, large size of families, polygamy; social tensions and armed conflicts,
- Prevalent cultural beliefs: attitudes towards raising children (e.g. assumptions that an extent of physical or verbal violence may be useful for child rearing)
- Lack of awareness: regarding appropriate child rearing practices and the harm that some might provoke (e.g. shaking babies)
- Role of the media and programs which sometimes encourage violence (e.g. scenes of violence and child participation in armed conflicts)
- Legislation: lacks provisions that target the protection of children. In cases where those laws are present they may not be adequately enforced. Also, reporting of violence against children is not compulsory in most of the countries in the MENA region

7.6.1 *The Paucity of Data*

Most studies refer the scarcity of data on violence against children to a number of reasons, such as the sensitivity of the issue—especially when it occurs in certain contexts such as the family—bit also the tendency to under report violence against children and the lack of awareness of its negative consequences, etc. Finally the issue attracts minimal attention from researchers and investigators, except recently, despite the abundance of studies addressing violence in the community in general in the last decade. Some of the country reports mention that such data are not available because of lack of field studies and epidemiological research on part of relevant bodies.

7.6.2 *The Refugees' Issues*

Half of the world's refugees are children.[33] Many refugee children spend their entire childhoods in displacement, uncertain about the future. Children—whether refugees,

[33]"Child Protection from Violence, Exploitation and Abuse - MENA Region." UNICEF.org. United Nations Children's Fund, n.d. Web. <http://www.unicef.org/protection/MENA.pdf>

internally displaced or stateless—are at greater risk than adults of violence, abuse, neglect, and exploitation. They may experience and witness disturbing events, or separate from their families. At the same time, family and other social support networks may be weakened and education may be disrupted. These experiences can have a profound effect on children—from infancy and childhood through adolescence.

7.6.3 The Gender Burden

During emergencies and in displacement, girls and boys may face particular gender-related protection risks. The total number of refugees in MENA has doubled in 4 years, largely due to the Syria crisis. Since 2011, more than three million Syrian refugees have fled their country and sought refuge in the region. Every 30 min, 35 children become refugees in MENA. Over 1,530,000 Syrian refugees are children, leaving national child protection systems overburdened in refugee-receiving countries in the region—countries that have already experienced several waves of refugee influxes and situations of protracted displacement.

7.6.4 The Civil Society

In addition, despite progress in the legislative and programmatic fronts—with many of the governments of MENA countries working with civil society groups, international NGOs, regional bodies, donors and United Nations agencies to better protect children—child protection remains a serious issue every country of the region. The nature and extent of child protection issues varies country to country, and includes issues such as violence against children—whether at homes, schools or institutional settings—harmful practices, particularly female genital mutilation and early marriage, juvenile justice, exploitative child labor and birth registration. Children in Algeria, Iraq and the Occupied Palestinian Territories have been exposed to political violence and conflicts; in Western Sahara, they have been affected by the deteriorating humanitarian situation.

7.6.5 The Problem of Education

Free basic education is guaranteed by law in all the countries of the Middle East and North African (MENA) region (except for Oman). A number of countries have even enacted penalties for guardians who do not enroll children of compulsory school age. However, compulsory education is generally not enforced across the region, and there are few effective measures to prevent student absences.

The right to education is also enshrined in regional human rights instruments. The African Charter on Human and People's Rights, adopted by the then Organization of African Unity in 1981, specifically stipulates that 'every individual shall have the right to education', and similarly Article 11 of the African Charter on the Rights and Welfare of the Child, adopted in 1990, recognizes that 'every child shall have the right to an education'. The Arab Charter on Human Rights, which came into force in 2008, also guarantees every citizen free education at least through the primary level, without discrimination of any kind. Civil society groups and the United Nations High Commissioner for Human Rights have expressed their deep concern that the right to education is limited to child citizens. As a result of certain policies and practices in some countries of the MENA there are groups of children that do not have access to education, based on their nationality or their citizenship/residency status (e.g. children of stateless persons, refugees, internally displaced persons and migrant families), geographic location (e.g. rural areas), economic situation (low income families), physical or other disability, minority groups, etc....

The MENA countries have committed more resources to education and are spending more public expenditure per pupil at all levels of educations than other developing countries at a similar level of per capita income. However, most of the MENA countries are spending more per pupil in secondary than primary education and, to a greater extent in tertiary than secondary education. This pattern of resource allocation favors children in families of higher income group, who are likely to send their children to university, as noted by the World Bank.

Chapter 8
The Prohibition of Violence in the Laws of Arab Countries

8.1 Abstract

Sadly, in the context of numerous uprises and social conflicts, many countries halted the implementation of child protective acts and procedures, in relation with armed conflicts and social instability. Cases of child sexual abuse, trafficking and exploitation have increasingly been reported in media and an expanding social network in the Arab region, linking more armed conflicts, social instability and child trafficking.

8.2 Country Profiles

Bahrain passed a Child Act in 2012, which includes a special chapter on the protection of children from abuse. Abuse is defined as: "Any act or omission that would lead to direct or indirect harm to the child (thus) preventing the proper, safe and healthy upbringing of the child, including physical, psychological or sexual abuse, neglect or economic exploitation". The law also provides definitions for each type of abuse addressed.

Since 1995, the Tunisian Child Protection Code has prohibited all forms of violence against children in their various settings, and has made it compulsory all professionals and citizens to report on threats to children to Child Protection Delegates.

Algeria's government reviewed a draft of Child Protection Act in the context of strengthening the legal system related to the rights of the child.

Sudan's constitution and the Child Act of 2010 have all prohibited the practice of torture, abuse or neglect. The Child Act includes strong penalties and comprehensive solutions for child abuse and protection from violence. It obligates any person who believes that a child's right has been violated to notify the authorities. In addition,

B. Gerbaka et al., *Child Sexual Abuse, Exploitation and Trafficking in the Arab Region*, Child Maltreatment 13, https://doi.org/10.1007/978-3-030-66507-4_8

several states have successfully issued laws to banning and criminalizing female genital mutilation.

In Iraq, the regional government of Kurdistan approved a law against domestic violence in 2011. The government of Iraq also issued Law 28/2012, which prevents the manufacturing and importing of children's toys that incite violence. It has also sought to issue a set of bills including the Draft Law on Child Protection in Iraq, the Draft Law on a Parliament for Children, the Draft Law on the Child Welfare Authority and the Anti-trafficking Law.

Oman drafted a Child Act, which includes a special section on the protection of children. In addition, several laws were enacted to prohibit all forms of physical and psychological violence, including corporal punishment, humiliation, neglect and exploitation within the family and residential institutions.

In 2012, Palestine ratified the amendments made on the 2004 Child Act. Article 68 of the amended law stipulates that: "No child may be subject to physical or psychological torture or to any treatment that is cruel or degrading to human dignity." The law also obliges professionals and child care takers to report abuse to the Child Protection Guide. Draft laws were also prepared for family protection and the protection of juveniles as well as the establishment of the National Council for Childhood under the umbrella of the Ministry of Social Affairs.

Qatar continues efforts to revise its Draft Child Act. In 2010 two decrees were issued to amend certain provisions of Qatar's accession to the CRC and the Optional Protocol on the Sale of Children, Child Prostitution and Child Pornography and give these instruments the force of law. The legal age of marriage for both women and men is 18.

In 20,012, Yemen undertook a comprehensive legal review of national legislations and regulations on children, followed by drafting a set of laws on the rights of the child, to be integrated into a single law. It also indicated that in 2007 amendments were proposed to parliament on the Child Rights Act and the Penal Code particularly crimes of child exploitation (sexual exploitation, child trafficking, begging).

8.3 Sexual Violence Against Children and Relevant Laws

Violence increasingly affects the lives of children in the Arab region. Younger children are at special risk, having less ability to speak up and seek support and also greater chances of suffering irreversible emotional and health damage. Hidden and socially accepted sexual violence against children (FGC, EMC) remain confronted with passivity or even active opposition.

Arab States have made significant progress towards universal primary education, with the average net enrolment ratio continuing to rise, from nearly 79% in 1999 to 83% in 2005.

However, these rates may be inflated due to low birth registration rates in rural areas. In addition, it is important to highlight that attendance rates are significantly lower than enrolment rates in many countries. Despite improvements in access to primary education, the number of out-of-school children remains high. More than six million children in the region were out of school in 2005, with almost half of the children, mainly girls, located in Iraq, Morocco, Saudi Arabia and Yemen.

Despite significant government spending and the advances in access to education, the average level of education youth receive is still lower in the MENA region than other developing countries with a similar level of per capita income. School progression and retention rates show a disturbing trend in many of the MENA countries with high drop-out and absenteeism at the secondary level. This has been attributed to poverty, economic necessity to find employment and low quality of education. With the exception of Iraq, Morocco and Yemen, the MENA region is largely on track to achieving the Millennium Development Goal of achieving gender parity in access to primary education by 2015.

The UN also states that gender disparities concern not only access to school but also participation in learning process; in nearly all MENA countries with data, boys repeat more than girls, showing that once girls have access to school, they do as well or better than boys. Overall though, strong gender disparities persist—three out of five children not enrolled in primary school in the region in 2005 were girls. Indeed, girls who have little schooling generally come from low-income communities and tend to marry early and begin childbearing at a young age. UNICEF has also noted its concerns that education systems in the region largely reproduces and reinforces the wider social discrimination and economic/political disparities experienced by girls and women in many countries of the region.

The Rome Statute's definition of sexual slavery includes situations where persons are forced to domestic servitude, marriage or any other forced labor involving sexual activity, as well as the trafficking of persons, in particular women and children. Sudan has seen a resurgence of slavery since1983, associated with the Second Sudanese Civil War. Slavery in Sudan predates Islam, but continued under Islamic and civil legislation.

8.4 Status of Arab States Ratification of CRC and the Optional Protocols

The ratification of LAS member states of all international rights of the child conventions has represented one of the most important priorities of joint Arab action for the advancement of the rights of the child over the past two decades. All Arab states have ratified the CRC, with the exception of Somalia, which has signed only. The Palestinian Authority signed and ratified the CRC in 1995, long before the United Nations granted the State of Palestine non-Member Observer State status in 2012.

This international legal commitment to the rights of the child has also been reflected by most Arab states joining or ratifying the two Optional Protocols (Table 1, Annex 2: The status of Arab states' ratification of the Convention and its' two protocols). Three countries (The United Arab Emirates, Comoros, and Mauritania) have not yet joined the Optional Protocol on the involvement of children in armed conflict, and two countries (Somalia and Lebanon) have signed but not ratified this protocol. Only two Arab countries (The United Arab Emirates and Somalia) have yet to join the Optional Protocol on the sale of children, child prostitution, and child pornography. The United Arab Emirates has indicated that it has established committee of relevant parties to study the possibility of joining the Optional Protocols.

As for the third Optional Protocol (OP3) of the CRC on a communications procedure, Morocco confirmed that it signed the protocol without any additional details. Other countries are studying the protocol. In Yemen, the Council of Ministers has agreed to join and referred the matter to the House of Representatives for discussion and approval. OP3 is also under review in the Sultanate of Oman, where the country's position will be determined after the enactment of the new Child Act. Bahrain formed a committee, chaired by the Foreign Ministry, to review the protocol and collect the views of relevant bodies on accession. Similarly, the Sudanese National Council for Childhood formed a technical committee to study OP3 and refer it to the concerned authorities.

While the completion of Arab commitments to the CRC enshrines and legitimizes its position within human rights mechanisms, it is yet to include the Optional Protocols or the withdrawal of reservations, due to the absence of official follow-up by Arab states to review reservations, consider their withdrawal and into taking steps towards ratification or accession. Seven countries (Bahrain, Sudan, Comoros, Lebanon, Libya, Mauritania, and Yemen) have not made any formal reservations on the provisions of the CRC, whereas the reservations were made by the other countries on articles that they consider to be in conflict with Islamic Shari'a law, their constitutions, or their laws (Table 2, Annex 3: Reservations by some Arab states on CRC: reasons and current status).

There are several forms of reservations by Arab countries; some are general statements while others are specific reservations or clarifications regarding articles 2, 4, 6, 7, 9, 13, 14, 16, 17, 20, 21, 30, and 40, on the basis that they are incompatible with Islamic Shari'a Law or the existing laws in these states. Eight states expressed reservations on Article 14 on freedom of thought, belief, and religion; on the basis that Islam is the country's constitution. Also, seven states entered reservations on Article 21 on adoption, on the basis that it is not allowed in Islam. As for Article 7 on birth registration, 4 countries have made reservations. In addition, 3 countries have reservations on Article 20 on foster care. Morocco withdrew its' reservation on Article 14 on October 17th 2006, and replaced it with an explanatory declaration stating that: "The Kingdom of Morocco interprets the provisions of the first paragraph of Article 14 of the CRC in the light of the constitution of October seventh, 1996, and other specially relevant national laws: Chapter six of the constitution which states that Islam is the religion of the state, and that the state guarantees for its' citizens the right of freedom of worship. Article 54 of Law 03–70 (Family Code) which states in its' sixth paragraph that children have the right to religious guidance and to an upbringing based on ethical conduct by their parents. In accordance with this statement, the Kingdom of Morocco confirms its' commitment to human rights as they are universally recognized and to the objectives of this convention." Egypt, Syria, and Oman also withdrew their reservations on Article 21. Egypt and Syria also withdrew their reservations on Article 20.

The position of Arab states towards maintaining reservations on some articles of the CRC and withdrawing others indicates that most of these countries have made reservations on a number of articles, based on the belief that their content or potential implications are not consistent with Islamic Shari'a. This position reflects the failure of the official authorities to periodically review the provisions of the convention, since the phrasing of these articles is nonbinding.

This is clear, for example, in Article 21, where a reference was made to countries that allow adoption—a clear expression that it is non-binding to countries that do not allow adoption. This article also includes a reference to "Kafala", inserted during the CRC drafting process to reflect the Islamic mechanism of adoption. In addition, some other articles contain unbinding guidelines that do not indicate obligation, recognition, or pledging specific action, as in Articles 5 and 14: "State parties shall respect. . . .." This is an additional reason for removing reservations; as such articles allow state parties the option to incorporate them in a way that does not conflict with their national laws.

It would be beneficial for countries that still have reservations on some of the articles of the CRC to take into account the experience of Morocco with regards to the withdrawal of reservations on Article 14, and also the measures adopted by Egypt, Oman and Syria.

8.4.1 Reservations of Arab States on the Two Optional Protocols

United Nations documents indicate that there is limited number of reservations on the two Optional Protocols by several Arab countries.

8.4.1.1 Optional Protocol on the Involvement of Children in Armed Conflict

The Sultanate of Oman made a general reservation arising from its reservation on the CRC. Based on paragraph 2 of Article 3 of the protocol on the involvement of children in armed conflict, the following countries have made a declaration stating that their military laws are in harmony with the requirements of the protocol, since the minimum age of voluntary recruitment in their armed forces is 18: Bahrain, Tunisia, Algeria, Saudi Arabia, Sudan, Syria, Iraq, Qatar, Kuwait, Libya, Egypt, Morocco, and Yemen. Syria also attached an explanatory statement.

8.4.1.2 Optional Protocol on the Sale of Children, Child Pornography, and Child Prostitution

Both Syria and Kuwait made reservations on Article 3, paragraph 5, on the need to take measures to ensure that all those involved in the adoption process act in accordance with the applicable international legal instruments. Syria attached a supplementary reservation on Article 3, paragraph 1B (2) on adoption. Data on the reservations of Arab states on this Optional Protocol indicate that Qatar withdrew its' reservation on 18 June, 2008, without being bound by any provisions that are inconsistent with Islamic Shari'a. Oman made a general reservation expressing the view that its' ratification of the Optional Protocol would be constraining by its reservations on the CRC.

An overall analysis of the reservations of some Arab countries on the Optional Protocols in contrast to the CRC, allows the following conclusions:

- The reservation of Syria on Article 3.1. (a) ii of the Optional Protocol of the CRC on the sale of children, child prostitution, and child pornography as regards to adoption, and in contrast with the withdrawal of its' reservations on Articles 20 and 21 of the CRC leads to the conclusion that this withdrawal also applies to the provisions of the Optional Protocol.
- The withdrawal of the general reservations of the Sultanate of Oman to the CRC may apply to the two protocols.
- On the second of April 2008, Qatar withdrew its' reservations on the Optional Protocol on the sale of children, child prostitution, and child pornography.

In conclusion, while most Arab countries have ratified the two optional protocols they are currently reviewing the Optional Protocol on a communications procedure. The CRC and its Optional Protocols represent a general framework for the civil, political, cultural, and social rights of the child, within a complete and integrated vision that prioritizes the best interests of the child. The reservations of Arab countries on the convention affect the spirit of this fundamental principle in one way or another, and thus the application of the provisions of the convention and the protocols requires placing a unified framework in the Arab region for the full recognition of the rights of the child.

The CRC approach is based on the importance and equal value of all the rights of the child, without fragmentation. This makes it necessary for Arab countries which still maintain reservations on some of the articles and Optional Protocols of the CRC to review these reservations according in line with the principle of the best interests of the child and to take practical steps to:

- Speed up the completion of reviewing national laws on the rights of the child to harmonize them with the provisions and spirit of the CRC
- Convene consultations involving specialists and stakeholders from various bodies to review other instruments related to child protection, including the Optional Protocol on a communications procedure;

- Promote the coordination, follow-up, exchange of experiences and communication between Arab bodies and institutions concerned with childhood, on various topics related to the rights of the child;
- Complete the ratification of international conventions related to international law on the rights of the child and withdraw reservations on some of the articles of the CRC, particularly as several of these reservations conflict with the basic mandatory principles of the convention representing the core or minimum inalienable rights. Examples of this are the child's right to life, right of survival, right to nondiscrimination on the basis of sex or birth, the principle of the child's best interest, and respect of the child's right to freedom of expression;
- Fill the gaps regarding state reservations on the articles of the CRC and the lack of consistency of legislation with the convention and its' optional protocols especially on issues related to adoption, foster care, alternative care, the definition of a child, and VAC

The issue of withdrawing reservations continues to be a major concern of the International Committee on the Rights of the Child, which it recalls in all of its' concluding observations thus reflecting the importance of this question for realizing the rights of the child. Also, the declaration by the Conference on the Rights of the Child in Islam, co-sponsored by the Organization of Islamic Conference, called on its member states Arab countries to withdraw their reservations on the convention due to the lack of contradiction with Islamic Shari'a. The declaration also called on Arab countries to join the supplementary protocols.

The Women, Family, and Childhood Department in the League of Arab States has worked on including the issue of the necessity of withdrawal of reservations on its' agenda. In addition, several recommendations were issued by the meetings of the Arab Childhood Committee in these regards. The department also organized several activities in this regards, the last of which was a workshop.[1]

The supplementary optional protocol of the CRC also mentions a communication procedure on the complaint-filing procedure. The commitment of Arab countries to secure children's rights and provide a safe environment for their growth and development led them to join the rest of the world in the course of ratification and accession of the CRC and its' optional protocols on the involvement of children in armed conflicts, the sale of children, child prostitution, and child pornography. They are invited today to join the third protocol on a communication procedure complaint-filing, as a clear sign of their commitment towards children in the Arab region as rights holders who are capable of demanding their rights, and of holding accountable those responsible for violating them through the use of an international mechanism that provides them with an opportunity for equity that their countries are not able to provide. Joining the protocol also confirms that Arab countries ensure children's freedom to express their opinions and ensures their protection against all forms of abuse, violence, and violations, and also work on ensuring that violations against

[1]The Optional Protocols of the International CRC and the Ombudsman Mechanism", Doha 2012.

children do not go unpunished, and on the provision of appropriate compensation for child victims.

The International Committee on the Rights of the Child, in its' concluding observations on national reports on the situation of children provided by Arab countries, urged these countries to work on establishing independent monitoring structures to monitor violations against children and to punish those who perpetrate them, and encouraged the presence of national institutions for human rights based on the Paris principles that ensure accountability in the area of child rights' violations. Up until now this kind of institution is non-existent in Arab countries and children are still deprived of full opportunities for redress and justice, therefore the ratification of the third protocol has an added significance as a step towards finding delicate, sensitive, and safe complaint and reporting mechanisms for children. This also came as a recommendation for countries in the Comparative Arab Report on the Implementation of the Recommendations of the UN Secretary General's Study on Violence against Children's first version. Until the date of preparation of this report, Morocco is the only Arab country, which has signed the third optional protocol. Yemen has also taken several steps towards its' ratification, through the approval of the Cabinet, and its' referral to the House of Representatives for the completion of legal and constitutional procedures. Sudan has also formed a technical committee to study the protocol and forward its' recommendations on ratification to the relevant references. In the Sultanate of Oman, it is currently being studied, and the position of the Sultanate will be determined after the enactment of the Child Act. As for Bahrain, a committee has been formed headed by the foreign ministry to review the protocol and gather opinions of relevant bodies on joining it.

According to a paper presented during the workshop "Optional Protocols of the International Convention on the Rights of the Child and the Ombudsman mechanism": "Ratification of the protocol does not posit an extra burden on states, in addition to the fact that it does not affect their national sovereignty, since domestic jurisdiction and the depletion of domestic equitable measures is fully respected, and their fulfillment is required before the application of international procedures for complaint-filing. Side by side with and through the efforts of national children's rights' institutions and with the support of advice, reporting, and complaints on behalf of the child, the third optional protocol will enhance national abilities of Arab countries to address issues of violence against children, and ensure that their commitment to children's rights is at the same level as the commitment shown by the ratification of other international conventions that include the work of international mechanisms designed to compensate for damage caused by violations".

8.5 Legal Procedures Adopted to Prohibit Corporal Punishment and Sexual Violence and Intimidation

Jordan modified the civil service system to strengthen penalties on those working with children who use physical violence against them. Violators are barred from further employment in any department where children are present. In 2007, instructions were issued to regulate student discipline in government schools. Bahrain's Council of Ministers issued a decree setting a common framework for reviewing the performance of schools and kindergartens. The National Authority of Qualifications and Quality Assurance and Training is designated to monitor and evaluate the educational performance of students and the presence of a safe and violence-free environment in schools.

Tunisia reviewed its penal law in 2010 adding a section on corporal punishment of children prohibiting individuals with authority over children from exercising violent behaviour towards them whatever the reason and requiring the use of alternative measures for child upbringing. However, there is no explicit text that punishes parents for committing violence against their children, except in cases where this violence is excessive, results in a fall, or leads to death.

Algeria, since 1994, considers violence to be a crime punishable by law. Legal measures were taken to prohibit the practice of all forms of VAC, whether verbal or physical, through ordinances that were further reinforced by a 2008 trend setting law on education that prohibits inflicting physical violence against students.

In 2011 Saudi Arabia's Ministry of Education in 2011 prepared guidelines for schools aimed at eliminating the use of violence against children and containing the harm this inflicts on children, through forming school based teams to provide guidance and ensure a safe and healthy educational environment.

Sudan implemented a prohibition of corporal punishment in Khartoum schools through ministerial directives. Administrative staff and educational guides monitor compliance and, in cases where violations are committed, a legal and administrative inquiry is held. In the event of harm being inflicted, police units intervene to protect the family and child.

In Iraq strict instructions are issued by the Ministry of Education, prohibiting violence in all forms against children in schools. The school carries the responsibility for any physical or psychological harm that befalls a child while at school.

In Oman, the Ministry of Education undertook several steps intended to limit the exposure of children to harm, including the revision of regulations and legislations related to education, updating guidelines for student and parent-teacher associations, referring cases of sexual or physical assault to the concerned authorities, and holding perpetrators accountable.

In the State of Palestine, suggested modifications to the Child Law include alterations to the executive regulations, which would upgrade the current referral and follow-up systems being applied through child protection networks.

A Child Protection Guide is responsible for initiating complaints against persons threatening the child and total confidentiality is ensured in all cases.

In Qatar, the Supreme Education Council has introduced a number of measures to prohibit violence in schools. Also, in 2001, a decree was issued by the Minister of Education barring school staff from inflicting psychological harm, offences and personal humiliation while guiding the student. The Ministry is implementing strict penalties on those violators, including possible expulsion from work.

Lebanon issued ministerial decrees prohibiting violence in schools, but these are non-binding to the private sector.

8.6 Measures Against Perpetrators of Crimes of Violence

Measures taken against perpetrators of crimes of violence and sexual abuse of children should prevent them from working with children, as is the case in Jordan, Tunisia, Algeria, Saudi Arabia, Sudan, Syria, Oman, Qatar, Kuwait, Libya, Egypt, Morocco, and Yemen. Legal decrees prohibit perpetrators of violence against and sexual abuse of children from returning to work with children.

Some measures adopted include dismissal from work, or preventing the perpetrator from working with children in the future. Some countries also take action to ensure enforcement of other legal punishments. Bahrain indicates that the country has no explicit provisions preventing abusers from working with children, but the special procedures of the Civil Service Bureau prevent recruitment of recidivist perpetrators. In Lebanon, there is no explicit provision preventing abusers from working with children; such decisions are left to judges. In Egypt, measures begin with pre-requisites for employment in accordance with the labor law, requiring publication of the criminal act in a newspaper, to prevent recruitment of ex-offenders or persons in conflict with the law. Government institutions have inspectors at the departments of legal affairs to investigate negligence and violations committed by staffers against children. Private foundations are also subject to the justice system and accountability in accordance with the labor law. These measures allow for dismissal of employees who commit violations and soil the foundation's reputation in terms of professional standards and honor. Other punishments include arrest, imprisonment and prohibition from interaction with children. Child protection strategies are already set in some countries and are in the process of development in others, whereas some countries still struggle with safety issues to comfort their child protection policies. Less is known about other Arab countries who did not yet share information about their child protection strategies. Since 2003, international organizations have been thoroughly involved in different stages of those processes, including the development of national and regional policies in response to the UNSV, mainly in the setting of a sustained support and stable national structures, in order to improve child protection policies as well as child friendly processes. In a significant step to respond to the UN questionnaire on VAC, 9 countries have submitted a report at that time: Egypt, Sudan, Syria, Yemen, Qatar, Kuwait, Morocco, Palestine and Algeria. Lebanon had a catch-up report. Arab countries, however, have difficulties providing enough data regarding the situation of violence against children in their respective context. Also, available studies do not cover all countries in the region.

8.7 How Did the Middle-East Arab Region Address CSA

8.7.1 Tradition, Change and Economic Progress

The concepts of the need to protect children, and that children have a sexual developmental trajectory, are universally held tenets in all of the world's cultures and religions. Although a particular child-rearing practice may have a long history within a culture (i.e. the practice is 'customary' or 'traditional')—this is not sufficient to assert that the practice is neither harmful nor abusive to children: prone sleeping and co-sleeping being negative ones, kangarooing being is a positive, FGM being a consensual but negative one [in Soudan, close to 95% of adult female have been genitally mutilated]. Parents, families, societies, cultures, ethnic and religious groups raise children is a manner that they believe to be beneficial to their children. However, review of practices in the light of a developing evidence-base can allow for the evolution of new and beneficial child protective attitudes and practices within families and society.

Based on an evolving evidence-bases of effective practices to prevent, identify, investigate and treat suspected child sexual abuse, professionals in different cultures can help individuals and societies rethink and reframe behaviors and practices relevant to the care of children and treatment of perpetrators. Although 'Western' economic 'progress' provides some protection to children from death and morbidity directly associated with poverty, the cultural changes associated with economic progress are not always in the best interests of children.[2] The social isolation of careers for children (often women) that can be associated with 'Western' economic 'progress' may have adverse side effects and can be 'concomitants' of child abuse and neglect, including child sexual abuse. During periods of rapid social changes [social riots, armed conflicts, displacement of populations, etc.] all members of a culture are vulnerable, but due to their dependence, children are particularly vulnerable at those times. It is increasingly recognized across all nations and cultures that children are the most important component of 'human capital'. There are strong economic reasons to protect children from sexual abuse—for this reason alone.

ISPCAN supports individuals, organizations and societies who hold resources and/or expertise in the prevention, identification, investigation and treatment of child sexual abuse to facilitate the protection of children in less resourced areas across the globe. It is important that this support is sensitive to local national, cultural, ethnic and religious traditions, practices and beliefs—provided that such traditions,

[2] May-Chahal, C. and Herczog, M. Child Sexual Abuse in Europe. Germany: Council of Europe Publishing, 2003. 14

practices and beliefs do not lead to child harm. In this regard, the relevant international UN instruments can provide some guidance. Whatever the local national, cultural, ethnic and religious traditions if they result in child sexual abuse or exploitation - it is appropriate that they be vigorously challenged.

8.7.2 The First Regional Consultation

The 2005 Regional Consultation, which was organized to contribute to the United Nations Secretary-General's Study on Violence against Children, highlighted that violence against children constitutes a problem throughout the MENA region and takes many forms. To almost all states in the region, the Committee on the Rights of the Child has recommended legislative reforms to better prohibit all forms of violence against children, including corporal punishment within the family and in alternative care settings.

While there is general recognition that violence and abuse against children occurs at home, at work, in schools, and in institutional settings, none of the countries have comprehensive data and information on its prevalence and nature. In many of the countries, the Committee on the Rights of the Child has expressed its concerns about the lack of sufficient information about child abuse and ill-treatment, and UNICEF is working with national governments to put in place comprehensive data collection and monitoring systems. Efforts by the governments of the region have shown an increasing willingness to discuss issues such as violence and child abuse—Oman and Saudi Arabia have organized a national workshop on child abuse and neglect, Syria has held high level conferences on violence against children, paving the way for a national plan of action.[3]

8.7.3 The Regional Approach

All the countries under review have taken legislative steps to address violence against children. Tunisia's Child Protection Code is one of the most comprehensive in the region—it shields children from violence, neglect and abuse through the establishment of child protection mechanisms, namely, through the establishment of a body of "delegates for childhood protection" able to investigate and intervene on behalf of children in difficult situations which may threaten the security and development of the children. Qatar has also facilitated the establishment of foundations which run national hotlines, provide face to face counseling services, and liaise with the police, the courts and the Ministry of Interior. However, as adolescents and

[3]Barakat, Mouta and Iman Ezz. 2003. Violence Towards Child Survey Study in the Basic Schooling Education in Syria. UNICEF. Damascus.

children who participated in the regional consultation indicated, even where laws and policies against violence exist, the means of enforcing them are weak. Very few countries have effective and comprehensive national systems for the detection, reporting, referral and intervention for children victims of abuse, especially domestic abuse. The consultation also confirmed that in general, most violence—especially sexual violence and abuse—against children remains hidden away inside the family circle or in the confines of the school. Laws in some of the countries also make reporting by children difficult. For example, under the Jordanian penal code, complaints from a child can only be accepted if they are supported by the parents or guardian. In Egypt and Lebanon, for example no periodic reports are available regarding child deaths due to violence, because such crimes usually happen as individual cases and do not represent a phenomenon; moreover, they are often attributed to accidental injuries. Thus, there are no government reports on child deaths suspected to be secondary to violence. In 2009 however, a child deaths review team was created in Lebanon, and one is on its way in Jordan. In this perspective, a child protection unit was also installed in the same premises.)

In Syria the reply to the UNSV admits the widespread prevalence of violence against children, whether in the home, at school, on the street or at the work place. The reported cases of violence do not represent however the whole reality due to lack of accurate monitoring mechanisms. Also there is lack of media coverage of the issue.

Palestine did not report an estimate of the problem, and refers to the absence of such statistics. Also there is poor monitoring of crimes committed against children or of complaints associated with that type of violence.

8.7.3.1 Concerning the Gulf Region[4]

"The Meeting of Experts in the Region of Gulf Cooperation Council" on the maltreatment of children, held in the Kingdom of Saudi Arabia in 2004, agreed on the presence of cases of child maltreatment in all countries of the region.

In Yemen, although the government of did not undertake any national surveys during the last decade addressing the issue of violence against children in particular, still there are some studies which address family violence in general. Also, there is a public system that officially investigates causes of death, including deaths of children. A periodic monthly report is published, describing a summarized statistical review of deaths which are known or suspected to be as a result of violence.

In Qatar, no previous surveys have been made regarding the prevalence of violence against children; there is, however, a report that shows the total number of cases of violence against children as given by relevant state bodies.

[4]Al-Mahroos, F. et al., "Child Abuse: Bahrain's Experience", Child Abuse & Neglect, Volume 29, Issue 2. February 2005. Pages 187–193.

Kuwait stated that violence does not constitute a phenomenon in the country; therefore there are no available statistics on that matter. Also there are no governmental bodies specialized in addressing violence against children in particular. There are, however, administrations and bodies within state ministries which are concerned with all human rights issues who undertake the follow up of all human rights issues and the defense against any violation of those rights, including children's rights and any form of violence that children might face.

8.7.3.2 Concerning North Africa

Sudan indicates that some research and surveys have been done concerning the market children, domestic laborers, child labor and juvenile justice, but did not report the findings of those surveys.

Algeria has s system of fact finding and research which allows official investigation of cases of child deaths by the security authorities and the police once the issue is addressed in a legal investigation and reports statistics regarding child deaths due to violence. A forensic death certificate is needed for such an investigation. The legal security authorities and the police have to periodically submit a statistical report on deaths and send it to relevant bodies and ministries.

8.7.3.3 Concerning the Whole Region

Several reports on violence against children in different countries of the MENA and Gulf regions (Iran, Jordan, Lebanon, Yemen and North Africa) have indicated the prevalence of different forms of violence (physical, verbal, sexual, neglect) at the home or at school. However, the size of the problem is yet not clarified in most of the countries. Useful tools in this perspective include:

- The I-CAST questionnaires (Lebanon 2006, 2007, 2008; Egypt 2006)
- Definitions of CAN, that need to be integrated within the provisions of law as being in accordance with:
  - The provisions of the CRC
  - The professionals' descriptions, mainly in the health sector
  - The societies' culture and awareness.

The Marrakech Declaration (2010) emphasizes the "importance of updating and developing the database on indicators on the situation of children in Arab states as a reference for planning, policy formulation and program design, while emphasizing the importance of conducting periodic studies on the situation of children in the Arab region in cooperation with relevant regional and international organizations".[5]

In its concluding observations on the reports of most Arab states, the CRC highlighted the limited progress made in the establishment of a comprehensive centralized system for data collection covering all areas of the convention, and particularly information related to groups of marginalized children. It noted that data documented and produced based on scientific methodologies is almost non-existent. In particular, data on cases of violence, abuse and exploitation is missing, and this certainly hinders the development of effective policies, plans and programs that can ensure the rights of the child. Gathering data according to gender, age, geographical location and marital status would provide policy makers and program planners with more realistic and scientific knowledge. It would enable more effective and realistic follow-up, monitoring and evaluation.

The Comparative Arab Report on Implementing the Recommendations of the UN Secretary-General's Study on VAC (2010) noted the lack of available data indicating the extent, nature and patterns of violence in the region.

Reporting of sexual violence is particularly missing, as the topic is still frequently considered a social taboo that is difficult to detect and report. This is particularly true if the sexual violence occurs within the child's family or community. The absence of available and accessible monitoring and reporting mechanisms on the local and national levels, and the absence of an integrated system for the protection of children is a key current priority. A lack of quantitative and qualitative information must not hinder programming and policy-making processes, nor make programs and activities related to prevention and protection from violence isolated from a cumulative systematic context.

Furthermore, existing assessment processes that frequently lack clear checklists and indicators must be improved. Institutes and universities in Arab states may provide actors involved in safeguarding the rights of the child with the required scientific competencies and research methodologies. They can also contribute to raising awareness about violence, in all its forms, through making it a topic of social discussion and research material in multiple forums. It is noticeable however that Arab universities and academic institutes are not adequately familiar with children's issues in general and issues of violence and abuse in particular. It should also be noted that within the region there are no certificates of specialization in child protection or the rights of the child. In some cases, the document [rights of the child] is incorporated into other specialties. Attempts to strengthen research capacity have been noted in some academic institutions through the establishment of a network on the initiative of Child Watch. The small numbers of studies that do exist have been funded primarily by outside donors, since states in the region, like Jordan, Syria, Oman, Palestine, Lebanon and Yemen. A few additional studies have

[5]Dr. M. Al Zagheer and Judge Johnny Elkazy, "Comparative review of the Arab States reservations on the CRC and the two Optional Protocols", Women, Family and Childhood Department, League of Arab States, 2012.

been disseminated by associations or research centers around the world, and are not part of a research plan designed to shape national decisions and policies.

On the regional level there is poor attention given to the production of data on the situation of children. The Arab Council for Childhood and Development stopped issuing its annual report in 2007, which previously contained development indicators for Arab children. Furthermore, even this report did not contain adequate child protection indicators.

In many states, individual governmental ministries gather information within its own area of focus, without the coordination of a national mechanism. This is the case in The United Arab Emirates, Djibouti, Oman, Palestine, Lebanon, Egypt and Yemen. Bahrain, Tunisia and Yemen referred utilizing UNICEF's ChildInfo database, which is a statistical mechanism that helps in data collection from different concerned ministries and structures on childhood indicators.

The process of collecting data on VAC should be an absolute priority in an area where social and cultural determinants hinder acknowledging the topic in public discussion.

The UN Study on VAC has encouraged many Arab states to respond by implementing some of its recommendations in order to formulate policies, design assistance on Violence-Related Information Management Systems programs, and amend legislation. However, the responses of states remain unsystematic and are not based on facts or data proven by national studies or research on the prevalence, causes and patterns of violence. The exposure of specific populations to increased risk is therefore unknown, resulting in lack of suitable development programs and preventive interventions.

In addition, information on cases requiring specialized services is incomplete and is not exchanged through a uniform case management system. This hinders the evaluation and monitoring process as well as the use of data to improve services according to ethical and scientific standards.

Part IV
Definitions, Types and Impacts of Sexual Abuse

Chapter 9
The Definitions and Their Consequences

9.1 Abstract

Key elements of the definition of CSA typically include an act against a child including sexual touching or fondling, intrusion or penetration (genital contact), indecent exposure, or other forms of sexual acts in which children are used to provide sexual gratification for the perpetrator (English 1998). Child sexual abuse or child molestation is a form of child abuse in which an adult or older adolescent uses a child for sexual stimulation. Other forms of child sexual abuse include engaging in sexual activities with a child (whether by asking or pressuring, or by other means), indecent exposure (of the genitals, female nipples, etc.), child grooming, or using a child to produce child pornography.

In their studies, Finkelhor and Pereda et al. presented data as broad (non-contact) and narrow (contact).[1] The problem, however, is how one determines these categories when measurement of CSA differs. For example, it would appear that the extremely high rates of narrow CSA of boys (60%) and girls (53%) in South Africa compared to other countries is due at least in part to the fact that Madu and Peltzer (2001)[2] included sexual kiss along with genital fondling and penetration in the category of contact abuse.

These categories are too broad if informative comparisons globally are to be made in the future. As such, while comparability to the prior reviews is a goal, one contribution of this study is to begin the process of encouraging greater specificity, enabling more meaningful comparisons. Categories of child sexual abuse of boys and girls include:

- all noncontact and contact sexual abuse including hugs combined;

---

[1]CSEC second World Congress Yokohama Conference. Commercial Sexual Exploitation of Children: The Situation in the Middle East/North Africa region. Summary. 2001.

[2]http://www.csecworldcongress.org/PDF/en/Yokohama/Background_reading/Regional_analyses/Summary situation in MEast & NAfrica_EN.pdf

B. Gerbaka et al., *Child Sexual Abuse, Exploitation and Trafficking in the Arab Region*, Child Maltreatment 13, https://doi.org/10.1007/978-3-030-66507-4_9

- non-contact child sexual abuse only—including exhibition, propositions, etc.;
- contact child sexual abuse only—including all sexual touching-fondling and/or penetration-rape (oral, anal, vaginal);
- Contact child sexual abuse—including only the abuse of sexual touching-fondling;
- Contact child sexual abuse—including only the abuse of penetration-rape.

Such definitions have also been updated in the 2017 WHO INSPIRE strategies in the context of the 2016 UN Global Partnership to End Violence on children.

9.2 Definitions of Sexual Violence in the INSPIRE Strategy

Any form of sexual abuse, assault, seduction and exploitation including:[3]

(i) Rape,
(ii) Attempted rape,
(iii) The inducement or coercion of a child to engage in any unlawful or psychologically harmful sexual activity including unwanted comments and advances [physical fondling as victims or actors or watchers; verbal seduction an attraction]
(iv) The use of children in [commercial and non-commercial] sexual exploitation and sexual trafficking;

---

[3] *Physical violence*. This includes fatal and non-fatal physical violence. The Committee is of the opinion that physical violence includes:

(a) All corporal punishment and all other forms of torture, cruel, inhuman or degrading treatment or punishment; and
(b) Physical bullying and hazing by adults and by other children.

1. Children with disabilities may be subject to particular forms of physical violence such as:

(a) Forced sterilization, particularly girls;
(b) Violence in the guise of treatment (for example electroconvulsive treatment (ECT) and electric shocks used as "aversion treatment" to control children's behaviour); and
(c) Deliberate infliction of disabilities on children for the purpose of exploiting them for begging in the streets or elsewhere.

2. *Corporal punishment*. In general comment No. 8 (para. 11), the Committee defined "corporal" or "physical" punishment as any punishment in which physical force is used and intended to cause some degree of pain or discomfort, however light. Most involves hitting ("smacking", "slapping", "spanking") children, with the hand or with an implement—a whip, stick, belt, shoe, wooden spoon, etc. But it can also involve, for example, kicking, shaking or throwing children, scratching, pinching, biting, pulling hair or boxing ears, caning, forcing children to stay in uncomfortable positions, burning, scalding, or forced ingestion. In the view of the Committee, corporal punishment is invariably degrading. Other specific forms of corporal punishment are listed in the report of the independent expert for the United Nations study on violence against children (A/61/299, paras. 56, 60 and 62).

(v) The use of children in audio or visual images of child sexual abuse, including virtual exposure and online sexual exploitation;
(vi) Child prostitution, sexual slavery, sexual exploitation in travel and tourism, trafficking for purposes of sexual exploitation (within and between countries), sale of children for any [including sexual] purposes
(vii) Forced [Child brides] marriage; and any type of inducement, coercion or arrangement of a child into [a forced] marriage or into living in couple.

9.3 Clinical/Research Definitions

Child sexual abuse vary in their wordings; academics and practitioners have struggled with definitions of what is a 'child', what is 'sexual', what is 'abuse', and even what is 'harm'.

There is however, a consistent concept that has arisen from decades of practical clinical experience and what is conveniently called: evidence-based research: that children are inherently vulnerable to physical and mental harm when involved in sexualized interactions before they are developmentally mature; and that the risk of these harms is greatly increased by factors such as the concurrent use of threat or force, the degree of physical intrusion, the duration, the degree of subterfuge and coercion.[4]

One widely used working definition of sexual abuse is that: *'sexual abuse' involves any sexual activity where consent is not, or cannot be, given*. This includes sexual contact that is accomplished by force or threat of force, regardless of the age of the participants, and all sexual contact between an adult and a child, regardless of whether there is deception or the child understands the sexual nature of the activity. The wordings of Article 19 of the CRC and its global comment 13 serve as a general and global reference to CSA.

Sexual contact between a teenager and a younger child can also be abusive if there is a significant disparity in age, development, or size rendering the younger child incapable of giving consent. The sexual activity may include sexual penetration, sexual touching, or noncontact sexual acts such as exposure or so called voyeurism.

---

[4]Dong, M., Anda, R., Dube, S., Giles, W. and Felitti, V. The relationship of exposure to childhood sexual abuse to other forms of abuse, neglect, and household dysfunction during childhood. Child Abuse & Neglect 2003; 6: 625–639.

9.4 Criminal Definitions[5]

Child sexual abuse terminology commonly derives from pre-existing criminal laws addressing sexual crimes more generally. As the pervasiveness of child sexual abuse has become apparent, many criminal statutes have been amended and new civil statutes enacted which define child sexual abuse in order to establish accountability and assure treatment when CSA occurs.

Criminal definitions usually specify different forms of sexual abuse, breaking down the behavior into different categories. Thus "sexual intercourse" can include degrees of penetration and different levels of mental intent. "Sexual contact" laws can specify which parts of the body are included and identify activities that are lawfully a legitimate form of child care even though intimate in nature. Similarly "exhibitionism" and "sexual exploitation" are often separately defined in a detailed fashion.

9.5 Definitions of Sexual Assault and Sexual Exploitation

Sexual assault and sexual exploitation include the following:

- Sexually exploiting children for commercial purposes.
- Exploiting children by making audio or visual recordings of cases in which they are sexually assaulted.
- Child prostitution, sexual slavery, sexual exploitation in travel and tourism, trafficking of children [inside countries and between them] and selling them for sexual purposes or for forced marriage.
- Forcing or coercing the child to partake of any illegal or psychologically detrimental sexual activity. Many children experience sexual harm that does not involve physical force but that still constitutes an assault on the self, is based on exploitation, and can lead to trauma/shock.

9.6 Broader Additions on Sexual Abuse

In addition to honor violence and early marriages, children are also being exposed to incest, sexual exploitation and abuse by adults in their close social environment. In this research project, we have chosen to classify all sexual activities by adults directed towards children as "abuse" and hence an act of violence. Children are unable to give consent to, or even understand, sexual relations with adults.

[5]Wortley, Richard; Stephen Smallbone (2006). Situational Prevention Of Child Sexual Abuse, Volume 19 of Crime prevention studies. Criminal Justice Press. p. 192.ISBN 1881798615.

Consensual sex between teenagers is not included in our definition of sexual abuse in this report. Since sexual relationships outside wedlock are associated with strong religious taboos in this mostly Muslim setting, sexual abuse in the MENA region is a particularly problematic topic for children.

Rape and sexual harassment against girls and women in Lebanon fall under gender-based societal violence. Because this topic is one of the undeclared taboos it is difficult to find statistics on these two types of violence in Lebanon. Nevertheless, sources from the Directorate General of Interior Security Forces illustrated that girls and women are subjected to sexual violence in far greater percentages than the different forms of violence perpetrated against men. The Directorate categorizes crimes, committed in the Lebanese society under the following categories: rape, sexual harassment, injury and incapacitation, confinement, confinement or abduction, kidnapping, kidnapping by parents, battering and harm, defloration, murder, attempted murder.

9.7 Definition of Harmful Practices

This category includes as examples, the following:

- Corporal punishment and all other forms of cruel and degrading treatment.
- Female genital mutilation.
- Amputating of limbs, shackling, wounding, burning and cauterizing.
- Adopting violent and degrading rituals in order to initiate an individual into a certain group, force-feeding children, fattening, and virginity tests (inspecting girls' genital organs).
- Forced marriage and early marriage.
- "Honor" crimes and acts of violence in the name of "retribution" (when conflict between different groups expands to include aggression against the children of certain parties) and incidents of death or violence in connection with dowries.
- Accusations of "magic" and related harmful practices such as "charms/fetishes".
- Cutting out the tongue and pulling out the teeth.

9.8 Definitions of Violence Through Information Technology and Communications[6]

The risks to children entailed in information technology and media cover the following interrelated areas[7,8]:

- Sexual assault on children performed with the purpose of producing visual and audio recordings is facilitated by the internet and other information technology and communications media.[9]
- Taking photographs or fake photographs (photo-shop)and morally offensive video tapes of children, or of people mocking children or a group of children, producing such photographs or allowing them to be taken, distributing or displaying them, having them in one's possession, or advertising them.
- Children as users of information technology and communications.
- Children, as receivers of information may be exposed to commercial ads, spam email, promotional ads, personal information, aggressive or violent content, incitement to hatred, prejudice, racism, pornography or undesired or deceptive content that is actually or potentially harmful.
- Children while communicating with others through information technology and media can be exposed to bullying or harassment, "seduction" and/or coercion, deception or persuasion that induces them to meet persons outside of the internet, and "luring" them to perform sex and/or provide personal information.
- Children may become involved as perpetrators in bullying others or harassing them, playing games adversely affect their psychological development, producing and downloading inappropriate sexual content, or providing misleading information and advice, and/or illegally downloading content, committing piracy or gambling or financial fraud and/or terrorism.

The effects of child sexual abuse can include depression and post-traumatic stress disorder anxiety, complex post-traumatic stress disorder, propensity to further victimization in adulthood and physical injury to the child, among other problems. Sexual abuse by a family member is a form of incest and can result in more serious and long-term psychological trauma, especially in the case of parental incest.[10]

---

[6]http://iiicongressomundial.net/congresso/arquivos/Rio%20Declaration%20and%20Call%20for%20Action%20-%20FINAL%20Version.pdf

[7]Wortley, Richard; Stephen Smallbone. "Child Pornography on the Internet". Problem-Oriented Guides for Police No. 41: p17. "The children portrayed in child pornography are first victimized when their abuse is perpetrated and recorded. They are further victimized each time that record is accessed."

[8]Sanderson, Christiane (2004). The seduction of children: empowering parents and teachers to protect children from child sexual abuse. Jessica Kingsley Publishers. p. 133.ISBN 184310248X.

[9]kdeniz, Yaman (2008). Internet child pornography and the law: national and international responses. Ashgate Publishing, Ltd.. p. 11. ISBN 0754622975.

[10]Klain, Eva J.; Heather J. Davies, Molly A. Hicks, ABA Center on Children and the Law (2001). Child Pornography: The Criminal-justice-system Response. National Center for Missing & Exploited Children. "Because the children depicted in child pornography are often shown while engaged in sexual activity with adults or other children, they are first and foremost victims of child sexual abuse.

Chapter 10
The Impacts and Consequences of CSA

10.1 Abstract: The Impact of Sexual Abuse on Children

In undertaking investigations and planning interventions, it is important to recognize that there are a range of different kinds of abusive and sexually harmful behaviors towards children, including[1]:

- *Adult males who perpetrate severe forms of sexual abuse* both within and outside the family with evidence of violent, sexually coercive actions against children, peers and adults.
- *Adult male abusers who perpetrate abuse against known children* within the family and social context, who have higher levels of abusive experiences themselves.
- *Internet offenders* who access pornographic material—this can be a solo activity, or as part of a complex international network of individuals who are responsible for creating and using pornographic material involving children.
- *Older children and young people* boys and girls who are described as showing 'reactive' patterns of sexually harmful behavior.
- *Older children and young people* who abuse in a coercive fashion against children, peers and adults, both within and outside the family. They have often experienced high level of maltreatment and adversity, and may have co-morbid disorders such as Attention Deficit, and Learning Difficulties.
- *Young people* who are recognized as being responsible for coercive sexual behaviors, or involving younger children in sexually harmful activities. They are young people with high rates of sexual abuse themselves and associated adversity.

[1]Russell, D. Sexual Exploitation: Rape, Child Sexual Abuse, and Workplace Harassment. Newbury Park: Sage Pub. 1984.

B. Gerbaka et al., *Child Sexual Abuse, Exploitation and Trafficking in the Arab Region*, Child Maltreatment 13, https://doi.org/10.1007/978-3-030-66507-4_10

- *Adult Female sexual abusers* who have been historically less recognized than males, and less well researched. However they do represent a significant minority of close to 5%.
- *Adult women* offend against children or young people, their own or in their social context as sole offenders, or in combination with a co-offender.
- *Recognizing Family contexts*. There is no one pattern of family context described which can be recognized as characteristic of the setting for sexually abusive behavior.

10.2 Psychological Effects[2]

Child sexual abuse may result in short, mid and long-term harms, including bio-behavioral alterations and psychopathology in later life. Indicators and effects include depression, anxiety, eating disorders, poor self-esteem, somatization, sleep disturbances, and dissociative and anxiety disorders including post-traumatic stress disorder. While children may exhibit regressive behaviors such as thumb sucking or bedwetting, the strongest indicator of sexual abuse is sexual acting out and inappropriate sexual knowledge and interest. Victims may withdraw from school and social activities and exhibit various learning and behavioral problems including cruelty to animals, attention deficit/hyperactivity disorder (ADHD), conduct disorder, and oppositional defiant disorder (ODD). Teenage pregnancy and risky sexual behaviors may appear in adolescence. Child sexual abuse victims report almost four times as many incidences of self-inflicted harm, especially when it affects children with special needs.[3]

The USA National Institute of Drug Abuse found that "Among more than 1400 adult females, childhood sexual abuse was associated with increased likelihood of drug dependence, alcohol dependence, and psychiatric disorders. The associations are expressed as odds ratios: for example, women who experienced non genital sexual abuse in childhood were 2.83 times more likely to suffer drug dependence as adults than were women who were not abused. Furthermore, a well-documented, long-term negative effect is the repeated or additional victimization in adolescence and adulthood.[4] A causal relationship has been found between childhood sexual abuse and various adult psychopathologies, including crime and suicide, in addition

[2]Haj-Yahia, M. and Tamish, S. The rates of child sexual abuse and its psychological consequences as revealed by a study among Palestinian university students. Child Abuse & Neglect 2001; 25: 1303–1327.

[3]Anda, R., Felitti, V., Bremner, J., Walker, J., Whitfield, C., Perry, B., Dube, S. and Giles, W. The enduring effects of abuse and related adverse experiences in childhood. European Achieves of Psychiatry and Neuroscience 2006; 256/3:174–186.

[4]Melissa A. Polusny; Victoria M. Follette (1995). "Long-term correlates of child sexual abuse: Theory and review of the empirical literature". Applied and Preventive Psychology. Elsevier Ltd. 4 (3): 143–166.

to other risk-taking behaviors like alcoholism and drug abuse. Males who were sexually abused as children more frequently appear in the criminal justice system than in a clinical mental health setting.[5] A study comparing middle-aged women who were abused as children with non-abused counterparts found significantly higher health care costs for the former. Intergenerational effects have been noted, with the children of victims of child sexual abuse exhibiting more conduct problems, peer problems, and emotional problems than their peers. There is no identified specific characteristic pattern of symptoms, but there are several hypotheses about the causality of these associations. Almost 51% to 79% of sexually abused children exhibit psychological symptoms. The risk of harm is greater if the abuser is a relative, if the abuse involves intercourse or attempted intercourse, or if threats or force are used. The level of harm may also be affected by various factors such as penetration, duration and frequency of abuse, and use of force. The social stigma of child sexual abuse may compound the psychological harm to children, and adverse outcomes are less likely for abused children who have supportive family environments.

10.2.1 An Increase in Dissociation and Posttraumatic Stress Disorder (PTSD)

Child sexual abuse, especially chronic abuse starting at early ages, has been found to be related to the development of high levels of dissociative symptoms, including amnesia for abuse memories. When severe sexual abuse (penetration, several perpetrators, lasting more than one year) had occurred, dissociative symptoms were even more prominent. Besides dissociative identity disorder (DID) and posttraumatic stress disorder (PTSD), child sexual abuse survivors may present borderline personality disorder (BPD), Body dysmorphic disorder (BDD) and eating disorders such as bulimia nervosa.

10.2.2 What Does Research Tell Us?

Because child sexual abuse often occurs alongside other possibly confounding variables, such as poor family environment and physical abuse, some scholars argue it is important to control for those variables in studies which measure the effects of sexual abuse. In 1998, Martin and Fleming state that "In most cases, the fundamental damage inflicted by child sexual abuse is due to the child's developing capacities for trust, intimacy, agency and sexuality, and that many of the mental

[5]Understanding child sexual abuse: education, prevention, and recovery. American Psychological Association Retrieved 30 October 2012.

health problems of adult life associated with histories of child sexual abuse are second-order effects." Other studies have found an independent association of child sexual abuse with adverse psychological outcomes.[6] For example, Kendler et al. found tin 2000 hat most of the relationship between severe forms of child sexual abuse and adult psychopathology in their sample could not be explained by family discord, because the effect size of this association decreased only slightly after they controlled for possible confounding variables. Their examination of a small sample of CSA-discordant twins also supported a causal link between child sexual abuse and adult psychopathology; the CSA-exposed subjects had a consistently higher risk for psychopathologic disorders than their CSA non-exposed twins. Furthermore, a meta-analysis by Bruce Rind et al. generated in 1998 much obvious controversy by suggesting that child sexual abuse does not always cause pervasive harm, that some college students reported such encounters as positive experiences and that the extent of psychological damage depends on whether or not the child described the encounter as "consensual." Of course, the study was criticized for flawed methodology and conclusions. The US Congress condemned the study for its conclusions and for providing material used by pedophile organizations.[7]

10.3 Physical Effects

10.3.1 Genital and Vital Injuries

Depending on the age and size of the child, and the degree of force used, child sexual abuse may cause internal lacerations and bleeding. In severe cases, damage to internal organs may occur, which, in some cases, may cause death.[8]

10.3.2 Genital and General Infections

Child sexual abuse may cause infections and sexually transmitted diseases. Due to a lack of sufficient vaginal fluid, chances of infections may higher depending on the age and size of the child. Vaginitis has also been reported.

---

[6]Nelson EC, Heath AC, Madden PA, et al. (February 2002). "Association between self-reported childhood sexual abuse and adverse psychosocial outcomes: results from a twin study". Archives of General Psychiatry. 59 (2): 139–145.

[7]US Congress (1999). "Whereas no segment of our society is more critical to the future of human survival than our children" (PDF). 106th Congress, Resolution 107.

[8]Anderson, James; Mangels, Nancie; Langsam, Adam (2004). "Child Sexual Abuse: A Public Health Issue". The Justice Professional. 17: 107.

10.3.3 Neurological and Cognitive Damages

Research shows that traumatic stress caused by sexual abuse, induces notable changes in brain functioning and development. Various studies have suggested that severe child sexual abuse may have a deleterious effect on brain development. In 1998, Ito et al. found "reversed hemispheric asymmetry and greater left hemisphere coherence in abused subjects"[9] Teicher et al. found in 1993that an increased likelihood of "ictal temporal lobe epilepsy-like symptoms" in abused subjects[10]; Anderson et al. recorded in 2002 abnormal transverse relaxation time in the cerebellar vermis of adults sexually abused in childhood; Teicher et al. also found that child sexual abuse was associated with a reduced corpus callosum area; various studies have found an association of reduced volume of the left hippocampus with child sexual abuse; and Ito et al. found increased electrophysiological abnormalities in sexually abused children.[11]

Some studies indicate that sexual or physical abuse in children can lead to the overexcitation of an undeveloped limbic system.[12] Teicher et al. used the "Limbic System Checklist-33" to measure ictal temporal lobe epilepsy-like symptoms in 253 adults. Reports of child sexual abuse were associated with a 49% increase to LSCL-33 scores, 11% higher than the associated increase of self-reported physical abuse. Reports of both physical and sexual abuse were associated with a 113% increase. Male and female victims were similarly affected. Navalta et al. found in 2006 that the self-reported math Scholastic Aptitude Test scores of their sample of women with a history of repeated child sexual abuse were significantly lower than the self-reported math SAT scores of their non-abused sample. Because the abused subjects verbal SAT scores were high, they hypothesized that the low math SAT scores could "stem from a defect in hemispheric integration." They also found a strong association between short-term memory impairments for all categories tested (verbal, visual, and global) and the duration of the abuse.

[9] Ito Y, Teicher MH, Glod CA, Ackerman E (1998). "Preliminary evidence for aberrant cortical development in abused children: a quantitative EEG study". The Journal of Neuropsychiatry and Clinical Neurosciences. 10(3): 298–307. PMID 9706537.

[10] Teicher MH, Glod CA, Surrey J, Swett C (1993). "Early childhood abuse and limbic system ratings in adult psychiatric outpatients". The Journal of Neuropsychiatry and Clinical Neurosciences. 5 (3): 301–6. PMID 8369640.

[11] Neumann, D.A., Houskamp, B.M., Pollock, V. and Briere, J. The long-term sequelae of childhood sexual abuse in women: A meta-analytic review. Child Maltreatment 1996; 1: 6–16.

[12] Ito Y, Teicher MH, Glod CA, Ackerman E (1998). "Preliminary evidence for aberrant cortical development in abused children: a quantitative EEG study". The Journal of Neuropsychiatry and Clinical Neurosciences. 10(3): 298–307. PMID 9706537.

10.4 The Offenders

10.4.1 Demographics

Offenders are more likely to be relatives or acquaintances of their victim than strangers.[13] A 2006–07 Idaho study of 430 cases found that 82% of juvenile sex offenders were known to the victims (acquaintances 46% or relatives 36%).[14]

More offenders are male than female, though the percentage varies between studies (see female child molesters). The percentage of incidents of sexual abuse by female perpetrators that come to the attention of the legal system is usually reported to be between 1% and 4%.[15] Studies of sexual misconduct in US schools with female offenders have shown mixed results with rates between 4% and 43% of female offenders. In 1993, Maletzky found that among 4402 convicted pedophilic offenders, 0.4% were female.[16] Another study of a non-clinical population found that, among those in their sample that had been molested, as many as a third were molested by women. In U.S. schools, educators who offend range in age from "21 to 75 years old, with an average age of 28".[17]

In the Netherlands, the Dutch national spokeswoman on human traffic and sexual violence against children, 3% of the convicted perpetrators are women, 14.58% of the victims are boys and "most victims were abused by a family member, friend or acquaintance." One in six perpetrators is himself underage.

10.4.2 Typology of Perpetrators

Early research in the 1970s and 1980s began to classify offenders based on their motivations and traits. Groth and Birnbaum (1978) categorized child sexual offenders into two groups, "fixated" and "regressed". Fixated were described as having a primary attraction to children, whereas regressed had largely maintained

[13]Fergusson, DM; Lynskey, MT; Horwood, LJ (October 1996). "Childhood sexual abuse and psychiatric disorder in young adulthood: I. Prevalence of sexual abuse and factors associated with sexual abuse". J Am Acad Child Adolesc Psychiatry.

[14]Joint Submission by The Office of the Governor C.L. Butch Otter, Governor and The Office of the Attorney General Lawrence Wasden, Attorney General (January 2008). "The Prosecution of Child Sexual Abuse in Idaho July 1, 2006 – June 30, 2007".

[15]M. S., Denov (1 Aug 2003). "The myth of innocence: sexual scripts and the recognition of child sexual abuse by female perpetrators". The Journal of Sex Research. 40 (3): 303–314. doi:https://doi.org/10.1080/00224490309552195

[16]Tomeo, Marie E.; Templer, Donald I.; Anderson, Susan; Kotler, Debra (2001). "Comparative data of childhood and adolescence molestation in heterosexual and homosexual persons". Archives of Sexual Behavior. 30 (5): 535–41. doi:https://doi.org/10.1023/A:1010243318426. PMID 11501300.

[17]Shakeshaft, C, "Educator Sexual Misconduct: A Synthesis of the Literature", U.S. Department of Education, 2004, p.24–25.

relationships with other adults, and were even married. This study also showed that adult sexual orientation was not related to the sex of the victim targeted, e.g. men who molested boys often had adult relationships with women.[18]

Holmes and Holmes expanded in 2002 on the types of offenders and their psychological profiles:

- Situational—does not prefer children, but offend under certain conditions.
- Regressed—Typically has relationships with adults, but a stressor causes them to seek children as a substitute.
- Morally Indiscriminate—All-around sexual deviant, who may commit other sexual offenses unrelated to children.
- Naive/Inadequate—Often mentally disabled in some way, finds children less threatening.
- Preferential—has true sexual interest in children.
- Mysoped—Sadistic and violent, target strangers more often than acquaintances.
- Fixated—Little or no activity with own age, described as an "overgrown child".

10.4.2.1 Persons Who Sexually Abuse Children

It has been suggested that four 'pre-conditions' must exist for an individual to sexually abuse a child. The abuser must:

- have the motivation to sexually abuse;
- be able to overcome internal inhibitors;
- be able to overcome external inhibitors; and
- be able to overcome the resistance of the child.

Offender characteristics have not proven an especially fruitful avenue for screening or preventing child sexual abuse. Despite popular conceptions, no 'profile' of a child sexual offender has been established with sufficient specificity and/or sensitivity to be of practical use as a screening mechanism.

There is reported resistance (both active and passive) to the establishment of systems that help to prevent, identify and treat child sexual abuse in all countries, cultures and ethnic and religious groups. Such findings are also noted in the Arab region [Jordan in 2005, Yemen in 2007, KSA in 2009, etc.] This resistance is noticed at the level of individuals and families, but also includes professional, educational, sporting and religious agencies—often for complex issues of philosophy, history or tradition. In addition, self-identified groups of individuals who wish to have sexual contact with children, justify their behavior using strategies to 'normalize' and 'legitimize' their sexually abusive behavior in the eyes of the public and officials.

---

[18]Groth, A. Nicholas; Birnbaum, H. Jean (1978). "Adult sexual orientation and attraction to underage persons". Archives of Sexual Behavior. 7 (3): 175–81. doi:https://doi.org/10.1007/BF01542377. PMID 666571.

10.4.3 Criminalization

The fact that child sexual abuse has long been perceived in most countries as a criminal act has meant law enforcement and judicial processes have played a significant role in the initial response to child sexual abuse. Where a child has been sexually abused by someone outside of the immediate family (i.e. extra-familial sexual abuse)—especially by someone who has an organizational duty of care, who is involved in trafficking children (or their images) for prostitution or financial gain—there is universal agreement across all nations, cultures and religions that law enforcement and judicial process have a substantial and primary role. The application of a criminal approach to abuse within the immediate family (i.e. intra-familial sexual abuse) has been more controversial.[19] The main reason for controversy is that interfamilial abuse may concern more than children on one side, and also children outside the family circle. Notwithstanding the important role that a criminal response to suspicions of child sexual abuse played when child sexual abuse is first identified as a cultural concern, over time most countries identify that a 'therapeutic' perspective is important to the subsequent health and well-being of affected children and their families.

Proponents of this less-punitive approach argue for a distinction between intra-familial and extra-familial child sexual abuse. Individuals favoring a therapeutic view also work to understand the origins of sexually abusive behavior in adults or in the sexually harmful behavior of young people. There is evolving evidence that many forms of intra-familial child sexual abuse can be managed at least in part through child protection services. This may ensure that a child is protected, treated, and other relevant services provided for the child and family to test whether the family can provide a safe environment for the child and, when necessary, determining whether the child needs a long-term alternate placement or not,[20] and in which conditions: inside the larger family circle such as grandparents or within institutions [Sectoral or State].

10.4.4 Prevention of Offense and Treatment

Published research on treatment of abused and neglected children has become more rigorous and more prevalent in the past decade. The research includes studies that report positive treatment results for children who suffer physical abuse, sexual

[19]This is based on ideas that somehow incest is different from other forms of CSA and this is largely not true. Some incest fathers/stepfathers are abusing children outside of their home. Some rape adult women.

[20]Data on offenders suggests that intrafamily offenders do not reoffend even without treatment, in which case it is the act of reporting to the justice system and not the CPS system that has the effect; available data is not affirmative on this point.

abuse, and/or are neglected. Many types of Evidence-Based Practice (EBP) are now available, including Trauma-Focused Cognitive Behavioral Therapy [TF-CBT], Parent-Child Interaction Therapy, and Abuse Focused-Cognitive Behavioral Therapy.[21] Given that as many as one of three cases of child sexual abuse result from abusive contact between a child and an older minor—an essential finding of the past 20 years is that youth who perpetrate child sexual abuse must be treated. With appropriate treatment, this group (i.e. children who sexually abuse other children) has much lower recidivism rates than do untreated minors or adults.

The best way to protect children is to prevent offenders from harming children by targeting risk, preventing relapse, and encouraging offenders to live a 'Good Life' (Beech et al. 2009). In addition to risk management and relapse prevention, we need to mention effective treatment of offenders. Counseling of children affected by child sexual abuse must include all persons in the household.

10.4.5 Essential Processes in all Cultures and Countries

Data collection is an important element in the social reaction to the incidence of child sexual abuse and sexual exploitation in any society regardless of the cultural components of that society. Systems for data collection need to be developed. Once child sexual abuse and sexual exploitation is acknowledged by society, responses to the problem need to be developed—including protective systems, policies and laws, appropriate curriculum & training, and a capacity building process for all professionals concerned. While acknowledging the national commitments towards the UN Convention on the Rights of the Child in general and Article 19 in particular, national programs need to take into consideration specific factors such as:

- legal definitions and concepts of child sexual abuse and sexual exploitation;
- specific types of child sexual abuse and sexual exploitation in some cultures; and
- differences in implementation capacities in each country and region.

In the context of child sale and sexual exploitation, countries need to sign the optional protocol of the Convention on the Rights of the Child. In the Arab region, armed conflicts have created large and deep spaces that increase child sale, sexual

[21]It is important to point out that all these evidence based interventions have been largely on one ethnic group of children and none have long follow-ups. Available data is not in a position yet to say with confidence that these interventions are the best ones globally. They are promising but CPS need to be more cautious in recommending them without further research and cultural modification. For example in the TF-CBT model, repeatedly going over the trauma is a critical part. In a culture where talking about sexual things to anyone is a taboo, a socially acceptable model needs to be promoted. Also, in some cultures, purification rituals might be more effective than desensitization in reducing anxiety around memories of the CSA? Any intervention needs to learn more than we currently know about the use of these specific interventions in diverse cultural contexts. Within the arab region, such types of therapies are in the process of implementation and evaluation.

and complex exploitation and human trafficking. The implementation of such protocols needs a mechanism of follow up by the League of Arab States and the UN agencies. It is noted that the level of development of countries is directly affected by their commitment to child protection and well-being, including minorities.

Professionals can play an important role in prevention, training, reporting, rehabilitation and data collection, for the purpose of capacity building of the child protection system at the national level. This is particularly important in countries where there are gender discrimination issues and where professionals are valued and respected in the society.

Children need also to be part of the process in a meaningful way, especially in education and child friendly reporting systems. Cases of severe maltreatment can be associated with child sexual abuse and sexual exploitation. Corporal punishment, emotional abuse and threats can therefore be antecedent or contextual to sexual offending. Best practices in parenting can provide guides for safe child care earlier in life, with proper and timely detection of groups at risk, either in child and parents, through visits to professionals or through home visitations.

10.4.6 Causal Factors

It is important to highlight that causal factors of child sex offenders are not known conclusively.[22] The experience of sexual abuse as a child was previously thought to be a strong risk factor, but research does not show a causal relationship, as the vast majority of sexually abused children do not grow up to be adult offenders, nor do the majority of adult offenders report childhood sexual abuse. The existence of a cycle of sexual abuse is therefore not established. Almost 25 years ago in 1996, there was greater belief in the theory of a "cycle of violence", because most of the research done was retrospective—abusers were asked if they had experienced past abuse. Even the majority of studies found that most adult sex offenders said they had not been sexually abused during childhood, but studies varied in terms of their estimates of the percentage of such offenders who had been abused, from 0 to 79%. More recent prospective longitudinal research—studying children with documented cases of sexual abuse over time to determine what percentage become adult offenders—has demonstrated that the cycle of violence theory is not an adequate explanation for why people molest children. Offenders may use cognitive distortions to facilitate their offenses, such as minimization of the abuse, victim blaming, and excuses.[23]

[22]Pedophilia. Psychology Today. Sussex Publishers, LLC. 7 September 2006.

[23]Ward, Tony; Hudson, Stephen M.; Marshall, William L. (1995). "Cognitive Distortions and Affective Deficits in Sex Offenders: A Cognitive Deconstructionist Interpretation1". Sexual Abuse: A Journal of Research and Treatment.

10.4.7 The Social Perspective of Pedophilia

Pedophilia is a condition in which an adult or older adolescent is primarily or exclusively attracted to prepubescent children, whether the attraction is acted upon or not. A person with this attraction is called a pedophile. In law enforcement, the term pedophile is sometimes used to describe those accused or convicted of child sexual abuse under sociolegal definitions of child (including both prepubescent children and adolescents younger than the local age of consent); however, not all child sexual offenders are pedophiles and not all pedophiles engage in sexual abuse of children. For these reasons, researchers recommend against imprecisely describing all child molesters as pedophiles.

The term pedocriminality (De: Pädokriminalität; Fr: pédocriminalité) is a controversial term which originated in the 1980s and has been used by organizations such as UNICEF, UNHRC, the World Health Organization and the Council of Europe to refer to child sexual abuse and sexual violence used against children, child prostitution, child trafficking and the use of child pornography. The term "cyber-pedocriminality" has been used to refer to the activities of viewers of child pornography online.[24]

10.4.8 Why Is There Recurrence? Recidivism[25]

Recidivism rates for sex offenders are lower than for the general criminal population. Estimated rates among child sex offenders vary. One study found that 42% of offenders re-offended (either a sex crime, violent crime, or both) after they were released. Risk for re-offense was highest in the first 6 years after release, but continued to be significant even 10–31 years later, with 23% offending during this time. A study done in California in 1965 found an 18.2% recidivism rate for offenders targeting the opposite sex and a 34.5% recidivism rate for same-sex offenders after 5 years.[26]

---

[24]Child Abuse Negl. 2010 Aug;34(8):570–5. doi: 10.1016/j.chiabu.2010.01.011. Epub 2010 Jun 2.

[25]Perry, B. Incubated in terror: neurodevelopmental factors in the 'cycle of violence' In J. Osofsky editor, Children in a Violent Society. NY: Guilford Press, 1997. Pp. 124–149. http://www.childtrauma.org/index.php/articles

[26]Frisbie, Louise Viets (1965). "Treated Sex Offenders Who Reverted to Sexually Deviant Behavior". Federal Probation. 29: 52.

10.4.9 Child and Young Adolescent Offenders

When a prepubescent child is sexually abused by one or more other children or adolescent youths, and no adult is directly involved, it is defined as child-on-child sexual abuse. The definition includes any sexual activity between children that occurs without consent, without equality, or due to coercion,[27] whether the offender uses physical force, threats, trickery or emotional manipulation to compel cooperation. When sexual abuse is perpetrated by one sibling upon another, it is known as "intersibling abuse", a form of incest. Unlike research on adult offenders, a strong causal relationship has been established between child and adolescent offenders and these offenders' own prior victimization, by either adults or other children.

According to a 2010 UNICEF report, 46% of Congolese schoolgirls confirmed that they had been victims of sexual harassment, abuse, and violence committed by their teachers or other school personnel.[28] In Mozambique, a study by the Ministry of Education found that 70 percent of female respondents reported knowing teachers who use sexual intercourse as a necessary condition to advance students to the next grade. Another survey by Promundo found that 16% of girls in North Kivu said they had been forced to have sex with their teachers. According to UNICEF, teachers in Mali are known to use "La menace du bic rouge" ("the threat of the red pen") or bad marks if girls do not accept sexual advances. According to Plan International, 16% of children in Togo, for instance, named a teacher as responsible for the pregnancy of a classmate.

10.4.10 The Case of Incest

Incest between a child or adolescent and a related adult is known as child incestuous abuse,[29] and has been identified as the most widespread form of child sexual abuse with a huge capacity to damage the young person. One researcher stated that more than 70% of abusers are immediate family members or someone very close to the family. Another researcher stated that about 30% of all perpetrators of sexual abuse are related to their victim, 60% of the perpetrators are family acquaintances, like a neighbor, babysitter or friend and 10% of the perpetrators in child sexual abuse cases are strangers. A child sexual abuse offense where the perpetrator is related to the child, either by blood or marriage, is a form of incest described as intrafamilial child sexual abuse.[30] The most-often reported form of incest is father–daughter and

---

[27]Shaw JA, Lewis JE, Loeb A, Rosado J, Rodriguez RA (December 2000). "Child on child sexual abuse: psychological perspectives". Child Abuse & Neglect.

[28]Abuse of power. Foreignpolicy.com. 14 April 2014. Retrieved 20 April 2014.

[29]Trusiani, Jessica. "Working with Survivors of Child Incestuous Abuse". Rutgers University.

[30]Russell, D. The Secret Trauma: Incest in the Lives of Girls and Women. Basic Books, Inc. New York, 1986.

stepfather–daughter incest, with most of the remaining reports consisting of mother/stepmother–daughter/son incest. Father–son incest is reported less often; however it is not known if the actual prevalence is less or it is under-reported by a greater margin. Similarly, some argue that sibling incest may be as common, or more common, than other types of incest: Goldman and Goldman reported that 57% of incest involved siblings[31]; Finkelhor reported that over 90% of nuclear family incest involved siblings[32]; while Cawson et al. show that sibling incest was reported twice as often as incest perpetrated by fathers/stepfathers.[33] Prevalence of parental child sexual abuse is difficult to assess due to secrecy and privacy[34]; some estimates state that dozens of million globally have been victimized by parental incest as children.[35]

[31]Goldman JD, Padayachi UK (May 1997). "The prevalence and nature of child sexual abuse in Queensland, Australia". Child Abuse & Neglect. 21 (5): 489–98. doi:https://doi.org/10.1016/S0145-2134(97)00008-2. PMID 9158908.

[32]Finkelhor, D. (1979). Sexually victimised children. New York: Free Press.

[33]Cawson, Pat; Wattam, Corinne; Brooker, Sue (2000). Child Maltreatment in the United Kingdom: A Study of the Prevalence of Child Abuse and Neglect. London: National Society for the Prevention of Cruelty to Children. ISBN 978-1-84228-006-5.

[34]Finkelhor, David; Ormrod, Richard (May 2001). "Child Abuse Reported to the Police" (PDF). Juvenile Justice Bulletin. U.S. Office of Juvenile Justice and Delinquency Prevention.

[35]Turner, Jeffrey S. (1996). Encyclopedia of relationships across the lifespan. Westport, Conn: Greenwood Press. p. 92. ISBN 0-313-29576-X.

Chapter 11
Commercial Sexual Exploitation of Children and Trafficking

11.1 Abstract

Commercial sexual exploitation of children (CSEC) is defined by the Declaration of the First World Congress against Commercial Sexual Exploitation of Children, held in Stockholm in 1996, as "sexual abuse by an adult accompanied by remuneration in cash or in kind to the child or third person(s)." CSEC usually takes the form of child prostitution or child pornography, and is often facilitated by child sex tourism. CSEC is particularly a problem in developing countries of Asia. In recent years, new innovations in technology have facilitated the trade of Internet child pornography.[1]

United Nations definition of "trafficking in persons"

An international consensus was created in December 2000, when countries adopted the United Nations Protocol to Prevent, Suppress and Punish Trafficking in Persons, Especially Women and Children. The U.N. Protocol was the first international legal instrument to define trafficking in persons and to provide for a comprehensive approach to combat the problem. Today, it remains the primary reference tool for countries in implementing their national policies to combat trafficking in persons and in developing frameworks of international cooperation in this field. The U.N. Protocol entered into force on 25 December 2003, when 20 countries deposited their instruments of ratification. As of August 2013, 157 countries are parties to the U.N. Protocol.

Article 3(a) of the U.N. Protocol states:

"Trafficking in persons" shall mean the recruitment, transportation, transfer, harboring or receipt of persons, by means of the threat or use of force or other forms of coercion, of abduction, of fraud, of deception, of the abuse of power or of a position of vulnerability or the giving or receiving of payments or benefits to achieve the consent of a person having control over another person for the purpose of exploitation. Exploitation shall include, at a minimum, the exploitation of the prostitution of others or other forms of sexual exploitation, forced labor or services, slavery or practices similar to slavery, servitude or the removal of organs.5

[1] *"What we do – Commercial sexual exploitation of children"*. unicef.org. *Retrieved 23 March 2015.*

B. Gerbaka et al., *Child Sexual Abuse, Exploitation and Trafficking in the Arab Region*, Child Maltreatment 13, https://doi.org/10.1007/978-3-030-66507-4_11

Furthermore, Sex trafficking is considered a violation of human rights and a form of sex discrimination, as nearly all victims are female. Sexually exploited women and girls are often experience various violations, including but not limited to forced sex with pimps and customers, beatings, and forced abortions. Sexual exploitation is hugely underreported because victims fear stigmatization, are threatened with violence and deprivation of food or money, lack faith in institutions, or have limited access to legal services or knowledge about how to navigate them.[2]

11.2 Types

Child sexual abuse includes a variety of sexual offenses, including[3]:

- Sexual assault—a term defining offenses in which an adult uses a minor for the purpose of sexual gratification; for example, rape (including sodomy), and sexual penetration with an object. Most U.S. states include, in their definitions of sexual assault, any penetrative contact of a minor's body, however slight, if the contact is performed for the purpose of sexual gratification.
- Sexual exploitation—a term defining offenses in which an adult victimizes a minor for advancement, sexual gratification, or profit; for example, prostituting a child, and creating or trafficking in child pornography.
- Sexual grooming—a term defining the social conduct of a potential child sex offender who seeks to make a minor more accepting of their advances, for example in an online chat room.

11.3 Disclosures

Children who received supportive responses following disclosure had less traumatic symptoms and were abused for a shorter period of time than children who did not receive support. In general, studies have found that children need support and stress-reducing resources after disclosure of sexual abuse. Negative social reactions to disclosure have been found to be harmful to the survivor's well-being. One study reported that children who received a bad reaction from the first person they told, especially if the person was a close family member, had worse scores as adults on general trauma symptoms, post-traumatic stress disorder symptoms, and

[2]Clift, Stephen; Simon Carter (2000). Tourism and Sex. Cengage Learning EMEA. pp. 75–78. ISBN 1855676362.

[3]CSEC second World Congress Yokohama Conference. Commercial Sexual Exploitation of Children: The Situation in the Middle East/North Africa region. Summary. 2001. http://www.csecworldcongress.org/PDF/en/Yokohama/Background_reading/Regional_analyses/Summary situation in MEast & NAfrica_EN.pdf

dissociation. Another study found that in most cases when children did disclose abuse, the person they talked to did not respond effectively, blamed or rejected the child, and took little or no action to stop the abuse. Non-validating and otherwise non-supportive responses to disclosure by the child's primary attachment figure may indicate a relational disturbance predating the sexual abuse that may have been a risk factor for the abuse, and which can remain a risk factor for its psychological consequences.[4]

The American Academy of Child and Adolescent Psychiatry provides guidelines for what to say to the victim and what to do following the disclosure. Asa Don Brown has indicated: "A minimization of the trauma and its effects is commonly injected into the picture by parental caregivers to shelter and calm the child. It has been commonly assumed that focusing on children's issues too long will negatively impact their recovery. Therefore, the parental caregiver teaches the child to mask his or her issues."

In many jurisdictions, abuse that is suspected, not necessarily proven, requires reporting to child protection agencies, such as the Child Protection Services in the United States. Recommendations for healthcare workers exist; those include primary care providers nurses, who often encounter suspected abuse and are advised to firstly determine the child's immediate need for safety. A private environment away from suspected abusers is desired for interviewing and examining. Leading statements that can distort the story are avoided. As disclosing abuse can be distressing and sometimes even shameful, reassuring the child that he or she has done the right thing by telling and that they are not bad and that the abuse was not their fault helps in disclosing more information. Dolls are sometimes used to help explain what happened. For the suspected abusers, it is also recommended to use a nonjudgmental, nonthreatening attitude towards them and to withhold expressing shock, in order to help disclose information.

11.4 Consequences of Trafficking in Persons

Trafficking is a crime against the human being and against State security that has both long- and short-term effects on the victim and State institutions.

11.4.1 Harm to Victims

A victim may suffer from both physical and psychological harm. Even if eventually rescued, the trauma suffered by victims of trafficking is long lasting and may never

[4]ECPAT Regional Consultation on the Commercial Sexual Exploitation of Children in North Africa. 12–13 June 2003. Rabat. Morocco.

fully dissipate. Victims of trafficking generally work in substandard conditions, under increased risk of injuries or death while on the job because of unregulated and unsafe working conditions or lack of proper health care.

Workers in the construction industry may suffer exposure to dust, chemicals, and other hazardous materials that can cause respiratory infections, scabies, tuberculosis, and other diseases associated with overcrowded, unsanitary conditions. Victims of sexual exploitation are more susceptible to contracting HIV/AIDS or other sexually transmitted diseases, but they rarely report these diseases for fear of stigmatization and of retaliation by the traffickers, thus aggravating their health.

Among the most common psychological consequences of trafficking are depression, memory loss, dizziness, suicidal thoughts, and many forms of shame, grief, fear, distrust, and self-hatred. Some victims may also experience post-traumatic stress disorder characterized by flashbacks, intrusive thoughts, dissociation, hopelessness, and other symptoms.

11.4.2 A Crime Against the State

Trafficking in persons also undermines the legitimacy of the State, whose goal is to promote the rule of law and the respect of human rights. Traffickers are often criminals who not only violate the rights of the victims but also commit crimes against the State, such as violations of immigration, tax, and business laws. In transnational trafficking in persons, the destination country often suffers an unlawful crossing of its borders, and the country of origin suffers an unlawful loss of its people and a disruption to its social fabric.

11.4.3 Economic Impact

Trafficking in persons is an illegal criminal activity that fuels the black market and encourages money-laundering practices. The lost tax revenue to the government, deriving from tax evasion, and the law enforcement costs of detecting and combating money laundering are just two of the most obvious negative economic impacts of trafficking in persons. In countries with a large number of trafficked children, various reports have proved the long-term negative impact on the economy from the decreased productivity of these children by the time they reach adulthood.

11.5 Consequences and Effects of Child Labor

The integration of a child in the labor market at a very young age has serious physical, societal and psychological repercussions. It also creates an environment that facilitates deviation, leading him or her to end up in correctional facilities. According to the statistics of the criminal security department, during the period 2008–09, 286 children were arrested for begging, 62 girls for prostitution and 222 boys for selling cigarettes. The focus groups and interviews led for the purpose of this research confirmed that many of the children in correctional facilities were working children.

Hence, it would seem that about 90% of the children in these correctional facilities are victims of child labor, and a proportion of them work for their parents who are supposed to offer them a safe environment. And although the results of this study may not be generalized, they do, however, present a clear picture of the dangers of child labor and its negative effects. Some of the worst effects or risks of child labor are the following.

11.5.1 Sexual Harassment

Working children are more exposed than others to sexual harassment because they spend most of their time outside the home and the safety of his/her family. If it is not the work environment itself that the child is exposed to, then it is on the streets while he/she is returning home. Considering that about 58% of the children in the sample work for more than nine hours per day, this entails that they work until very late at night, some children even work until early morning. This necessarily exposes these children to all forms of harassment, and especially sexual harassment. Some of the children discussed how their friends were raped by their employers, and some discussed harassment they suffered themselves. Even some of the employers reported cases of the children working for them being harassed.

11.5.2 Begging and Exploitation

Some children face problems with their families and it sometimes reaches the point where they are thrown out of the house or run away, thus finding themselves on the streets without any protection. In such cases, children are often caught within gangs who lure them by promising a place to stay and food in exchange for their "services". When interviewing some of the children caught by these gangs, most of them came from broken homes, were exposed to violence, and some were even tied with chains by their fathers or step-mothers. They ran away from this environment to the streets. The only available option to them on the streets was often joining such gangs, who made the children work and abide by their conditions, which included informing the police whatever the gang made them memorize.

According to some organizations that work in the care and rehabilitation of these children, the main problem stems from the fact that many of these children do not have any identification papers, and when they join the gangs they are immediately trained as to how best to deal with the police if they are ever caught. They are told to give a fake name and give the name of the gang leader as their father. So when they are released, it is done under a fake name, and hence the fake father [head of the gang] may come and claim he lost the family papers, and so the child is registered under his name, which allows him to take the child back. Gangs are sometimes home to dozens of children in one room, during which time they may be subject to all forms of persecution and harassment. They are required to bring back minimal amounts of money daily. If they were unable to collect that amount, then they would not be allowed to return to the shelter until they did, even though they would have to work until very late at night. Otherwise, the child would be often beaten by his "boss". Even if the child came back with the required amount, worse dangers awaited as they would go to sleep at night, and often the child would be molested and sexually harassed and raped by gang members. Based on the interviews with the children who worked for these gangs, it appears that most of them were raped by the gang leader or his son, or even by other children like him. In fact, the older children assault the younger ones, especially the younger girls among them.

11.5.3 Smoking and Drug Abuse

It was previously shown that more than a quarter of the children in the sample smoked and 10 per cent of them took drugs, such as sniffing or drinking gas, drinking alcohol and smoking weed.

Most of these children ended up in correctional facilities.

Smoking, drinking and drug abuse obviously require money that the child does not always have, especially if he or she is working for someone or being exploited by a gang that takes all of his or her earnings. This leads many children to steal to have enough money to buy their addictive substances.

11.5.4 Health Problems

The most serious of injuries that may occur to the children are those that happen as a consequence of handling machinery for which they are not sufficiently experienced. The results of the interviews show that 6 per cent of the children suffered from injuries due to falling or dropping such equipment.

Discouraging demand for trafficking victims is increasingly at the heart of many anti-trafficking policies focusing on preventing the crime. For instance, article 9 (5) of the U.N. Protocol makes it clear that addressing the demand for the services of trafficking victims is an essential part of effectively preventing and combating trafficking in persons. The article states: States Parties shall adopt or strengthen legislative or other measures, such as educational, social or cultural measures, including through bilateral and multilateral cooperation, to discourage the demand that fosters all forms of exploitation of persons, especially women and children, which leads to trafficking.3

11.6 Types of Victims

Often, victims of trafficking do not readily identify themselves as such. For example, individuals tricked into forced labor through the imposition of extortive "fees" may require education, or those who are psychologically attached to a sex trafficker as a "boyfriend" may require counseling before they understand that they are being exploited and their human rights are being violated. Under international, regional, and national legislation, different types of victims of trafficking can be identified. Broadly, victims can be divided into five main categories: victim, derivative victim, potential victim, vulnerable victim, and presumed victim. An individual often falls under more than one of these categories.

11.6.1 Victim

The term "victims of crime" has been defined in article A(1) of the United Nations Declaration of Basic Principles of Justice for Victims of Crimes and Abuse of Power as "[p]ersons who, individually or collectively, have suffered harm, including physical or mental injury, emotional suffering, economic loss or substantial impairment of their fundamental rights, through acts or omissions that are in violation of criminal laws operative within Member States." Likewise, article 1(a) of the Council of Europe Framework Decision on the Standing of Victims in Criminal Proceedings in defines a victim as "[a] natural person who has suffered harm, including physical or mental injury, emotional suffering or economic loss, directly caused by acts or omissions that are in violation of the criminal law of a Member State."

A similar definition of "victim" is present in article 1 of the Egyptian anti-trafficking law, which defines a victim of trafficking as "a natural person who suffered any material or moral harm, in particular bodily, psychological or mental harm; or economic loss if the harm or loss was caused directly by one of the crimes stipulated in this law." A reference to this type of victim is included in article 1 of the Iraqi law, which states, "The victim means the person who suffered from material or moral damage caused by one of the crimes stipulated in this law."

Article 586(1) of the Lebanese law states: For the purpose of this law, a victim of trafficking means any natural person who is subject to trafficking in persons or who is reasonably considered as such by the competent authorities irrespective of whether the perpetrator of the crime was identified or arrested or tried or charged.

Article 1 of the Syria's law also defines "victim": A victim of trafficking is a person against whom the act of trafficking was committed or was subject thereto.

11.6.2 Derivative Victim

Article A(2) of the United Nations Declaration of Basic Principles of Justice for Victims of Crime and Abuse of Power includes in the definition of "victim," when appropriate, the family members of the victim. It states: The term "victim" includes, where appropriate, the immediate family or dependents of the direct victim and persons who have suffered to assist victims in distress or to prevent victimization.

11.6.3 Potential Victim

A potential victim is a person who is part of a risk group and is vulnerable to becoming a victim of trafficking. Common examples of potential victims in the Middle East and North Africa (MENA) region are street children in Egypt. Traffickers often target this risk group because of its vulnerability, which is caused by lack of economic opportunities and limited access to information and social services.

11.6.4 Vulnerable Victim

The definition of "vulnerable victim" takes into account the fact that a victim of trafficking is, most frequently, vulnerable. The *travaux préparatoires* to the U.N. Protocol state that "[t]he reference to the abuse of a position of vulnerability is understood to refer to any situation in which the person involved has no real and acceptable alternative but to submit to the abuse involved."185

This qualification of a vulnerable victim is relevant when establishing guidelines for the status of a victim of trafficking and the types of benefits he or she may receive from the State. It is crucial to understand that victims of trafficking, as vulnerable victims, are in a situation in which they have no choice but to submit to exploitation and, therefore, cannot be held liable for criminal acts that may be committed under duress or as a result of their being trafficked.

11.6.4.1 Best Practice

In United States V. Veerapol, the court applied the vulnerable victim enhancement doctrine, which affirms that crimes committed against a susceptible victim warrant an enhanced penalty for the offender. The court stated that a person from a foreign country coming to the United States who does not know the language or the culture is a vulnerable person. In this case, the wife of the Thai ambassador recruited girls from Thailand to work in her house and in the restaurant she owned in Los Angeles. She was convicted of trafficking and given an enhanced penalty because the victims were deemed to be vulnerable persons.

11.6.5 Presumed Victim

A presumed victim is a person who has already been trafficked but has not been identified as a victim of trafficking. Such a person falls outside the protection of the legal system.

11.6.5.1 When the Victim Is a Child

Some basic considerations must be made when the victim is a child. Article 6.4 of the U.N. Protocol states that "[e]ach State Party shall take into account, in applying the provisions of this article, the age, gender and special needs of victims of trafficking in persons, in particular the special needs of children, including appropriate housing, education and care."187 In addition, according to the U.N. First Aid Kit for use by Law Enforcement First Responders in Addressing Human Trafficking, first responders must "assume that a child's needs and capacities are different from those of adults and that it is unlikely that children can make informed decisions. If children agree to certain actions and decisions, it may simply be because they feel overwhelmed" and "even if your legislation indicates otherwise, you should assume that all persons below the age of 18 are children, especially if the child in question is not from your country, as that is the international standard."

11.6.5.2 Best Practice

Acknowledging the various typologies of victims and the difficulties that law enforcement officers can face in identifying victims of trafficking among various populations of vulnerable groups, the Jordanian National Strategy for the Prevention of Trafficking in Persons, adopted in December 2012, urges the State to formulate and implement training programs for law enforcement personnel and members of civil society on methods for identifying both victims and those negatively affected by the crime.

11.6.6 The Islamic Law Perspective

The holy Qur'an lays out certain regulations and mechanisms to lend additional support to women and children, especially orphans, who are considered more vulnerable than other groups, and states that believers are to do good to parents, kinfolk, orphans, the needy, neighbors, strangers, wayfarers, and slaves. Women and children are granted special protection by Islam, and believers are required to provide assistance to the needy and those in distress.

Some contend that the failure to do so is a sin because of a generally accepted principle of Islamic law: "whoever neglects an obligation is legally liable for the consequences of that neglect." This protection is granted to all, as the Qur'an 5:32 states: "If anyone kills a person, it would be as if one has killed all of humanity; if anyone saves a person, it would be as if one has saved all of humanity."

11.7 Indicators of Victims of Trafficking

11.7.1 Physical and Other Indicators of Victims of Trafficking

Victims of human trafficking may have been physically beaten or treated poorly. As a result, physical indicators may exist that can assist law enforcement officials in identifying potential victims.

These indicators may include (a) visible marks, scratches, and bruises from physical abuse; (b) torture scars, such as cigarette burns; (c) a sickly appearance as a result of malnutrition; and (d) brands and tattoos depicting ownership of the victim. There are additional signs that law enforcement officials should look for to assess whether a person is a victim of trafficking. For example, they should consider whether someone is trying to speak on behalf of the victim; whether the victim is in possession of his or her personal or travel documents, money, or other personal property; and whether the potential victim appears to be sleeping and working in the same location.190 Other useful clues are the potential victim's ability to leave the work premises freely; his or her terms of employment (including the number of working hours, vacations, and sick days); and the existence of appropriate safety measures and sanitation in the workplace.

11.7.1.1 Best Practice

The U.S. Department of Homeland Security's Blue Campaign initiative provides indicators that law enforcement officials should look for in determining if a person is a victim of trafficking:

- Is the victim in possession of his or her identification and travel documents?
- Was the victim coached on what to say to law enforcement and immigration officials?
- Was the victim recruited for one purpose and then forced to engage in another job?
- Is the victim's salary taken away to pay off a smuggling or transportation fee?
- Was the victim forced to perform sexual acts?
- Does the victim have freedom of movement?
- Has the victim or his or her family been threatened with harm if the victim attempts to escape?
- Has the victim been threatened with deportation or law enforcement action?
- Has the victim been harmed or deprived of food, water, sleep, or medical care?
- Can the victim freely contact family and friends?
- Is the victim a juvenile engaged in commercial sex?
- Is the victim allowed to socialize or attend religious service?

Law enforcement should be aware of certain signs of trafficking that are typical of child victims, such as (a) having no access to their parents or guardians, (b) looking intimidated and behaving in a way that does not correspond with behavior typical of children their age, (c) having no friends of their own age outside of work, (d) having no access to education, (e) having no time for playing, (f) living apart from other children and in substandard accommodations, (g) eating apart from other members of the "family," (h) receiving only leftovers to eat, (i) being engaged in work that is not suitable for children, (j) travelling unaccompanied by adults, and (k) travelling in groups with people who are not relatives.

11.7.2 Understanding the Victim's State of Mind

All victims have undergone some form of trauma as result of their trafficking. Victims may be repeatedly told by the trafficker that law enforcement is not to be trusted; therefore, victims may initially be suspicious of those trying to help them. Because many trafficking victims are in the country illegally, they are often reluctant to come forward for fear of being arrested and deported. Despite being a victim of trafficking, they sometimes believe that their present situation is better than where they came from. Additionally, many also fear for their families back home, because their traffickers have threatened to hurt their family members if they try to escape or cooperate with law enforcement. Nearly all victims are unaware of their rights.

Furthermore, some victims do not self-identify with being a victim. For instance, if the perpetrator provides them with shelter, food, and "stable employment," the victims may not realize that they have been trafficked.

11.7.3 Effective Communication with Victims of Trafficking

Trafficking victims may initially be hesitant to cooperate with law enforcement officials. For this reason, it is imperative that police officers be particularly sensitive when communicating with victims. It is important to convey to the victim that first and foremost they are safe now, and no one will hurt them. Police officers must also help victims understand that they are in fact victims and not criminals. Finally, because most victims are unaware of their rights, law enforcement officers must explain what rights victims have, what assistance they are entitled to, and how they may receive such assistance.

11.8 Regional Legal Frameworks

Since the passage of the U.N. Protocol in 2000, many countries around the world have adopted comprehensive anti-trafficking laws to combat human trafficking in compliance with the legislative mandate of the U.N. Protocol. The region covered here includes Morocco, Algeria, Tunisia, Egypt, Jordan, Lebanon, Syria, Palestine, Sudan, Yemen, Iran, Saudi Arabia, Kuwait, Bahrain, Qatar, the United Arab Emirates, Djibouti, Iran, Iraq, Libya and Oman.[5] These countries are very different in terms of political structures, economic welfare, and social development. But they have in common ratification of the United Nations *Convention on the Rights of the Child* (CRC) with no reservations on Articles 34 and 35, which cover the right of children not to be exploited for sexual purposes.[6]

In the Arab world alone, 12 States have adopted comprehensive anti-trafficking laws: Bahrain, Djibouti, Egypt, Iraq, Jordan, Kuwait, Mauritania, Oman, Qatar, Saudi Arabia, Syria, and the United Arab Emirates. Algeria and Lebanon have

---

[5]http://www.unicef.org/events/yokohama/backgound8.html#_edn2

[6]This summary is based on the situation analysis written by Dr. Najat M'jid for the Arab-African Forum against Commercial Sexual Exploitation, Rabat, Morocco, 24–26 October 2001. This regional consultation in preparation for the 2ndWorld Congress against Commercial Sexual Exploitation of Children brought together representatives of 65 countries in the Middle East and Africa. Bibliographical references are available in the source document (in French): *Rapport sur la situation de l'exploitation sexuelle des enfants dans la région MENA*, 10 septembre 2001, available on the regional consultation website:http://perso.respublica.fr/forum_ese. Papers prepared for regional consultations in preparation for the second World Congress are not endorsed by the Congress co-organizers but remain working documents feeding into regional discussions.

adopted anti-trafficking provisions in their penal codes. The remaining States Members of the Arab League continue to use existing laws to prosecute trafficking cases.

11.9 The Situation in the Middle East/North Africa Region[7,8]

Trafficking in persons is a complex crime that affects many spheres of law and criminal justice. Since the passage in 2000 of the United Nations Protocol to Prevent, Suppress and Punish Trafficking in Persons, Especially Women and Children, supplementing the United Nations Convention against Transnational Organized Crime1 (hereafter U.N. Protocol), international legal experts have been debating to which discipline trafficking in persons belongs.[9]

Today, many experts agree that the human rights approach to trafficking in persons is the most appropriate because it recognizes the trafficked person as a

[7]This summary is based on the situation analysis written by Dr. Najat M'jid for the Arab-African Forum against Commercial Sexual Exploitation, Rabat, Morocco, 24–26 October 2001. This regional consultation in preparation for the second World Congress against Commercial Sexual Exploitation of Children brought together representatives of 65 countries in the Middle East and Africa. Bibliographical references are available in the source document (in French): Rapport sur la situation de l'exploitation sexuelle des enfants dans la région MENA, 10 septembre 2001, available on the regional consultation website: http://perso.respublica.fr/forum_ese. Papers prepared for regional consultations in preparation for the second World Congress are not endorsed by the Congress co-organizers but remain working documents feeding into regional discussions.

[8]Report of the SR on the sale of children, child prostitution and child pornographyhttp://arabnews.com/saudiarabia/women_day/article306363.ece?comments=al

[9]1949 Convention: Asserting the dangers of prostitution.

In 1949, the United Nations adopted the Convention for the Suppression of the Traffic in Persons and of the Exploitation of the Prostitution of Others. Article 1 of the convention stipulates that "[t]he Parties to the present Convention agree to punish any person who, to gratify the passions of another: (1) Procures, entices or leads away, for purposes of prostitution, another person, even with the consent of that person; and (2) Exploits the prostitution of another person, even with the consent of that person."109 The ethical imperative underlining the convention is clearly stated in the Preamble: Prostitution and the accompanying evil of the traffic in persons for the purpose of prostitution are incompatible with the dignity and worth of the human person and endanger the welfare of the individual, the family and the community.110

4.B.2.3. ICCPR: Prohibition against slavery, servitude, or forced labour.

Article 8 of the International Covenant on Civil and Political Rights of 1966 further criminalizes all forms of slavery that may be considered trafficking and mandates: "1. No one shall be held in slavery; slavery and the slave-trade in all their forms shall be prohibited. 2. No one shall be held in servitude. 3. (a) No one shall be required to perform forced or compulsory labour."111

4.B.2.4. CEDAW: Suppression of trafficking in women

A special protection warranted to women was recognized in the United Nations Convention on the Elimination of All Forms of Discrimination against Women of 1979, which, in article 6, calls on States to take legislative and other measures to suppress all forms of trafficking in women and exploitation of prostitution of women.112.

4.B.2.5. CRC: Call for prevention of trafficking in children

victim entitled to human rights and, as such, entitled to protection and assistance if those human rights have been violated, regardless of the sex, age, or nationality of the victim. Children may be subject to sexual abuse in the family or school or in the different institutions. However, the term sexual exploitation is used to refer to childhood prostitution and their use in pornographic activities. The same applies to trafficking in children where the child is transferred from one person to another in exchange for money. This is usually done in order to use those children in different forms of domestic labor, agricultural labor and also in sex tourism.

Traffickers use a variety of techniques to recruit their victims, ranging from kidnapping to the simple promise of a low-wage job. Traffickers intentionally seek out the weakest and most vulnerable members of society in order to exploit them for personal gain, frequently by taking advantage of conditions of poverty, economic collapse, civil unrest, and social upheaval. Often, the trafficker gains the confidence of the victim through a combination of physiological means. At times, unscrupulous employment agencies deceive workers into entering abusive work situations, and what first appears as a legitimate job can easily turn into forced labor or sexual exploitation. Women and children are especially vulnerable to trafficking and are often trafficked by their own communities, by their families, and in public places of business and commerce. Promise of an immediate payment may lead families to sell their children to traffickers.

Laws in all countries of the Middle East and North Africa region prohibit sexual exploitation of children and the production of pornographic material in the context of prohibiting prostitution and sexual exploitation in general. As for sexual abuse, many countries do not have specific laws that protect children subject to rape. The penalty is usually a severe one in case the victim is under age. The rapist may be spared the penalty, if he agrees to marry the victim and in many cases the girls are forced to marry their rapists.

The Convention on the Rights of the Child of 1989 grants protection for children from trafficking in article 35: States Parties shall take all appropriate national, bilateral and multilateral measures to prevent the abduction of, the sale of or traffic in children for any purpose or in any form.113

4.B.2.6. Migrant Workers Convention: Prohibition against slavery, servitude, or forced labour

The protection of migrant workers from exploitation is provided for in the International Convention on the Protection of the Rights of All Migrant Workers and Members of Their Families of 1990 in article 11, which states:

(1) No migrant worker or member of his or her family shall be held in slavery or servitude; (2) No migrant worker or member of his or her family shall be required to perform forced or compulsory labour.114

4.B.2.7. ILO Convention No. 189: Decent Work for Domestic Workers

In June 2011, the International Labour Organization adopted Convention No. 189 concerning decent work for domestic workers. The convention is revolutionary in that it grants domestic workers status equal to other workers. Specifically, article 3 provides: Each Member shall, in relation to domestic workers, take the measures set out in this Convention to respect, promote and realize the fundamental principles and rights at work, namely: (a) freedom of association and the effective recognition of the right to collective bargaining; (b) the elimination of all forms of forced or compulsory labour; (c) the effective abolition of child labour.115

In the regional conference on Commercial Sexual Exploitation of Children in North Africa (ECPAT), organized in Rabat, Morocco in June 2003, the five participating countries submitted a report regarding the situation of sexual exploitation of children and suggested recommendations to address this phenomenon (23). Lebanon is also, by nature, a place for sexual tourism, where legislation is not tackling directly internet crimes, sexual exploitation, extra-territoriality, aggravating conditions for sexual abuse, etc. On the same subject, an International Conference on Effective Strategies for the Prevention of Child Online Pornography Trafficking and Abuse was held in Bahrain, March 2009.[10] Reports from Arab countries agree that it is

---

[10]Regional law prohibiting trafficking in persons

4.C.1. Arab Charter on Human Rights

Articles 9 and 10 of the 2004 Arab Charter on Human Rights clearly prohibit trafficking in persons. In particular, article 9 states: No one shall be subjected to medical or scientific experimentation or to the use of his organs without his free consent and full awareness of the consequences and provided that ethical, humanitarian and professional rules are followed and medical procedures are observed to ensure his personal safety pursuant to the relevant domestic laws in force in each State Party. Trafficking in human organs is prohibited in all circumstances .116 Article 10 of the Arab Charter states:

1. All forms of slavery and trafficking in human beings are prohibited and are punishable by law. No one shall be held in slavery and servitude under any circumstances.

2. Forced labour, trafficking in human beings for the purposes of prostitution or sexual exploitation, the exploitation of the prostitution of others or any other form of exploitation or the exploitation of children in armed conflict are prohibited.117

4.C.1.1. Distinction between slavery and trafficking

It is important to notice that the Arab Charter distinguishes between slavery and trafficking in human beings but prohibits both. Although slavery requires exercising the right of ownership over another, trafficking is about control or undue influence rather than buying and selling. Trafficking is therefore conventionally viewed as a form of modern-day slavery.

4.C.1.2. Prohibition of prostitution and exploitation of the prostitution of others

The Arab Charter also distinguishes between prostitution and exploitation of the prostitution of others, prohibiting both forms of trafficking. Prostitution is prohibited by the domestic law of Arab countries. Unlike the Arab Charter, the U.N. Protocol prohibits only exploitation of the prostitution of others.

4.C.1.3. Prohibition of all forms of trafficking including forced labour

Although Article 10(b) of the Arab Charter does not explicitly use the term "labour trafficking," it makes it clear that "all forms of trafficking" are prohibited, including "forced labour."118

4.C.1.4. Abolition of specific forms of trafficking

The Arab Charter highlights specific forms of trafficking, including the exploitation of children in armed conflict, trafficking in human organs, and medical or scientificexperimentation.119 In doing so, the Arab Charter recognizes the significance of these forms of exploitation and establishes that they all must be abolished.

4.D. Arab laws prohibiting trafficking in persons: General principles and specific rules

The countries of the Arab world can be divided into three groups on the basis of the status of their trafficking laws. The first group encompasses those countries that have already enacted comprehensive anti–trafficking legislation: Bahrain, Djibouti,

Egypt, Iraq, Jordan, Kuwait, Mauritania, Oman, Qatar, Saudi Arabia, Syria, and the United Arab Emirates. The countries that enacted provisions in penal codes to prosecute cases of trafficking in persons are Algeria and Lebanon. Comoros, Libya, Morocco, the Palestinian Authority, Somalia, Sudan, Tunisia, and Yemen use existing legislation to prosecute cases of trafficking. Various legal principles characterize these laws and offer a valuable comparative prospective of the current status

difficult to obtain accurate data and information regarding the prevalence of sexual exploitation. Police records also do not provide an estimate of the size of the problem. The prevalent form of sexual exploitation in the North Africa region is child prostitution; child trafficking is associated more with economic exploitation than with sexual exploitation since it is associated with child labor in areas such as domestic labor. The sectors most at risk are street children beggars and domestic laborers. Forced early marriage, especially in Egypt, Mauritania and Chad are considered a form of sexual exploitation, as are the child trafficking in Iraq and the problem of smuggling children inside the state of Libya for the purpose of prostitution and slave trade.

Responses to violence against children in the community: Arab professionals provide expertise to decision makers about the condition of children in such settings, where problems are too big for one Arab country, including living conditions and social challenges, sexual and commercial exploitation of humans and organs, humanitarian assistance and support, as well as access to education and control of frontiers, arm smuggling and corruption.[11]

Sex trafficking is considered a violation of human rights and a form of sex discrimination, as nearly all victims are female. Sexually exploited women and girls are often experience various violations, including but not limited to forced sex with pimps and customers, beatings, and forced abortions. Sexual exploitation is hugely underreported because victims fear stigmatization, are threatened with violence and deprivation of food or money, lack faith in institutions, or have limited access to legal services or knowledge about how to navigate them.[12]

---

of anti-trafficking legislation in the Arab world. These principles are the non-punishment of the victim, the statute of limitations, the prosecution of demand, the aggravating circumstances, and the issue of extraterritoriality.

4.D.1. Principle of non-punishment of the victim

4.D.1.1. Principle of non-punishment

Recognition of trafficked persons as victims requires the application of the principle of non-criminalization, according to which the law must excuse such persons from original liability for acts committed as a result of being trafficked, including illegal entry, falsification of travel documents, or prostitution, if criminalized in the country.

Although the U.N. Protocol treats the trafficked person as a victim, it does not specifically provide for the principle of non-criminalization. Similarly, many domestic laws are silent on the issue, thus denying victims protection from liability for crimes committed as a consequence of being trafficked. States should ensure that trafficked persons are not prosecuted for immigration law violations or for their involvement in activities that are a direct result of being a trafficked person. States must ensure, in particular, that legislation prevents trafficked persons from being prosecuted, detained, or punished for the illegality of their entry or residence or for their involvement in activities that are a direct result of that situation. Non-liability provisions ensure that victims of trafficking are not prosecuted or punished for offences they commit.

[11] http://www.unicef.org/events/yokohama/backgound8.html#_edn1

[12] http://en.wikipedia.org/wiki/Sexual_slavery#cite_note-finkelhor1994-12
http://en.wikipedia.org/wiki/Sexual_slavery#cite_note-hobbs-13
http://en.wikipedia.org/wiki/Sexual_slavery#cite_note-O-14
http://en.wikipedia.org/wiki/Sexual_slavery#cite_note-sheldon20-15

Commercial sexual exploitation of children (CSEC) constitutes a contemporary form of slavery. A declaration of the World Congress against Commercial Sexual Exploitation of Children, held in Stockholm in 1996, defined CSEC as: 'sexual abuse by the adult and remuneration in cash or kind to the child or a third person or persons. The child is treated as a sexual object and as a commercial object. 'CSEC includes the prostitution of children, child pornography, child sex tourism and survival sex, where a child engages in sexual activities to have access to needs, such as food, or shelter or even education. The prostitution of children is a form of commercial sexual exploitation of children, most often for the financial benefit of an adult. In many parts of the world, child prostitution is tolerated and ignored by the authorities. Child pornography refers to images or films depicting sexually explicit activities involving a child; as such, child pornography is a visual record of child sexual abuse. Abuse of the child occurs during the sexual acts and the production of child pornography,; such effects on the child are compounded by the wide distribution and lasting availability of the photographs. Child sex tourism (CST) is a travel to a foreign country for commercially facilitated child sexual abuse.[13] Mental and physical consequences include disease (including HIV/AIDS), drug addiction,

---

[13]The Islamic Law Perspective

The Qur'anic legislation is the first law to recognize the principle of nonpunishment of the victim of a crime, especially when linked to trafficking for the purpose of sexual exploitation. In accordance with the Qur'an, Surah 24:33, "But force not your maids to prostitution when they desire chastity.... But if anyone compels them, yet, after such compulsion, is Allah, Oft-Forgiving, Most Merciful [to them]."120

4.D.1.2 Two models of non-punishment: Duress and causation

Countries follow two main models when establishing the principle of non-punishment of the illegal acts committed by victims of trafficking: the duress model and the causation model. In the duress model, the person is obliged to prove that he or she was compelled to commit the offences. In the causation model, the principle applies when the individual can prove that the offence was directly connected or related to being trafficked.

Duress model: This model is followed by the criminal code of Lebanon, which provides, in article 586(8), that "a victim shall be exempt from punishment if (s)he was compelled to commit acts punishable by law or if (s)he violated the conditions of residency or work."121

Causation model: An example of this model is present in the Egyptian anti-trafficking law, according to which a victim of trafficking in persons is not punishable for the commission of any crime that is the direct result of having been trafficked. In particular, article 21 states: The victim shall not be criminally or civilly liable for any of the crimes of human trafficking as long as the crime occurred or was directly related to being a victim.122

4.D.1.3 Principle of non-punishment in Arab legislation

The Arab Model Law on Combating Human Trafficking of 2012 provides for the principle of non-punishment in Article 27 by stating that "the victim shall not be criminally or civilly liable for any of the crimes of human trafficking as long as the crime occurred or was directly related to being a victim."123 Article 28 also stipulates that victims "shall be exempt from all the penalties stipulated in the laws regarding violations of immigration, nationality and residency as long as they are directly related to their status as victims."124 At the domestic level, only four laws in the Arab world explicitly specify that a victim of trafficking should not be punished. This principle is expressed in several ways and is sometimes referred to as a principle of non-criminalization, immunity, excuse, non-liability, or (more accurately) nonpunishment.

4.D.1.3.1 Egypt

pregnancy, malnutrition, social ostracism, and possibly death. The Rome Statute also recognizes rape, sexual slavery, enforced prostitution, forced pregnancy, enforced sterilization, "or any other form of sexual violence of comparable gravity" as crime against humanity if widespread or systematic. Sexual slavery is an example of crime against humanity as in Bosnia and Herzegovina, Sudan and Darfour, under the rubric of torture and enslavement.[14]

11.10 Routes of Trafficking in Persons in the MENA Region

Trafficking routes can be international, regional, and domestic. The following are the main routes in the MENA region:

The Egyptian law provides for the principle of non-punishment of a victim in article 21, by stating that "[t]he victim shall not be criminally or civilly liable for any of the crimes of human trafficking as long as the crime occurred or was directly related to being a victim."125

4.D.1.3.2. Qatar

An identical provision appears in article 4 of the Qatari law.126 Additionally, article 25 of the Qatari law specifically exempts a victim from all penalties stipulated in Law No. 4 of 2009 regarding violations of entry, residency, and kafala laws (sponsorship rule laws) by aliens.127

4.D.1.3.3. Lebanon

Article 586(8) of the criminal code of Lebanon provides that "a victim shall be exempt from punishment if (s)he was compelled to commit acts punishable by law or if (s)he violated the conditions of residency or work."128

4.D.1.3.4. Jordan

Similarly, the Jordanian law gives public prosecutors the authority not to pursue investigation or prosecution of a victim of trafficking for any of the crimes stipulated in the trafficking law. However, it must be noted that the authority is discretionary, and the law does not provide any guidance on when it should be exercised.129

[14]International Labour Organization Convention Concerning the Prohibition and Immediate Action for the Elimination of the Worst Forms of Child Labour

A further international convention that sheds light on the meaning and scope of trafficking in persons is the International Labour Organization (ILO) Convention Concerning the Prohibition and Immediate Action for the Elimination of the Worst Forms of Child Labour Convention of 1999. The convention includes trafficking in children in the definition of "worst forms of child labour" and states in article 3: For the purposes of this Convention, the term "the worst forms of child labour" comprises: (a) all forms of slavery or practices similar to slavery, such as the sale and trafficking of children, debt bondage and serfdom and forced or compulsory labour, including forced or compulsory recruitment of children for use in armed conflict; (b) the use, procuring or offering of a child for prostitution, for the production of pornography or for pornographic performances; (c) the use, procuring or offering of a child for illicit activities, in particular for the production and trafficking of drugs as defined in the relevant international treaties; (d) work which, by its nature or the circumstances in which it is carried out, is likely to harm the health, safety or morals of children.36This convention has been ratified by all the MENA region countries.

- Regional trafficking from less affluent countries in North Africa to more affluent countries in the Gulf States
- International trafficking to all Arab countries and especially to the Gulf States, from Eastern Europe, the Caucasus, Central Asia, and South and Southeast Asia
- International trafficking from North Africa to Europe, the United States, and Canada
- Domestic trafficking between rural areas and the main cities in all countries of the MENA region

The root causes of trafficking are economic, social, cultural, legal, and political in nature. Populations that are rendered vulnerable by one or more of these factors are more likely to be trafficked. Traffickers intentionally target the weakest and most vulnerable members of society in order to exploit them. Among the major causes of trafficking are poverty and underdevelopment, social and cultural traditions, weak legal institutions, civil war and political unrest, and corruption.

People trafficked for any of the exploitative purposes defined by the U.N. Protocol may travel over international or domestic routes. They may be trafficked by individuals or organized criminal groups. Article 4 of the U.N. Protocol states, except as otherwise stated therein, that the offence of trafficking in persons occurs "where those offences are transnational in nature and involve an organized criminal group."[15]

[15]According to article 3(2) of the United Nations Convention against Transnational Organized Crime, the parent convention of the U.N. Protocol, international trafficking occurs when "[i]t is committed in more than one State; or is committed in one State but a substantial part of its preparation, planning, direction or control takes place in another State; or is committed in one State but involves an organized criminal group that engages in criminal activities in more than one State; or is committed in one State but has substantial effects in another State."75 Moreover, under article.

16 (extradition) and article 18 (mutual legal assistance), offences are considered transnational if the person sought is located in the territory of the requested State or if victims, witnesses, proceeds, instrumentalities, or evidence is located in the requested State. Article 2(a) defines "organized criminal group" as "a structured group of three or more persons, existing for a period of time and acting in concert with the aim of committing one or more serious crimes or offences established in accordance with this Convention, in order to obtain, directly or indirectly, a financial or other material benefit."76

Transnationality and the involvement of an organized criminal group are not required for the establishment of the crime of trafficking in persons in national legislation.

As article 34(2) of the United Nations Convention against Transnational Organized Crime states: The offences established in accordance with articles 5, 6, 8 and 23 of this Convention shall be established in the domestic law of each State.

Party independently of the transnational nature or the involvement of an organized criminal group.77

In summary, trafficking routes can be international, regional, and domestic. The following are the main routes in the MENA region:

• Regional trafficking from less affluent countries in North Africa to more affluent countries in the Gulf States

• International trafficking to all Arab countries and especially to the Gulf States, from Eastern Europe, the Caucasus, Central Asia, and South and Southeast Asia

11.11 Finding Solutions: Training Manual to Combat Trafficking in Persons

Economic factors are directly addressed in the U.N. Protocol, which mentions poverty, underdevelopment, and lack of equal opportunities as the main root causes of trafficking in persons. Economic vulnerability may also include unemployment and lack of access to opportunities, which make people want to migrate in search of better conditions. Even a normal, legitimate flow of economic migration from a poor country to a richer one provides opportunities for traffickers to victimize immigrants, who are more vulnerable having left their home areas.

According to article 3(2) of the United Nations Convention against Transnational Organized Crime, the parent convention of the U.N. Protocol, international trafficking occurs when "[i]t is committed in more than one State; or is committed in one State but a substantial part of its preparation, planning, direction or control takes place in another State; or is committed in one State but involves an organized criminal group that engages in criminal activities in more than one State; or is committed in one State but has substantial effects in another State." Moreover, under article 16 (extradition) and article 18 (mutual legal assistance), offences are considered transnational if the person sought is located in the territory of the requested State or if victims, witnesses, proceed, instrumentalities, or evidence is located in the requested State. Article 2(a) defines "organized criminal group" as "a structured group of three or more persons, existing for a period of time and acting in concert with the aim of committing one or more serious crimes or offences established in accordance with this Convention, in order to obtain, directly or indirectly, a financial or other material benefit."

Transnationality and the involvement of an organized criminal group are not required for the establishment of the crime of trafficking in persons in national legislation. As article 34(2) of the United Nations Convention against Transnational Organized Crime states:

The offences established in accordance with articles 5, 6, 8 and 23 of this Convention shall be established in the domestic law of each State Party independently of the transnational nature or the involvement of an organized criminal group.

11.12 Summarizing Challenges and Opportunities

All of the countries except Djibouti have adopted ILO Worst Forms of Child Labor Convention 182, and are thus committed to eliminating the exploitation of children in prostitution and pornography, and trafficking of children into hazardous labor.

• International trafficking from North Africa to Europe, the United States, and Canada
• Domestic trafficking between rural areas and the main cities in all countries of the MENA region

Most of the countries, too, adopted the 1996 Stockholm Declaration and Agenda for Action, which calls for national plans of action against commercial sexual exploitation of children (CSEC). These countries also have in common, however, a number of constraints that have hindered preparation of national plans of action. In all the countries of the region, there is cultural resistance to addressing the problem because the subject is largely taboo. Often the issue is dealt with more generally under headings such as 'violence' and 'trauma'. This means that there has been no regional consensus on defining CSEC in law; in some countries, for example, it is looked upon as an indecent act, in others as rape, although in all 20 countries there is some section of the penal code that can be invoked against sexual abuse and exploitation. This variously includes legal concepts as diverse as 'rape with deflowering' and 'encouragement to solicit'. Laws covering homosexuality, sexual harassment, pedophilia and 'acts against nature' are all part of the legal battery invoked in debate on CSEC in the region, and this lack of harmonization of approaches is at best confusing and at worst a hindrance to concerted action. Extraterritoriality does not appear to feature in laws in place in the region. Even when laws are invoked, moreover, sentences vary widely from a few months to 30 years imprisonment and in some cases only fines. Law enforcement is also patchy, and legal assistance is not always available to the victim. In some countries non-governmental organizations (NGOs) provide the only reliable source of legal advice. Similarly, although there have been moves to lift professional confidentiality in cases of sexual abuse identified by medical professionals in the region, there is very limited reporting by doctors as a result of ignorance of the law and poor coordination between medical and judicial sectors.

11.12.1 Legislative Reforms[16]

Social exclusion relates to a lack of access to social rights and prevents groups from receiving the benefits and protection to which all citizens should be entitled. Marginalization from social security derives from complex factors, including

[16]Arab Charter on Human Rights

The Arab Charter on Human Rights adopted by the League of Arab States in 2004 does not give a comprehensive definition of trafficking. However, article 9 prohibits trafficking in human organs and presumably trafficking for the use of "medical experimentation."40 In addition, article 10 prohibits "all forms of slavery and trafficking in human beings."41 Article 43 encourages ratifying States to interpret the Arab Charter in congruence with other international and regional human rights conventions, thereby encouraging States to interpret trafficking in persons as defined under the U.N. Protocol. Article 43 reads:

Nothing in this Charter may be construed or interpreted as impairing the rights and freedoms protected by the domestic laws of the States parties or those set forth in the international and regional human rights instruments which the States parties have adopted or ratified, including the rights of women, the rights of the child and the rights of persons belonging to minorities.42

2.B.2. Council of Europe

gender, ethnicity, and the low status of groups within societies. Such marginalization involves discrimination in education, employment practices, access to legal and medical services, and access to information and social welfare. Social exclusion is particularly important when discussing how to prevent revictimization and retrafficking. Trafficked persons face considerable obstacles on their return home, including the attitudes and biases within their own communities. Social and cultural practices are sensitive to context and therefore must be considered with special caution to avoid generalization. For example, cultural practices (such as arranged, early, or forced marriages) and other practices (such as temporary marriages, marriages by catalogue, or mail-order brides)—if they lack consent and they entail an element of exploitation—can all contribute to trafficking in persons. Furthermore, in many societies, cultural norms affect the manner in which women are treated, making gender-based discrimination a contributing factor to women's vulnerability to trafficking. In addition, women from certain societies who are trafficked into prostitution find it more difficult to reintegrate into their families and communities after being freed from exploitation.

In times of peace, States in MENA have demonstrated a strong commitment to protect the human rights of children by universally ratifying the Convention on the Rights of the Child (CRC), which serves as the foundation for recognizing and protecting child rights in international law and encompasses all children, including refugee children.

The MENA region also features near universal ratification of the Optional Protocol to the CRC on the Involvement of Children in Armed Conflict, as well as

---

In 2005, the Council of Europe adopted the Convention on Action against Trafficking in Human Beings, which, similarly to the U.N. Protocol, defines "trafficking" in Article 4 as the following: The recruitment, transportation, transfer, harbouring or receipt of persons, by means of threat or use of force or other forms of coercion, of abduction, of fraud, of deception, of the abuse of power or of a position of vulnerability or of the giving or receiving of payments or benefits to achieve the consent of a person having control over another person, for the purpose of exploitation. Exploitation shall include, at a minimum, the exploitation of the prostitution of others or other forms of sexual exploitation, forced labour or services, slavery or practices similar to slavery, servitude or the removal of organs.43

2.B.3. European Union

Expanding on the U.N. Protocol's definition of "trafficking in persons," Directive 2011/36/EU of the European Parliament and of the Council on Preventing and Combating Trafficking in Human Beings and Protecting Its Victims of 5 April 2011defines trafficking in article 2 as the following: The recruitment, transportation, transfer, harbouring or reception of persons, including the exchange or transfer of control over those persons, by means of threat or use of force or other forms of coercion, of abduction, of fraud, of deception, of the abuse of power or of a position of vulnerability or of the giving or receiving of payments or benefits to achieve the consent of a person having control over another person, for the purpose of exploitation. Exploitation shall include, as a minimum, the exploitation of the prostitution of others or other forms of sexual exploitation, forced labour or services, including begging, slavery or practices similar to slavery, servitude, or the exploitation of criminal activities, or the removal of organs.44 It is notable that this new definition includes in the act the transfer of control over those persons and explicitly refers to begging and criminal activities as forms of exploitation.

the Optional Protocol to the CRC on the Sale of Children, Child Prostitution and Child Pornography.

Yet, another possible purpose of exploitation in trafficking is pornography, which can be considered a form of sexual exploitation. As detailed in article 2(a), paragraph ii, of the *travaux préparatoires* of U.N. Protocol (negotiation text), sexual exploitation of a child includes "prostitution, sexual servitude or use of a child in pornography." In addition, article 2(c) of the Optional Protocol to the Convention on the Rights of the Child on the Sale of Children, Child Prostitution, and Child Pornography defines "child pornography" as "any representation, by whatever means, of a child engaged in real or simulated explicit sexual activities or any representation of the sexual parts of a child for primarily sexual purposes."

The International Centre for Missing and Exploited Children (ICMEC), an international non-governmental organization based in the United States is particularly active in the fight for children's rights. According to ICMEC, child pornography today has become a global crisis. In 2006, ICMEC published *The Child Pornography Model Legislation* in an effort to promote the harmonization of the law on child pornography. The model legislation details seven criminal offence objectives, including incorporating child pornography offences into the penal code; criminalizing the knowing possession of child pornography, regardless of the intent to distribute; criminalizing knowingly downloading or knowingly viewing child pornography images on the Internet and using the Internet to distribute child pornography; penalizing those who make known to others where to find child pornography; criminalizing the actions of parents or legal guardians who acquiesce to their child's participation in child pornography; criminalizing grooming offences; and punishing attempted crimes. Most States in MENA have also acceded to the International Covenant on Civil and Political Rights (ICCPR), which complements provisions in the CRC, and also recognizes the right of all children to be registered at birth, to acquire a nationality, and to enjoy child-specific protections in all situations. MENA is also host to regional human rights instruments addressing the protection of children, including the Covenant on the Rights of the Child in Islam, the African Charter on the Rights and Welfare of the Child, the Arab Charter on Human Rights, and the African Charter on Human and Peoples' Rights. Several States in the region have also ratified the 1951 Convention.

11.12.2 Countries with Anti-trafficking Provisions in Their Penal Codes

In 2009, Algeria amended its penal code to include the definitions of "organ trafficking," "trafficking in persons," and "migrant trafficking." It also added begging to the forms of trafficking in persons. Article 303 states: "Trafficking in persons" is defined as recruitment, transport, transfer, harboring or receiving one or many persons by means of threat or use of force or other forms of coercion, abduction, fraud, deceit, abuse of power or a situation of vulnerability, or by offering or accepting payment or benefits to obtain the consent of a person who has authority over another to the end of exploitation. "Exploitation" comprises exploitation of another's prostitution or any other form of sexual exploitation, exploiting another's begging, labor or forced services, slavery or practices similar to slavery, servitude or taking of organs. The Algerian law expands the U.N. definition by including other forms of exploitation, but it is, however, more restrictive than the U.N. Protocol in regard to the issue of consent and provides that consent of the victim is irrelevant only when illegal means are used without making a broader consent exception for children. Article 586(1) of the Lebanese law defines "exploitation" as entailing forcing a person to participate in one of the following acts: (a) acts punishable by law; (b) prostitution and exploitation of the prostitution of others; (c) sexual exploitation; (d) begging; (e) slavery or practices similar to slavery; (f) forced or compulsory labor, including recruitment, forced or compulsory recruitment of children in armed conflict; (g) forced involvement in terrorist attacks; and (h) removal of human organs or tissues.

11.12.3 Status of Refugees and Its 1967 Protocol

All states in the Middle East and North Africa (MENA) region[17] have ratified the United Nations Convention on the Rights of the Child (CRC).[18] A number of countries have made interpretative declarations or reservations on Articles 20 and 21 in relation to foster care for children and adoption, and reservation to Article 14 relating to freedom of religion. Kuwait, Saudi Arabia and Qatar have expressed general reservations with reservation with respect to all such articles as are in conflict with the provisions of Islamic law.[19] With the exception of Iraq, Saudi Arabia and

[17]Understanding Trafficking in Persons in the MENA region.

In providing special protection for children, the U.N. Protocol prescribes that the proof of means is irrelevant when children are trafficked. In these cases, only the act and the exploitative purpose must be proved. Article 3(c) reads, "The recruitment, transportation, transfer, harbouring or receipt of a child for the purpose of exploitation shall be considered 'trafficking in persons' even if this does not involve any of the means set forth in subparagraph (a) of this article."18 As a consequence of this provision, a child cannot give consent even if none of the means are used. Therefore, the consent of the child is, in every circumstance, irrelevant.

Certain forms of trafficking relate mainly to children. They include trafficking for the purposes of begging, illegal adoption, child sex tourism, and pornography.

[18]The Occupied Palestinian Territory is not party to the CRC - the Palestinian Authority is not a state and therefore cannot sign or ratify the CRC. This section covers Algeria, Bahrain, Egypt, Iraq, Jordan, Kuwait Libya, Morocco, Oman, Qatar, Saudi Arabia, Syria, Tunisia, and the United Arab Emirates.

[19]The Arab League Model Law to Combat the Crime of Trafficking in Persons uses a definition of "trafficking in persons" that follows the U.N. Protocol's definition. Article 1 defines trafficking as the following: Recruitment, transportation, transfer, harbouring or receipt of persons— within the

the United Arab Emirates, MENA countries have also acceded to the Optional Protocols of the CRC on the Involvement of Children in Armed Conflicts and on the Sale of Children [Illegal Adoption[20]], Child Prostitution[21] and Pornography.[22] None of the MENA countries have expressed reservations to reduce obligations to protect children from all forms of violence.[23] A variety of other international legal

---

State's borders or abroad—for the purpose of exploitation by means of threat or use force or other forms of coercion, abduction, fraud, deceit, abuse of power or a situation of vulnerability or need, by offering, promising or accepting payment or benefits to obtain the consent of a person who has authority over another. Exploitation shall include any of these acts that are committed against victims of human trafficking: acts of prostitution, all forms of sexual exploitation, forced labour or services, slavery or practices similar to slavery, begging, removal of organs, conducting scientific experiments and any other form of exploitation that is legally criminalized.47

[20]Adoption may be a form of trafficking if the child is exploited. In the absence of exploitation, adoption does not constitute a form of trafficking even if the child is being sold, although adoption in such a case would be illegal. Under article 1(d) of the Supplementary Convention on the Abolition of Slavery, the Slave Trade, and Institutions and Practices Similar to Slavery, the sale of children is considered slavery through the following: [A]ny institution or practice whereby a child or young person under the age of 18 years is delivered by either or both of his natural parents or by his guardian to another person, whether for reward or not, with a view of the exploitation of the child or young person or of his labour.20

Consequently, the sale of children in the name of inter-country adoption may be considered a practice similar to slavery. As stated in the *travaux préparatoires* of the U.N. Protocol, article 3(c), (Interpretative Notes), "Where illegal adoption amounts to a practice similar to slavery, it will fall within the scope of the Protocol."21 Further, in its preamble, the 1993 Convention on the Protection of Children and Co-operation in Respect of Inter-Country Adoption sets its objective: "To ensure that inter-country adoption takes place in the interest of the child and to prevent abduction, sale of, or traffic in children."22

[21]Cases of child sex tourism in the MENA region have been reported in Comoros, Egypt, Iraq, Morocco, Saudi Arabia, and Yemen.28

[22]Egypt claims it acceded to the Optional Protocol on the Involvement of Children in Armed Conflict, but there is no record in the UN Human Rights database.

[23]United Nations definition of "trafficking in persons"

An international consensus was created in December 2000, when countries adopted the United Nations Protocol to Prevent, Suppress and Punish Trafficking in Persons,

Especially Women and Children. The U.N. Protocol was the first international legal instrument to define trafficking in persons and to provide for a comprehensive approach to combat the problem. Today, it remains the primary reference tool for countries in implementing their national policies to combat trafficking in persons and in developing frameworks of international cooperation in this field. The U.N. Protocol entered into force on 25 December 2003, when 20 countries deposited their instruments of ratification. As of August 2013, 157 countries are parties to the U.N. Protocol.

Article 3(a) of the U.N. Protocol states: "Trafficking in persons" shall mean the recruitment, transportation, transfer, harbouring or receipt of persons, by means of the threat or use of force or other forms of coercion, of abduction, of fraud, of deception, of the abuse of power or of a position of vulnerability or the giving or receiving of payments or benefits to achieve the consent of person having control over another person for the purpose of exploitation. Exploitation shall include, at a minimum, the exploitation of the prostitution of others or other forms of sexual exploitation, forced labour or services, slavery or practices similar to slavery, servitude or the removal of organs.5

instruments have addressed trafficking[24] in persons as an element of their provisions. Alongside the U.N. Protocol, these provisions constitute an integral part of the international legal framework on trafficking in persons.[25]

11.12.4 United Nations Declaration on the Elimination of Violence Against Women

The United Nations Declaration on the Elimination of Violence against Women was adopted in 1993 and includes trafficking in persons in the definition of "violence against women." In particular, article 2 includes in that definition "rape, sexual abuse, sexual harassment and intimidation at work, in educational institutions and elsewhere, trafficking in women and forced prostitution."

In the current situation of unrest, Legal factors are manifested in the lack of access to the criminal justice system, which occurs either because (a) the trafficked person is a foreigner or lacks access to legal representation or (b) the system itself does not offer an appropriate remedy. In addition, insecurity may be fostered by the "double witness" or "corroborative evidence" rule, which disqualifies the evidence unless a witness's testimony is corroborated by another witness or other material evidence implicates the accused. A possible consequence of this rule is that victims of trafficking are not given a chance to be heard in court. Trafficking in children must be distinguished from trafficking in adults because the law often grants additional protection to the child victim of trafficking because of his or her high vulnerability. According to the United Nations Children's Fund (UNICEF), as many as 5.5 million children are victims of forced labor and child trafficking.

The U.N. Protocol recognizes the special status of children, in article 6(4), which states: Each State Party shall take into account, in applying the provisions of this article, the age, gender and special needs of victims of trafficking in persons, in particular the special needs of children, including appropriate housing, education and care.

[24]Since the passage of the U.N. Protocol in 2000, many countries around the world have adopted comprehensive anti-trafficking laws to combat human trafficking in compliance with the legislative mandate of the U.N. Protocol.

In the Arab world alone, 12 States have adopted comprehensive anti-trafficking laws: Bahrain, Djibouti, Egypt, Iraq, Jordan, Kuwait, Mauritania, Oman, Qatar, Saudi Arabia, Syria, and the United Arab Emirates. Algeria and Lebanon have adopted anti-trafficking provisions in their penal codes. The remaining States Members of the Arab League continue to use existing laws to prosecute trafficking cases.

[25]Office of the High Commissioner for Human Rights at the United Nations (OHCHR), www.ohchr.org

11.13 Some Responses and Examples of Action Against CSEC[26,27]

11.13.1 Countries' Reports

A national program to protect children's rights was begun in 1997 in **Jordan**, and includes awareness-raising campaigns against child abuse, as well as training for social workers. The program also covers psychotherapeutic care for abused children and a shelter for victims.

In 1995, **Tunisia** introduced a Code for the Protection of Children, including a rapid reaction task force to intervene in emergencies, under the direction of the Family Judge, to ensure that the provisions of the Code are used.

Morocco and **Yemen** recently established telephone hotlines for children at risk of or suffering abuse. Between January 2000 and September 2001, the Moroccan hotline received more than 200,000 calls, 40,000 of which came from children. As a result, 728 case files were opened, of which 48 involved cases of sexual abuse.

Also in **Morocco**, the NGO Bayti (Children on the streets) has developed targeted, participatory psychosocial approaches to the needs of children, socio-economic reinsertion alternatives, parenting programs and case management of children. ADFM (the Association of Women's Rights in Morocco) has established resource centers for women suffering violence; and the NGO Ennakhil helps women and children victims of sexual violence or in prostitution.

In **Lebanon**, Dar Al Amal, an NGO set up in 1970, takes care of women and children who have suffered sexual abuse; the Lebanese Society of Paediatrics created a club for the prevention of accidents and sexual harm to children.

In Soudan, during the presentation of a case decided on January 24, 2011, the defendants recruited a number of victims for the purpose of inducing them to sell their kidneys. One of the victims sold his kidney for US$6000, of which US$1000

[26]Child sex tourism amounts to trafficking when a person travels to a foreign country for the purpose of engaging in prostitution with children. Child sex tourism is not specifically defined in the Optional Protocol to the Convention on the Rights of the Child on the Sale of Children, Child Prostitution and Child Pornography. Article 2(b) does, however, provide a definition of "child prostitution": "the use of a child in sexual activities for remuneration or any other form of consideration."25 Article 10(1) states: States Parties shall take all necessary steps to strengthen international cooperation by multilateral, regional and bilateral arrangements for the prevention, detection, investigation, prosecution and punishment of those responsible for acts involving the sale of children, child prostitution, child pornography and child sex tourism. States Parties shall also promote international cooperation and coordination between their authorities, national and international non-governmental organizations and international organizations.26 Article 10(3) mentions: States Parties shall promote the strengthening of international cooperation in order to address the root causes, such as poverty and underdevelopment, contributing to the vulnerability of children to the sale of children, child prostitution, child pornography and child sex tourism.27

[27]"Commercial Sexual Exploitation of Children: MENA Region", Second World Congress Against Commercial and Sexual Exploitation, UNICEF, 24–26 October 2001

was given to the defendant. The court convicted the victim for selling a part of his body in return for a material benefit, violating Law No. 23 of 1977 in regard to human organs, and was sentenced to one year in prison. The court also sentenced the defendants to six months imprisonment in accordance with article 8 of the law on combating human trafficking.

In general, however, CSEC remains an issue that has not been sufficiently tackled in the region. Awareness-raising campaigns and activities are rare, probably because of the taboo nature of the subject. Mobilization of the private sector is not undertaken in a structured way. In Morocco, the tourism sector is beginning to promote ‘clean tourism’ and is looking into how it can combat sex tourism.

In relation to undertakings made through ratification and adoption of international instruments, there has been some action but not enough. Application of the CRC remains weak in most countries of the region. Prevention, protection, rehabilitation and reintegration programs are rudimentary; child participation is rare. This is to some extent a result of a lack of basic tools for action, especially good coordination among sectors dealing with children’s issues. There is also a shortage of professionals with field-level experience of CSEC (social workers, judges, doctors, teachers, law enforcement), and a lack of national strategies based on consultation and cooperation across sectors. Monitoring mechanisms are not in place, nor are the basic tools they need: indicators, surveys, disaggregated data.

Seven countries in the region—Algeria, Bahrain, Jordan, Libya, Occupied Palestinian Territory (OPT), Syria and the United Arab Emirates—have also ratified the Arab Charter on Human Rights, which includes specific articles protecting children from abuse, exploitation, and involvement in armed conflicts and violence.[28]

Following the ratification of the CRC, MENA countries have enacted or propose to enact laws to protect children from violence, abuse, neglect or exploitation. A number of countries have put in place comprehensive Child Laws that bring together legal provisions for the protection of the child. For example, Tunisia has adopted the Child Protection Code, Egypt is waiting for the Parliament to approve amendments to the 1996 Child Law, and Algeria has introduced a Bill on Child Protection which aims to establish a mechanism for protecting children against all forms of violence, ill- treatment, abuse and negligence.

In countries where no comprehensive child law has been introduced, specific laws have been adopted or amended to better promote child protection. In Jordan where the Parliament has yet to approve the 2004 Child Bills Act, amendments were introduced to Juvenile Act N. 24 of 1968 to guarantee protection and care for children who are exposed to abuse by one or both parents,[29] while Juvenile Act No. 11 mandates judges the right to inspect juvenile centers affiliated with the

[28]UNCHR. Trafficking and Forced Labor in United Arab Emirates. Geneva. 2003. www.antislavery.org/archive/submission. August 2003

[29]“Jordan Third Periodic Report”, Committee on the Rights of the Child, CRC/C/JOR/3, 2 March 2006

Ministry of Social Development every three months.[30] Oman is also in the processing of preparing draft Juvenile Law, which will increase the minimum age for criminal responsibility for nine to 14 years of age.[31] While welcoming these legislative reforms, the Committee on the Rights of the Child has consistently recommended MENA countries to expedite the adoption and enforcement of proposed laws, to strengthen efforts to provide better legal protection for children, and to ensure that relevant domestic laws are in full conformity with the principles and provisions of the CRC, through enacting new legislations and or amending existing ones.[32] Moreover, further research is necessary to evaluate the extent to which new or amended laws are enforced and programs are implemented, in order to better assess gaps between policies and practices at the national and local levels. In addition, despite progress in the legislative and programmatic fronts—with many of the governments of MENA countries working with civil society groups, international NGOs, regional bodies, donors and United Nations agencies to better protect children—child protection remains a serious issue every country of the region. The nature and extent of child protection issues varies country to country, and includes issues such as violence against children—whether at homes, schools or institutional settings—harmful practices, particularly female genital mutilation and early marriage, juvenile justice, exploitative child labor and birth registration.[33] Children in Algeria, Iraq and the Occupied Palestinian Territories have been exposed to political violence and conflicts, and in Western Sahara have been affected by the deteriorating humanitarian situation, including trafficking of persons and organs.[34]

While the majority of MENA countries have also acceded to the Optional Protocol of the CRC on the Sale of Children, Child Prostitution and Pornography, commercial sexual exploitation of children is still regarded as an issue of 'considerable delicacy' in the Middle East, reports ECPAT International. Governments of the region have participated in two conferences on sexual exploitation, the first in

---

[30]"NGOs Supplementary Report on the third Jordanian Official Report on CRC", National Center for Human Rights, Jordan, March 2006

[31]"At a Glance—Oman, the Big Picture", UNICEF website, http://www.unicef.org/infobycountry/oman.html

[32]For example, see Concluding Observations for Oman, Saudi Arabia and Syria.

[33]"Birth Registration" Child Protection Information Sheet, UNICEF, May 2006.

[34]In many States, a statute of limitations or prescription period sets forth the maximum time within which legal proceedings may be initiated with respect to certain events. This limitation is often an obstacle to filing a lawsuit in cases of human trafficking in the Arab world. For example, in Algeria, the crime of human trafficking is a misdemeanour.131 Consequently, and in accordance with article 8 of the Law of Criminal Procedures, the limitation period is three years. Although article 8 provides for exceptions in the application of the statute—"the public action shall not be extinguished by passage of time in cases of felonies and misdemeanours that are qualified as terrorist or destructive acts, as transnational organized crimes, as corruption, or as embezzlement of public funds"132—trafficking in persons is not among the qualifying crimes that warrant the exception. Contrary to the Algerian law, however, article 19 of the Arab League Model Law on Combating Human Trafficking provides that "criminal activities involving crimes of human trafficking that are mentioned in this law shall not be subject to a limitation."133

October 2001 and the second in December 2004, indicating a will to confront the issue.[35] Countries such as Morocco and Algeria have also amended the Penal Code

---

[35]The Islamic Law Perspective

Islamic law abolishes the statute of limitations in cases of trafficking in accordance with the tradition of the Prophet that "a right of a Muslim shall not be extinguished by passage of time."136

4.D.3. Aggravating circumstances

Broadly speaking, aggravating circumstances can be divided into three groups, depending on whether they refer to the trafficking offender, the victim of trafficking, or the act of trafficking itself.

The Gulf Cooperation Council Model Law to Combat Human Trafficking includes all three groups and, in article 4, provides for enhanced penalties for the following aggravating circumstances:

- If the perpetrator establishes, forms, organizes, or manages an organized criminal group that aims to commit crimes of human trafficking
- If the crime is committed against children, women, or people with special needs
- If the crime is accompanied by duress or deception of abuse of office
- If the perpetrator is carrying a weapon or threatening to use one
- If the perpetrator is the spouse of the victim; is his descendant, ascendant, or guardian; has authority over the victim; is a public official entrusted with the application of the law; seeks the assistance of others
- If the crime is committed by more than one person
- If the crime is committed by an organized criminal group
- If the crime is of an international or transnational nature137

4.D.3.1. Aggravating circumstances regarding the offender

The aggravating circumstances related to the offender vary greatly across the Arab region. At times, enhanced penalties are prescribed when the offence was committed within the framework of a criminal organization. Such is the case of article 2 of the anti-trafficking law of the United Arab Emirates, which states: Temporary confinement shall be sentenced onto those committing the crime of human trafficking stipulated in Article 1 of this law, for a period of not less than five years. The sentence of life in prison shall be passed for any of the following: if the perpetrator has organized, planned or operated an organized criminal group, or assumed leadership or called for others to join the group.

In other instances, the penalty is increased when the offender is a parent, sibling, guardian, spouse, partner, or person who exercises authority over the trafficked individual. Such is the case of the Algerian criminal code. The code specifies in article

303(4) that "[t[rafficking in persons is punishable by an imprisonment for three (3) to ten (10) years and a fine of 300,000 DA to 1000,000 DA."139 However, article 303(5) states: Trafficking in persons is punishable by imprisonment for ten (10) to twenty (20) years and a fine of 1000,000 DA to 2,000,000 DA if the infraction is committed under one of the following circumstances: when the perpetrator is a victim's spouse, relative, legal guardian, has authority over the victim or is public official whose position has facilitated the perpetration of the crime.140 Enhanced penalties will also be imposed if the offence is committed by a public official, as in article 6(4) of the Egyptian law, which provides for "life imprisonment and a fine not less than 100,000 pounds and not to exceed 500,000 pounds.. . . If the perpetrator was a public official or was assigned to carry out a public service and committed the crime by exploiting the office or public service."141

66 Understanding Trafficking in Persons in the MENA region.

4.D.3.2. Aggravating circumstances regarding the victim

Among Arab legislators, there is no consensus as to which victim warrants an enhanced penalty for the perpetrator. Some Arab anti-trafficking laws state that a penalty may be enhanced if the crime is committed against a child, a woman, or a person with special needs.142 Article 4 of the Saudi Arabian law enhances the penalty "if the crime is committed against a woman or people of special needs" or "if the crime is committed against a child, even if the perpetrator is not aware that

to better protect children from trafficking, prostitution and pornography. However, generally, National Plans of Action to address this issue have not been developed, and commercial sexual exploitation remains a sensitive issue not openly discussed or seriously addressed at the community or national level. National statistics on the extent and nature of commercial sexual exploitation are often inadequate. It is generally recognized nevertheless that the many of the countries are transit and destination states for child victims of trafficking, and that a large percentage of street children and domestic workers are at risk of commercial sexual exploitation—in Egypt, some estimate that up to 80 per cent of children living on the streets have been sexually exploited.

11.13.2 Protecting Children from Child Labor in the Context of Trafficking[36]

UNHCR addresses the underlying factors of child labor, such as poverty, social attitudes condoning the practice, and demand from economic sectors where child labor is prevalent. To help mitigate poverty, UNHCR also offers vocational training, literacy and life-skills opportunities, as well as cash assistance, food vouchers, and core relief items to refugee families who are socio-economically vulnerable. Furthermore, UNHCR works with governments to strengthen existing legal and policy frameworks for the protection of children from child labor, with a particular emphasis on the worst forms of child labor, and to ensure that children involved in child labor benefit from multi-sectoral services. More than two million Syrian refugees have received in-kind assistance, cash or vouchers, helping to reduce their economic vulnerability.[37]

---

the victim is a child."143 Article 8 of the Syrian law specifies that a penalty shall be enhanced "if the crime is committed against women or children or person[s] with special needs."144 Article 4 of Bahrain's law stipulates that aggravating circumstances in a crime of trafficking in persons include any victim who is "below fifteen years of age, a female or a person with special needs."145 The law in Jordan states in article 7(b)(2) that a penalty for the crime of human trafficking shall be enhanced "if the victim is a female, a minor, or a person with a disability."146 Similarly, article 15 of the Qatari law enhances the penalty "if the victim is a female, a child, a person with a disability, or incapacitated."147 Other laws are similar to the Egyptian law, which does not consider trafficking in women an aggravated circumstance but enhances the penalty to life imprisonment "if the victim was a child, was incapacitated or was a person with disabilities."148

[36]Report of the Special Rapporteur on trafficking in persons, especially women and children", Sigma Huda, Mission to Bahrain, Oman and Qatar, Human Rights Council, A/HRC/4/23/Add.2, 25 April 2007.

[37]The difference between trafficking in persons and smuggling of migrants is not always clear and, even in cases with a great deal of information, may be difficult to discern. Though both practices involve money, movement of people, and often the same routes, the lines between them are sometimes blurred. According to the Protocol against the Smuggling of Migrants by Land, Sea and Air supplementing the United Nations Convention against Transnational Organized Crime,

In Arab trafficking laws, there are two approaches In determining whether illegal means are necessary to establish a crime of trafficking. One is represented by the Egyptian law, follows the U.N. Protocol in defining “illegal means” broadly to include “exploitation of a position of vulnerability. The other is modelled by the Syrian anti-trafficking law, does not require illegal means to establish the crime of trafficking in persons. Article 4(1) of the Syrian law defines the crime by requiring acts and illegal purposes,68 whereas article 4(2) states that the criminal nature of the acts mentioned above shall not change whether they were committed by force or threat of force; by resorting to violence or persuasion; by exploitation of ignorance or vulnerability; by deception, fraud, or abuse of office; or by conspiring with or providing assistance to one who has authority over the victim.69 Furthermore, Article 4(3) states that “in all cases consent of the victim is irrelevant.”70 According to this model, illegal means are not elements in the crime of trafficking but are instead aggravated circumstances that may enhance the penalty.

11.13.3 Protecting Children from Trafficking and Exploitation[38,39]

In certain sub-regions of MENA, a high number of refugee children may travel alongside adults in mixed migratory movements.[40] These factors expose them to

“smuggling of migrants” means “[t]he procurement, in order to obtain, directly or indirectly, a financial or other material benefit, of the illegal entry of a person into a State Party of which the person is not a national or permanent resident.”73 Bearing in mind this definition, three key differences can be identified between migrant smuggling and trafficking: transnationality, exploitation, and source of profit.

[38]The relationship between the smuggler and the migrant usually ends once the migrant has crossed the border. Smuggling fees are paid in advance or on arrival. The smuggler has no intention of exploiting the smuggled person after arrival. The smuggler and the migrant are partners, albeit disparate, in a commercial operation that the migrant enters into willingly. Trafficking involves the ongoing exploitation of the victim in some manner to generate illicit profits for the trafficker. The trafficker’s intention is to maintain the relationship with the exploited victim to the final destination. Smuggling can become trafficking, for example, when the smuggler “sells” the migrant or deceives, coerces, or forces the migrant to work off transportation costs under exploitative conditions.

[39]“Violence against Children – Regional Consultation Middle East and North Africa”, United Nations Secretary-General’s Study on Violence against Children.

[40]To smuggle a person means to facilitate the person’s illegal border crossing and entry into another country. Trafficking in persons, in contrast, need not involve any border crossing. When it does, the legality or illegality of the border crossing is irrelevant. Thus, although smuggling of migrants is always, by definition, transnational, trafficking need not be.

risks of being sold, enslaved,[41] trafficked, or sexually or economically exploited,[42] as well as victims of organ trafficking.[43]

The Coalition for Organ Failure Solutions (COFS), a non-profit international health and human rights organization, estimates that there are at least hundreds of Sudanese victims of organ trafficking in Egypt as well as numerous others from Eritrea, Ethiopia, Iraq, Jordan, Somalia, and Syria. The total number of organ trafficking victims in Egypt is estimated to be in the thousands. In order to mitigate these risks, in Yemen and North Africa, UNHCR and partners advocate for child-sensitive reception facilities and alternatives to detention. The second of the four strategies to combat trafficking in persons in the Middle East and North Africa (MENA) region is to prosecute the crime by adopting and implementing anti-trafficking legislation and related laws. This chapter looks at relevant international,

---

[41]Various circumstances regarding the nature of the crime also warrant enhanced penalties. If the crime was committed using weapons or threatening to use weapons, the law of Jordan enhances the penalty from imprisonment of no fewer than six months or a fine of no less than 1000 dinars or not to exceed 5000 dinars, or both of these punishments, to a punishment of hard labour not to exceed 10 years or a fine of no less than 5000 dinars and not to exceed 20,000 dinars.151 The Bahraini law enhances the penalty "[i]f the crime is of a non-national nature,"152 or in other words, if it is cross-border in nature. Similarly, article 15(g) of the law of Qatar states that the penalty will be imprisonment not to exceed 15 years and a fine not to exceed 300,000 riyals if the crime "is transnational in nature."153 Finally, some countries impose strict sentences if the victim suffers serious injury or death as a consequence of being trafficked. Such is the case of the law of Bahrain, which enhances the penalty when "the victim suffers an incurable disease as a result of committing the crime."154 The law of Djibouti talks about actions that "caused the victim any type of medically proven physical, moral or mental harm."155 A sentence of life imprisonment and a fine of not less than 100,000 pounds and not to exceed 500,000 pounds are provided under the Egyptian law when "the crime resulted in the death of the victim or caused him to suffer a permanent disability or an incurable disease."156 However, the most severe of all penalties is prescribed by the recently passed Iraqi anti-trafficking law of 23 February 2012, which, in article 8, states, "If the act of human trafficking leads to death of the victim, the sentence shall be capital punishment."157

[42]On May 5, 2010, a Giza Criminal Court issued a sentence in the case known as the "marriage of a minor with a view to sexual exploitation." The accused, Suleiman bin Abdul Rahman, a 76-year-old man of Saudi nationality, was sentenced to 10 years of rigorous imprisonment and fined 100,000 pounds for marrying and sexually exploiting a 14-year-old Egyptian girl. The court also sentenced the marriage broker, the lawyer who created the marriage contract, and the parents of the girl for exploiting her and delivering her to the defendant in return for money.149

[43]Trafficking for the purpose of organ removal: This form amounts to trafficking that is carried out by means of a commercial transaction without the consent of the donor of the organ. In the MENA region, most organ "donations" originate from Egypt. The most common recipient countries are Saudi Arabia and Oman.

World Health Organization Guiding Principles on Human Cell, Tissue, and Organ Transplantation

The World Health Organization was instrumental in including the removal of organs within the forms of trafficking in persons. The Commentary to Principle 5 of the Guiding Principles on Human Cell, Tissue and Organ Transplantation adopted by the World Health Assembly on 21 May 2010 states: Payment for cells, tissues and organs is likely to take unfair advantage of the poorest and most vulnerable groups, undermines altruistic donation, and leads to profiteering and human trafficking. Such payment conveys the idea that some persons lack dignity, that they are mere objects to be used by others.37

regional, and domestic legislation which criminalize trafficking in persons and highlight the most important challenges to prosecuting trafficking in persons in the MENA region as well as the Gulf.[44]

In its comprehensive approach to trafficking, the U.N. Protocol treats slavery as one of the purposes of trafficking. In article 3(a), it states that trafficking in persons occurs "for the purpose of exploitation" and that "[e]xploitation shall include, at a minimum, the exploitation of the prostitution of others or other forms of sexual exploitation, forced labor or services, slavery or practices similar to slavery, servitude or the removal of organs."71 The U.N. Protocol therefore makes trafficking in persons a crime distinct from that of slavery and indicates that slavery or practices similar to slavery are one of the purposes for which victims are trafficked. However, given that slavery and practices similar to slavery constitute one of the exploitative purposes of trafficking, the prohibition of slavery remains an important element in combating trafficking in persons.

The clearest distinctions between slavery and trafficking in persons may be drawn between ownership and control and undue influence and exploitation. A victim of trafficking in persons may not be subject to "ownership," although he or she may be under the control of the trafficker, such as through physical or psychological coercion, deception or threats, as defined in the U.N. Protocol. Thus, the understanding of what constitutes "illegal means" has shifted in focus from the exercise of the power of ownership as conveyed in the 1926 definition of "slavery" in the Convention to Suppress the Slave Trade and Slavery to the exploitation of a position of vulnerability and the exercise of other forms of control. There is no distinguishable "face" of a trafficked victim. However, trafficked persons are always people who, because of poverty, war, natural disasters, gender, ethnic, origins, and other factors pertaining to their status or to specific circumstances, are susceptible to exploitation.

---

[44]Article 9 of the law of Oman does not consider trafficking in females to be an aggravated circumstance. But if the victim is a child or a person with special needs, it enhances the standard penalty of 3 to 7 years with a sentence of imprisonment lasting no fewer than 7 years nor exceeding 15 years, plus an increased fine. The Lebanese law considers a pregnant woman a vulnerable victim and enhances the penalty only in such cases. One may consider enhancing the penalty in trafficking cases that involve a female as an example of positive discrimination that is allowed under article 3 of the Training Manual to Combat Trafficking in Persons 67

Arab Charter on Human Rights.150 However, this proposition runs counter to the established principles in comparative models that focus on the conditions of vulnerability of females and males rather than gender as grounds for enhancing the penalty.

11.14 A Bill of Rights for Victims of Trafficking

Once a victim has been identified, he or she must be protected from further harm. Arab countries, to varying extents, have recognized a range of victims' rights in their anti-trafficking laws. For example, article 23 of the Egyptian trafficking law guarantees the following rights for victims of trafficking: the right to safety, the right to protection of one's inviolability and identity, the right to information, the right to be heard in court, the right to legal assistance, the right to personal security, the right to return to one's homeland, and the right of an Egyptian victim of trafficking abroad to be returned to Egypt. Also, article 22 of the Egyptian law explicitly stipulates the following: The State shall guarantee the protection of the victim and shall work to create the appropriate conditions for his assistance, health, psychological, educational, and social care; and rehabilitation and reintegration into the society, within the framework of liberty and human dignity. Bahrain's trafficking law provides a number of protective measures for trafficking victims that must be considered during investigations or court proceedings. These measures include the right to information, or to be informed of one's legal rights in a language one understands, and the right to medical and psychiatric care. In addition, Article 5 of the law explicitly states that "the victim shall be examined by a specialist physician if he so requests or if it transpires that he is in need of medical or psychiatric care" and that "admitting the victim into a medical or psychiatric center or a welfare center if it transpires that his medical or psychological condition or age so requires" shall occur in the stage of investigation or court proceedings with respect to a crime of trafficking in persons.196 The Syrian law also provides that victims of trafficking should be entitled to receive information regarding their legal rights "in a language that they understand." The Syrian law states that victims of trafficking have the right to privacy, including the right to withhold their name, location where they are receiving care, or any other information that may reveal their identities. Similar laws guaranteeing rights for victims of trafficking are found in Saudi Arabia and Oman. On the basis of these laws and international standards, the rights of victims can be summarized as follows:

- The right to safety
- The right to privacy
- The right to information
- The right to legal representation
- The right to be heard in court
- The right to compensation for damages
- The right to assistance
- The right to seek residence
- The right to recovery and reflection period
- The right to safe return to country of origin
- These rights entitle victims of trafficking to benefits that should be granted regardless of their immigration status or their willingness to testify in court.

11.14.1 Right to Safety

The right to safety is especially relevant in States where the law requires the victim of trafficking to testify against the traffickers or to cooperate in other ways with the authorities in the prosecution of trafficking cases. In such circumstances, the victim should be provided with protection from possible reprisals from traffickers as a prerequisite to coming forward and testifying. Derivative victims are likewise to be considered in these cases, because family members of traffickers' victims may also be targeted as part of any such reprisals. In this regard, article 6 of the U.N. Protocol provides that "[e]ach State Party shall endeavor to provide for the physical safety of victims of trafficking in persons while they are within its territory."

Likewise, the Office of the High Commissioner for Human Rights (OHCHR) "Recommended Principles and Guidelines on Human Rights and Human Trafficking" provides that States should ensure the following: Trafficked persons are effectively protected from harm, threats or intimidation by traffickers and associated persons. To this end, there should be no public disclosure of the identity of trafficking victims and their privacy should be respected and protected to the extent possible, while taking into account the right of any accused person to a fair trial. Trafficked persons should be given full warning, in advance, of the difficulties inherent in protecting identities and should not be given false or unrealistic expectations regarding the capacities of law enforcement agencies".

11.14.2 Right to Privacy

Victims of trafficking should be entitled to the right to privacy, in civil and religious settings.[45] Article 6(1) of the U.N. Protocol provides that States Parties "shall protect the privacy and identity of victims of trafficking in persons, including, inter alia, by making legal proceedings relating to such trafficking confidential."201 States should ensure that the names and identifying information of trafficked persons and their family members are not disclosed to the public.

---

[45]Illicit sale of children for the purpose of intercountry adoption does not constitute a form of trafficking in most countries of the Middle East because Islamic law does not recognize the institution of adoption in accordance with the Qur'an, which states in Surah XXXIII: 4–5: "... [N or] has He made your adopted sons your sons. Such is only your manner of speech by your mouths. But God tells you the Truth, and He shows the right way. Call them by (the names of) their fathers: that is juster in the sight of God."16 Islamic law recognizes Kafala, as an alternative to adoption. Kafala is a system of fosterage where a child may be placed under the guardianship of a family, but the child continues to retain his lineage. This explains why many countries of the Middle East that follow Islamic law had reservations regarding Article 21 of the 1989 Convention on the Rights of the Child, which recognizes adoption, because it is inconsistent with Islamic law. Unlike other regions where baby trafficking is prevalent, there is no demand for adopted children in the Middle East.

11.14.3 Right to Information

Victims of trafficking have the right to information. Accordingly, articles 6(2)(a) and 6(3)(b) of the U.N. Protocol provide that States Parties should make available to victims of trafficking "information on relevant court and administrative proceedings" and "information, in particular as regards their legal rights, in a language that the victims of trafficking in persons can understand."

11.14.4 Right to Legal Representation

Victims of trafficking must be granted the right to legal representation. Guideline 6 (5) of the OHCHR's "Recommended Principles and Guidelines on Human Rights and Human Trafficking" recommends "providing trafficked persons with legal and other assistance in relation to any criminal, civil or other actions against traffickers/ exploiters."

11.14.5 Right to Be Heard in Court

A victim of human trafficking should be entitled to be heard during all stages of criminal and civil proceedings. The U.N. Protocol provides in article 6(2)(b) that the States Parties should provide victims of trafficking in persons with "assistance to enable their views and concerns to be presented and considered at appropriate stages of criminal proceedings against offenders." Moreover, victims of trafficking should be provided with "information on relevant court and administrative proceedings.

"Under Egyptian law, implementation of the right to be heard in court requires that the victim's views should be considered and that he or she has "[t]he right to legal assistance, in particular the right to counsel." The court or public prosecutor may assign a lawyer in accordance with the rules prescribed in the criminal procedures law and should take the necessary measures to protect the victim's safety, as well as the safety of any witness testifying on the victim's behalf. This law also requires informing the victim of his or her rights in accordance with the relevant administrative, legal, and judicial regulations.

11.14.6 Right to Compensation for Damages

Victims of trafficking in persons have a right to compensation for the trauma and exploitation that they have suffered as a result of their being trafficked. In regard to compensation, article 6(6) of the U.N. Protocol states that "[e]ach State Party shall ensure that its domestic legal system contains measures that offer victims of trafficking in persons the possibility of obtaining compensation for damage suffered."

Article 14(2) of the United Nations Convention against Transnational Organized Crime states: When acting on the request made by another State Party in accordance with Article 13 of this Convention, States Parties shall, to the extent permitted by domestic law and if so requested, give priority consideration to returning the confiscated proceeds of crime or property to the requesting State Party so that it can give compensation to the victims of the crime or return such proceeds of crime or property to their legitimate owners. States around the world have addressed such obligations by developing five basic models of civil compensation of victims:

11.14.6.1 Mandatory Restitution

Some legal systems grant victims of trafficking the right to receive restitution for their losses.

11.14.6.2 Confiscation of Assets

Some anti-trafficking laws provide for forfeiture of assets in addition to imprisonment as the appropriate criminal sanction imposed on a trafficker. These laws thus provide that damages to victims of trafficking are to be paid out of the traffickers' property.

11.14.6.3 State Fund

In some legal systems, compensation to victims of trafficking is paid out of specially created State funds.

An early draft of the law of Bahrain provided that "a government fund shall be established" to provide for the necessary funding for implementing policies specified in the law. However, this provision was deleted in its entirety in the final version of the law. The Egyptian law provides for the establishment of a State fund "to assist victims of human trafficking" and "to provide financial assistance to the victims who have suffered harm resulting from any of the crimes stipulated in this law."211 It is significant to note that in addition to "[t]he proceeds of the fines sentenced for the crimes stipulated in this law, as well as the properties, objects, and means of transportation forfeited [which] shall be allocated directly to the fund," the law allows the fund to "accept contributions, grants, and donations from national and foreign entities."

11.14.7 Civil and Religious Actions[46]

Other legal systems recognize the right of a victim of trafficking to seek damages in a civil court. For instance, the law of Jordan provides that a person "injured because of one of the crimes stipulated in this law may seek compensation in accordance with the general principles in the laws in force." The law of Oman—in an attempt to enhance a victim's access to justice—provides that a victim of trafficking shall be exempted from the fees of a civil action that he or she files asking for compensation for the harm resulting from the exploitation. General rules regarding compensation may also apply to victims of trafficking. For example, article 3 of the Algerian Code of Criminal Procedure gives crime victims the right to file a civil action, and article 239 states that anyone who wants to use the right conferred by Article 3, and who claims to be a victim of a crime or misdemeanor, can file the civil action in the same session as the criminal proceeding already in progress. In addition, a person who suffers harm as a result of a crime may file a separate civil action asking for compensation in accordance with article 124 of the Algerian Civil Code, which provides that any act that causes harm to another gives rise to compensation. The law of Qatar provides in article 10 that the criminal court with jurisdiction to decide a case of human trafficking shall also have jurisdiction to decide a civil action that may arise as a result of the criminal action.

11.14.7.1 Punitive Damages

In some legal systems, victims are awarded not only damages to compensate for their losses or moral damage but also punitive damages, whose purpose is to reform or deter the perpetrator whose conduct damaged the victim.

[46]Islamic law also recognizes the right of a victim of a crime to compensation in accordance with the Islamic tradition of the Prophet, la darar wa la dirar, or "no injury and no inflicting of injury." According to this tradition, a person who causes harm should repair such harm—the basis for providing compensation for damage. As stated in the Majallah-el Ahkam-i-Adliya, "[A] person who does an act shall be held responsible if such act causes harm to another. The purpose of the principle of no injury or repaired harm is to achieve justice, a basic principle under Islamic law."218

11.14.8 Right to Provision of Services in Civil and Religious Jurisdictions[47]

Victims of trafficking should be entitled to assistance in the form of medical, psychological, legal, and social aid. In this regard, article 6(3) of the U.N. Protocol states: 3. Each State Party shall consider implementing measures to provide for the physical, psychological and social recovery of victims of trafficking in persons, including, in appropriate cases, in cooperation with non-governmental organizations, other relevant organizations and other elements of civil society, and, in particular, the provision of: (a) Appropriate housing; (b) Counselling and information, in particular as regards their legal rights, in a language that the victims of trafficking in persons can understand; (c) Medical, psychological and material assistance; and(d) Employment, educational and training opportunities. The right to "appropriate housing" is closely related to the right to security, and it imposes on States a duty to consider providing shelters for victims, operating them either directly or in cooperation with non-governmental organizations (NGOs) and international organizations. Within the shelters, various services may be provided, depending on the type of victim and the location of the shelters. The Gulf Cooperation Council Model Law to Combat Human Trafficking dictates that shelter should be provided for victims of trafficking. Most trafficking laws provide that victims of trafficking are entitled to accommodation in safe places such as shelters.

The Bahraini law, for example, allows for "admitting the victim into a special center for the provision of shelter or ... with a licensed authority to undertake providing accommodation thereto if it is found that this is required."

11.14.9 Right to Seek Residency

A victim of trafficking should be entitled to seek residency in the country of destination. The immediate return of the victims to their home countries may be unsatisfactory both for the victims and for the law enforcement authorities endeavoring to combat trafficking. For the victims, return might make them, their family, or their friends in the country of origin vulnerable to reprisals by the traffickers.

For law enforcement purposes, if the victims continue to live clandestinely in the country or are removed immediately, they cannot give information for effectively combating trafficking. The more confident the victims are that their rights and interests will be protected, the more information they will be able to provide.

Accordingly, article 7 of the U.N. Protocol states that "each State Party shall consider adopting legislative or other appropriate measures that permit victims of

[47]The right to assistance is covered by the Islamic principles of assistance to those in distress and those in need—victims of trafficking certainly find themselves often psychologically and physically traumatized and require medical and psychological aid.

trafficking in persons to remain in its territory, temporarily or permanently, in appropriate cases" and "shall give appropriate consideration to humanitarian and compassionate factors."

Paragraph 68 of the Legislative Guide for the Implementation of the Protocol to Prevent, Suppress and Punish Trafficking in Persons, Especially Women and Children, which supplements the United Nations Convention against Transnational Organized.

Crime, advocates adopting measures that provide victims of trafficking with some legal form of residency status: [T]here is no obligation to legislate measures relating to the status of victims.

However, in several countries where measures have been adopted for the temporary or permanent residence of victims of trafficking, such as Belgium, Italy, the Netherlands and the United States of America, such measures have had a positive effect on victims coming forward to testify against traffickers and on non-governmental organizations encouraging victims to whom they provide services to report incidents to the government.

Some states have made residency status contingent on the victim's testifying in court and, more broadly, cooperating with the authorities prosecuting the traffickers. However, it is more in line with a human rights-based approach to combating trafficking not to make residency status contingent on the victim's cooperation with the authorities. The right to seek residency is rarely present in Arab legislation. Article 15(7) of the Saudi Arabian law states that "if the victim is a foreigner and it is necessary for him to stay in the Kingdom during the investigation procedures, the prosecution or the competent court would assess the matter." Article 7 of the Bahraini law states that the minister of social development must form a "Committee for the Assessment of the Status of Foreigners Who Are Victims of Trafficking in Persons."228 The law is more detailed than the Saudi law in that it empowers the committee to examine the needs of a victim for repatriation to his or her country of origin or for a job if the victim must remain in Bahrain for an extended period. However, such employment recommendations are subject to review no less often than once every six months.

11.14.10 Right to Recovery and Reflection Period

Closely linked to the concept of residency status is the legislator's option, in the country of destination, of granting the victim a "recovery and reflection period." In its Toolkit to Combat Trafficking in Persons, the United Nations Office on Drugs and Crime highlights the importance of such a period: Granting a reflection period, followed by a temporary or permanent residence permit would ideally be granted to victims of trafficking regardless of whether the trafficked person is able or willing to give evidence as a witness. Such protection of the victim serves to raise his or her confidence in the State and its ability to protect his or her interests. Once recovered, a trafficked person with confidence in the State is more likely to make an informed decision and cooperate with authorities in the prosecution of traffickers.

Articles 6 and 8 of European Union Council Directive 2004/81/EC of 29 April 2004 include provisions regarding the residence permit issued to third-country nationals who are victims of trafficking in human beings or who have been the subject of an action to facilitate illegal immigration and who cooperate with the competent authorities. These provisions make a reflection period available to persons who are willing to cooperate with the authorities prosecuting cases of trafficking: Member states shall ensure that the third-country nationals [who are victims of trafficking in human beings or who have been the subject of an action to facilitate illegal immigration and who cooperate with the competent authorities] are granted a reflection period allowing them to recover and escape the influence of the perpetrators of the offences so that they can take an informed decision as to whether to cooperate with the competent authorities. During the reflection period . . . the third-country nationals concerned shall have access to [medical psychological treatment, translation services, and legal aid] and it shall not be possible to enforce any expulsion order against them. After the expiry of the reflection period, or earlier . . . Member States shall consider:

(a) the opportunity presented by prolonging the third-country national's stay on its territory for the investigations or the judicial proceedings, and(b) whether he/she has shown a clear intention to cooperate and (c) whether he/she has severed all relations with those suspected of [trafficking inhuman beings and illegal immigration].231However, the Council of Europe Convention on Action against Trafficking in Human Beings has made such a period a mandatory requirement for States Parties to the Convention regardless of the willingness of victims of trafficking to cooperate with the prosecuting authorities:

Each Party shall provide in its internal law a recovery and reflection period of at least 30 days, when there are reasonable grounds to believe that the person concerned is a victim. Such a period shall be sufficient for the person concerned to recover and escape the influence of traffickers and/or to take an informed decision on cooperating with the competent authorities. During this period it shall not be possible to enforce any expulsion order against him or her. This provision is without prejudice to the activities carried out by the competent authorities in all phases of the relevant national proceedings, and in particular when investigating and prosecuting the offences concerned. During this period, the Parties shall authorize the persons concerned to stay in their territory.232.

11.14.11 Right to Safe Return to Country of Origin

Just as victims of trafficking in persons should have the right to seek residency in the country to which they have been trafficked, they should likewise have the right to a dignified return to their country of origin. Countries should ensure that victims are returned only with their voluntary and informed consent. The assistance of NGOs and other mechanisms should be called into play to ensure that victims are protected from past and potential traffickers both while they are in transit and during their reintegration.

Article 8(1) of the U.N. Protocol provides that States Parties of which victims of trafficking are nationals or residents should "facilitate and accept, with due regard for the safety of that person, the return of that person without undue or unreasonable delay." Repatriation of victims "shall preferably be voluntary." Victims should be provided with all necessary assistance to ensure a dignified return. The repatriation of victims of trafficking may be regulated through international or bilateral treaties between countries of origin and countries of destination.

11.15 Procedural Protection of Victims of Trafficking

Procedural law is instrumental in ensuring that the rights of victims are guaranteed within the times prescribed by law. Effective procedural laws are also a reflection of a human rights approach to combating trafficking that strives to ensure that victims of trafficking do not endure any further abuse during the prosecution phase. In addition, procedural laws must take specific account of the special needs of child victims and child victim witnesses. A number of principles are therefore needed to ensure that procedural law is in harmony with the protections afforded by anti-trafficking legislation.

11.15.1 Witness Protection

Witness protection is critical to securing the safety of victims of trafficking who wish to testify against their traffickers. Moreover, the availability of strong witness protection mechanisms and procedural measures may be an important factor in a victim's decision to cooperate with the authorities prosecuting a case. The United Nations Convention against Transnational Organized Crime stipulates the following: [E]ach State Party shall take appropriate measures within its means to provide effective protection from potential retaliation or intimidation for witnesses in criminal proceedings who give testimony concerning offences covered by this Convention and, as appropriate, for their relatives and other persons close to them. Similarly, article 23 includes a provision on obstruction of justice and requires the criminalization of various forms of obstruction, including the use of physical force, threats, or intimidation.237 Protective measures must be in place, particularly during court proceedings. In this regard, the Council of Europe Convention on Action against Trafficking in Human Beings provides the following: [E]ach Party shall adopt such legislative or other measures as may be necessary to ensure in the course of judicial proceedings: A. the protection of victims' private life and, where appropriate, identity; B. victims' safety and protection from intimidation, in accordance with the conditions under its internal law and, in the case of child victims, by taking special care of children's needs and ensuring their right to special protection measures. Some States have enacted various witness protection mechanisms that are not necessarily specific to victims of trafficking but that can and should be applied to them. Other States, however, provide for specific protection related to the crime of trafficking. For instance, article 20 of the Qatari law states that "anyone who discloses or reveals the identity of the victim or that of the witness subjecting him to danger or causing him harm . . . shall be punished with imprisonment with a period of not more than 2 years and a fine not to exceed 50,000 Dinar. Also, article 23 of Egyptian Law No. 64 of 2010 provides for the protection of witnesses during court proceedings "to avoid any influence upon them" and calls upon the State to "take whatever measures [that are] required to conceal their identity." Similarly, article 10 of Iraqi Law No. 28 of 30 April 2012 mentions "providing the necessary protection of witnesses and victims." The double witness rule or the corroborative evidence rule disqualifies the evidence if there is only one witness. Under that rule the witness's testimony must be corroborated by another witness or by other material evidence implicating the accused. Some countries have applied the rule in criminal proceedings to deny victims of trafficking standing as a credible witness. Such rules must be examined and reconsidered to allow the experiences of trafficking victims to be heard in court even when some elements of their story cannot be corroborated.

11.15.2 Investigation and Court Proceedings

Should the victim decide to cooperate with the authorities in pursuing the prosecution of a trafficking case, he or she will have a right to protection from possible retaliation. Having such legislation in place affords much-needed security and peace of mind to victims of trafficking, who frequently fear intimidation and reprisals from traffickers. Paragraph 6(2b) on the U.N. Protocol provides for "assistance to enable [victims'] views and concerns to be presented and considered at appropriate stages of criminal proceedings against offenders, in a manner not prejudicial to the rights of the defense." The various procedural principles needed to provide such protection include privacy of victim witnesses, gender sensitivity, special protection for child victim witnesses, inadmissibility of past behavior, and avoidance of overreliance on victim testimony.

11.15.3 Privacy of Victim Witnesses

The protection of privacy in court proceedings is critical to ensuring the safety and security of a victim of trafficking who chooses to cooperate with the authorities prosecuting the case. The threat of intimidation or reprisals from traffickers targeting the victim or members of the victim's family may be heightened if the victim's identity is not protected during court proceedings. Security promised by privacy during investigation and court proceedings will consequently allow for more efficient disclosure of the offence of trafficking in persons. As a general rule, court proceedings should be open to the public and the media to promote confidence in the judicial system. However, in many trafficking-in-persons cases, in particular within cases involving sexual exploitation or children, the best way of doing justice is to declare the court proceedings closed.

11.15.4 Gender Sensitivity

Because victims of trafficking are often women, it is important to ensure that antitrafficking legislation adopts a gender-sensitive approach. For example, women (including women who are social welfare workers) should be involved at all stages of the proceedings concerning cases of trafficking, including the investigation and trial.

11.15.5 Child Victim Witnesses

Child victims are particularly vulnerable and therefore require extra measures of protection beyond those that should be afforded to adult victim witnesses. Children have special rights, needs, and vulnerabilities that must be considered when prosecuting trafficking cases involving child victim witnesses. Special interviewing techniques should be used when working with child victim witnesses, and special procedures should be implemented to spare them the trauma of testifying in court.

Some legal systems provide for audiovisual recording of hearings of children and others, allowing children to appear before the court by videoconference.

11.15.6 Inadmissibility of Past Behavior

Another important legislative consideration concerning procedural law is the inadmissibility of a trafficked victim's past behavior in court proceedings. This factor is particularly important in cases of sex trafficking.

11.15.7 Avoiding Overreliance on Victim Testimony

The OHCHR "Recommended Principles and Guidelines on Human Rights and Human Trafficking" provides that States, intergovernmental organizations, and

NGOs should consider the following: Providing law enforcement authorities with adequate investigative powers and techniques to enable effective investigation and prosecution of suspected traffickers.

States should encourage and support the development of proactive investigatory procedures that avoid over-reliance on victim testimony.

11.16 Importance of Participation in the Implementation of Prevention, Prohibition, and Prosecution Efforts

In the area of trafficking in persons, cooperation among the relevant government agencies, among countries when cases of trafficking have an international component, and among governments and civil society is essential in guaranteeing the implementation of all prevention, protection, and prosecution efforts. Cooperation among governments and civil society organizations is equally important to identifying victims of trafficking and to offering direct services, such as legal assistance, medical care, and psychological aid. Civil society organizations can also contribute to a dignified process of repatriation (if the victim so desires) and reintegration or of integration into society if the victim is granted resident status.

11.17 International Obligation of Cooperation with Civil Society

The U.N. Protocol stipulates that the States Parties should cooperate with nongovernmental organizations (NGOs) in adopting prevention measures to combat trafficking and measures of assistance and protection. According to article 9, "Policies, programs and other measures established in accordance with this articles hall, as appropriate, include cooperation with non-governmental organizations, other relevant organizations and other elements of civil society."246 Furthermore, article 6(3) of the U.N. Protocol states: Each State Party shall consider implementing measures to provide for the physical, psychological and social recovery of victims of trafficking in persons, including, in appropriate cases, in cooperation with non-governmental organizations, other relevant organizations and other elements of civil society, and, in particular, the provision of (a) Appropriate housing; (b) Counseling and information, in particular as regards their legal rights, in a language that the victims of trafficking in persons can understand; (c) Medical, psychological and material assistance; and (d) Employment, educational and training opportunities.

The Council of Europe Convention on Action against Trafficking in Human Beings also refers to civil society and calls on States to raise awareness about the role of civil society in identifying demand as a root cause of trafficking, to make available to victims contact information for NGOs in their country of origin to assist them when they return, and to adopt measures to protect NGOs offering assistance to victims of trafficking from retaliation or intimidation during criminal proceedings.

Article 5(6) regarding prevention of trafficking in human beings states: Measures established in accordance with this article shall involve, where appropriate, non-governmental organizations, other relevant organizations and other elements of civil society committed to the prevention of trafficking in human beings and victim protection or assistance. References to civil society are also present in three other articles. Article 10(1) addresses the identification of the victims reads: Each Party shall provide its competent authorities with persons who are trained and qualified in preventing and combating trafficking in human beings, in identifying and helping victims, including children, and shall ensure that the different authorities collaborate with each other as well as with relevant support organizations, so that victims can be identified in a procedure duly taking into account the special situation of women and child victims and, in appropriate cases, issued with residence permits under the conditions provided for in Article 14 of the present Convention. Article 12 (5) discusses the assistance of the victims:

Each Party shall take measures, where appropriate and under the conditions provided for by its internal law, to co-operate with nongovernmental organizations, other relevant organizations or other elements of civil society engaged in assistance to victims. Article 16(5), which addresses the repatriation and return of victims, reads: Each Party shall adopt such legislative or other measures as may be necessary to establish repatriation programs, involving relevant national or international institutions and non-governmental organizations. These programs aim at avoiding re-victimization. Each Party should make its best effort to favor the reintegration of victims into the society of the State of return, including reintegration into the education system and the labor market, in particular through the acquisition and improvement of their professional skills. With regard to children, these programs should include enjoyment of the right to education and measures to secure adequate care or receipt by the family or appropriate care structures.

11.17.1 Role of Law Enforcement in Working with NGOs

Law enforcement officials assigned to cases of human trafficking should have a list of appropriate local NGOs that can assist in protecting and rehabilitating the victim. Cooperation with NGOs is also a way for law enforcement to gather intelligence concerning trafficking rings and vulnerable victims in their community. NGOs may also assist law enforcement in identifying victims of trafficking. Victims may be more willing to tell their stories to NGOs, which are regarded as empathetic, rather than to law enforcement officers, who may be regarded as threatening. This situation is exacerbated in the case of trafficking victims who are in the country of destination illegally and who may fear deportation. In addition, NGOs may have accumulated expertise in victim profiling and in victims' typical behavior patterns, which may aid in identification. After a successful rescue, NGOs play a significant role when it comes to interacting with the victim.

NGOs may counsel victims and assist in reducing their trauma, as well as assisting in victims' interviews with law enforcement officials. NGOs are also better equipped to help rehabilitate victims; they provide them with the appropriate care and necessary assistance, such as medical and psychological care; they inform victims of their legal rights and the best paths for accessing justice; and they empower victims during the rehabilitation process. NGOs are the crucial link between victims and civil society, as well as law enforcement and civil society.

11.17.2 Models of Participation of Civil Society in Government Efforts to Combat Trafficking in Persons

Two main models serve to engage civil society organizations in government efforts to combat trafficking in persons: the representation model and the consultation model.

11.17.2.1 Representation Model

The representation model—the more inclusive model for the full partnership of civil society organizations in government anti-trafficking efforts—involves the inclusion of representatives of relevant NGOs on a national inter-agency body tasked with implementing anti-trafficking policies.

11.17.2.2 Consultation Model

The consultation model, conversely, engages NGOs on a consultative basis. In this model, the law mandates that the government regularly retain representatives of civil society organizations concerned with trafficking in persons as consultants. NGO participation can include testifying as part of parliamentary hearings aimed at policy development and refinement, consulting in research and investigations carried out by parliament, or providing independent expertise in policy evaluation.

11.17.3 Civil Society on Arab Committees to Combat Trafficking in Persons

The Gulf Cooperation Council Model Law to Combat Human Trafficking, while providing for coordination among State agencies, is silent about coordination between such State agencies and members of civil society. Similarly, the law of the United Arab Emirates makes it a function of the National Committee for Combating Human Trafficking to coordinate "between different state bodies including Ministries, Departments, Establishments and Authorities related to the combating of human trafficking," but it makes no reference to NGOs. Article 23 of the Omani law mandates that the National Committee for Combating Trafficking in Persons shall coordinate among all competent national authorities "and relevant international organizations to set up measures and procedures capable of combating transnational trafficking crimes."

The law of Jordan gives the National Committee to Protect from Human Trafficking the authority to cooperate with all agencies to implement programs for the physical, mental, and social rehabilitation of victims and those who are affected by the crime of human trafficking and to supervise the hosting of these persons in the places that were established for this purpose. NGOs are not represented on these national committees. The Saudi Arabian law is also silent regarding any role for NGOs.

The Syrian law is clearer with regard to the role of civil society, stating that "[t]he concerned authorities shall take measures to ensure providing victims of trafficking the appropriate protection ... in cooperation, whenever necessary, with official institutions, popular organizations, trade unions, and NGOs that are concerned with the issue."

The only reference in the Egyptian law to institutions other than the government is in article 26, which states that "the competent authorities shall provide care, education, training, and rehabilitation programs to the Egyptian victims, whether through governmental or non-governmental institutions."

In Bahrain, article 8 of the law on human trafficking calls for establishing the Committee for Combating Trafficking in Persons with the purpose of coordinating among government departments, but it does not call for coordination with civil society. Although the functions of the Bahraini committee do not include coordination with civil society, the law does require the minister of social development to nominate "representatives of three civil societies" to the committee, a model of civil society participation that should be applauded.

It should also be noted that Arab anti-trafficking laws address preventive measures only as a part of the functions of inter-agency task forces. These measures include (a) conducting research, (b) collecting information, (c) carrying out media campaigns, (d) participating in international conferences related to human trafficking, (e) amending existing legislation related to human trafficking, (f) creating a database of information and statistics on the subject, (g) conducting training programs for those who are in charge of implementing human trafficking legislation, and (h) ensuring the implementation of the law by the competent government authorities.

Again, these laws should allow for a civil society role in implementing these measures. In defining the functions of Arab inter-agency task forces, the Arab laws do not distinguish between coordination and reporting, nor do they emphasize reporting as one of the most important means of enforcement. For instance, Bahrain's law makes it a function of the Committee for Combating Trafficking in Persons to participate with the appropriate government authorities in preparing reports to be presented to U.N. committees, but it does not provide for a self-reporting mechanism where the committee itself would publish an annual or periodic report to be submitted to parliament. However, the Bahraini law entrusts the committee with submitting a report to the minister of foreign affairs on the implementation of international conventions to which the Kingdom is a party.

The law of the United Arab Emirates includes preparation of reports on the measures taken by the government to combat human trafficking as a function of the National Committee to Combat Human Trafficking, but it does not provide for the issuance of an annual report.

Additionally, for the reasons detailed in the previous sections, NGOs and other elements of civil society must be consulted in any report that assesses the scope of the problem and the appropriate responses.

11.17.4 Engaging the Five Elements of Civil Society

Civil society organizations combat trafficking in persons at the local, national, regional, and international levels. Civil society is composed of five main elements: non-governmental organizations, corporations, academia, media, and religious institutions. Each element has a separate but essential role to play in confronting and combating trafficking in persons in the Arab world.

11.17.5 Non-governmental Organizations

Non-governmental organizations combat trafficking in persons in a number of ways. Among the most common forms of activities undertaken by NGOs to fight trafficking are public awareness campaigns, advocacy, research, networking, provision of direct services, and policy development. "Five Years after Stockholm", ECPAT International, 2001, Thailand. **ECPAT** is a network of organizations and Individuals working together to eliminate the commercial sexual exploitation of children. Established in 1990. The acronym stands for *End Child Prostitution, Child Pornography and Trafficking of Children for Sexual Purposes*. ECPAT has Special Consultative Status with the Economic and Social Council of the United Nations (ECOSOC).

11.18 Finding a Solution to the Trafficking Problem: Past, Present and Future[48]

In addition to economic, social, and cultural factors, political instability, war, and conflict may contribute to trafficking in persons. These factors particularly affect transitional societies, where civil unrest, loss of national identity, and political instability may create a favorable environment for organized crime, including trafficking in persons. In such cases, the disruption of traditional community life, along with its protective framework, make people extremely vulnerable to exploitation. In cases of civil war and ethnic conflicts, often a single, targeted minority group suffers a complete breakdown of social mechanisms, thereby increasing its vulnerability.

Finally, the resulting displacement of people in cases of strife leads to their isolation, thus increasing the ease by which traffickers can victimize them. Corruption is a major contributing factor to the crime of trafficking in persons; it is both an underlying root cause and a facilitating tool. It is important to remember that trafficking in persons may thrive in no small part because of the implicit or explicit participation or inaction by public officials.

For example, a border control officer turns a blind eye to people without legal documents crossing the border accompanied by their trafficker. Moreover, cases have been reported in which officials accepted or extorted bribes or sexual services, falsified identity documents, discouraged trafficking victims from reporting their crimes, or tolerated child prostitution and other trafficking-in-persons activities in commercial sex sites. While looking for solutions, it is important to remember the diversity of treatment of women and children within MENA. In Yemen, child labor sits at 23%. However, it is much lower in places such as Bahrain, where it remains at 5 percent. Again, child marriage is much higher in certain regions rather than others. In Sudan and Yemen, child marriage is between 32 and 34 percent. Countries like Algeria, however, are much lower, around 2 percent.

Religion plays a key role in deciding the treatment of women and children and the determination of their rights. Islam and the Quran are interpreted in many different ways by each country. There are Sunnis and Shias throughout the region and within those branches are various sects, including Ismaili and Zayidi. In order for a solution to be found, it will be important to address each interpretation and the possible concerns that will follow.[49] Culture, also, is key in determining the treatment of

---

[48]"Making Children's Rights Work in North Africa: Country Profiles on Algeria, Egypt, Libya, Morocco and Tunisia", International Bureau for Children's Rights, August 2007, Canada.

[49]The Islamic Law Perspective

The illicit sale of children for the purpose of inter-country adoption does not constitute a form of trafficking in most countries of the Middle East because Islamic law does not recognize the institution of adoption in accordance with the Qur'an, which states in Surah 33:4–5: [Nor] has He made your adopted sons your sons. Such is only your manner of speech by your mouths. But God tells you the Truth, and He shows the right way. Call them by (the names of) their fathers: that is more just in the sight of God.23 Islamic law recognizes kafala as an alternative to adoption.

women and children. Some practices, such as those rooted in prescriptive scripture, arise from religion; others arise from long held traditions. Again, it is important to address these concerns while searching for a solution to the abuse and harassment of women and children. There is a need to improve the quality of education in the region. Education methods tend to focus on learning by rote education rather than on developing critical thinking, analytical and participation skills. Also, in a number of countries in the region, there is a mismatch between the education system and the labor market. Also, quantity and quality of school infrastructure are poor (lacking facilities for sports activities, play and for children with disabilities and special needs), classrooms are too few in numbers and educational materials are inadequate. In the late 1990s, several MENA countries adopted pedagogical reforms (student centered learning, competency-based curricula, and focus on critical thinking). However, despite these efforts, there is little evidence of a significant shift away from a traditional model of teaching.

The Committee on the Rights of the Child has also reiterated its serious concerns regarding the quality of education in the Middle East and North Africa region. The Committee has recommended reforms of curriculum and teaching methodology, with emphasis on critical thinking, child-centered teaching methods and human rights education.

Saudi Arabia, for example, recently took action to address these issues by passing legislation to officially criminalize domestic violence. Under this new law, perpetrators of physical or psychological abuse could face up to one year in prison and a fine of around $13,000.17

Child helplines offer several services to children, the foremost of which is to uphold their Right to be heard and the Right to have freedom from all forms of violence as enshrined in Articles 12 and 13 of the Convention on the Rights of the Child.[50]

Kafala is a system of fosterage where a child may be placed under the guardianship of a family, but the child continues to retain his lineage. This arrangement explains why many countries of the Middle East that follow Islamic law had reservations regarding article 21 of the 1989 Convention on the Rights of the Child, which recognizes adoption: adoption is inconsistent with Islamic law. Consequently, there is little demand for adopted children in the Middle East.24

[50]1 Article 121. States Parties shall assure to the child who is capable of forming his or her own views the right to express those views freely in all matters affecting the child, the views of the child being given due weight in accordance with the age and maturity of the child.2. For this purpose, the child shall in particular be provided the opportunity to be heard in any judicial and administrative proceedings affecting the child, either directly, or through a representative or an appropriate body, in a manner consistent with the procedural rules of national law.

U.N. Protocol

As previously mentioned, the U.N. Protocol is the first international convention that comprehensively addresses trafficking in persons; as such, it is the primary reference in regard to criminalizing human trafficking. Article 5 of the U.N. Protocol calls on States to criminalize any offence committed intentionally under article 3. The article also mandates that States should criminalize attempts to commit the crime and participation as an accomplice in the commission of the crime. Article 5 reads:

Children contacting child helplines are offered counseling services and if their needs are greater child helplines refer them to partner organizations. Child helplines do not operate in isolation, they have formal arrangements with other child focused organizations and governments in their areas of operation so as to be able provide holistic support to children in need of care and protection. In Africa 16 child helplines are operational in as many countries. Some offer their services at the national level while others are currently working in regional spaces and making efforts to scale up their operations with the support of the national governments, UNICEF, Plan and other international and regional non-governmental organizations. In Ghana a project is underway to establish a national child helpline. Similarly in Burundi, South Sudan, Djibouti and many other countries Child Helpline International is working towards setting up of helplines.

---

1. Each State Party shall adopt such legislative and other measures as may be necessary to establish as criminal offences the conduct set forth in Article 3 of this Protocol, when committed intentionally.

2. Each State Party shall also adopt such legislative and other measures as may be necessary to establish as criminal offences:

a. Subject to the basic concepts of its legal system, attempting to commit an offence established in accordance with paragraph 1 of this Article;

b. Participating as an accomplice in an offence established in accordance with paragraph 1 of this Article; and

c. Organizing or directing other persons to commit an offence established in accordance with paragraph 1 of this Article.106

For assistance in complying with article 5, reference must be made to the United

Nations Code of Conduct for Law Enforcement Officials of 1979, which comprises eight articles:

Training Manual to Combat Trafficking in Persons 57

Article 1. Law enforcement officials shall at all times fulfill the duty imposed upon them by law, by serving the community and by protecting all persons against illegal acts, consistent with the high degree of responsibility required by their profession.

Article 2. In the performance of their duty, law enforcement officials shall respect and protect human dignity and maintain and uphold the human rights of all persons.

Article 3. Law enforcement officials may use force only when strictly necessary and to the extent required for the performance of their duty.

Article 4. Matters of a confidential nature in the possession of law enforcement officials shall be kept confidential, unless the performance of duty or the needs of justice strictly require otherwise.

Article 5. No law enforcement official may inflict, instigate or tolerate any act of torture or other cruel, inhuman or degrading treatment or punishment, nor may any law enforcement official invoke superior orders or exceptional circumstances such as a state of war or a threat of war, a threat to national security, internal political instability or any other public emergency as a justification of torture or other cruel, inhuman or degrading treatment or punishment.

Article 6. Law enforcement officials shall ensure the full protection of the health of persons in their custody and, in particular, shall take immediate action to secure medical attention whenever required.

Article 7. Law enforcement officials shall not commit any act of corruption. They shall also rigorously oppose and combat all such acts.

Article 8. Law enforcement officials shall respect the law and the present Code. They shall also, to the best of their capability, prevent and rigorously oppose any violations of them.107

11.19 Conclusion

Trafficking in persons is unique: it is the only business that specializes in humans as merchandise. Thus, a large part of combating trafficking is the treatment of and aid for the victims. The victims must be protected from retaliation by their traffickers, from prosecution or deportation under the country's legal system, and from harm while they are recovering from their trauma. In addition, victims must be given support in pursuing justice, recovering, and reintegrating into society. Such support would entail providing victims with legal assistance in the prosecution of the traffickers and on matters related to their immigration status. Victims also have a right to be informed of their rights and to be treated as victims rather than criminals, despite any illegal activity in which they may have participated while they were being trafficked. Finally, various procedural law principles must be in place to ensure that the rights of the victims and of their families are duly guaranteed, in civil and religious laws.[51]

[51]Respect for the individual is the central precept of Islam—the warning against persecution of individuals is repeated 299 times in the Qur'an, and the phrase "justice and equality" appears at least 16 times. It may also be argued that equal protection is likewise a basic premise in Islamic legal theory. For example, the Prophet Muhammad declared in the Great Pilgrimage that "[a]ll Moslems are brothers unto one another" and that "[t]here is no superiority of an Arab over a non-Arab except as his devotion is concerned."173

Chapter 12
Female Genital Mutilation/Female Cutting/ Female *Circumcision*

12.1 Abstract

FGM is a manifestation of violence on girls and a fundamental breach of their rights; this custom is still practiced in a number of Arab countries, but does not include all Arab communities. Female genital mutilation (FGM) is one of the major forms of violence against girls and constitutes a clear violation of their rights. This traditional practice still exists in a number of Arab nations, although some countries, such as Jordan, Bahrain, Tunisia, Algeria, Syria, Palestine, Qatar, Morocco, and Lebanon, have all reported that such practices are not performed within their borders. Egypt has passed legislation criminalizing female circumcision and genital mutilation. In Yemen, the practice is prevalent in some coastal cities. The draft amendments to the Rights of the Child submitted to the country's House of Representatives include legal provisions on the prohibition of female genital mutilation. Other countries have not provided any information regarding this issue to the LAS. The practice is also found elsewhere in Asia, the Middle East, and among communities from these areas around the world.

12.2 Female Genital Mutilation/Cutting/Female Circumcision (FGM) in History

The United Nations Population Fund estimated in 2010 that 20 percent of women affected by FGM had been infibulated, a practice found largely in northeast Africa.[1]

A Greek papyrus from 163 B.C. mentions both boys and girls in Egypt undergoing circumcision and it is widely accepted to have originated in Egypt and the Nile

[1]"Frequently Asked Questions on Female Genital Mutilation/Cutting", United Nations Population Fund, April 2010.

B. Gerbaka et al., *Child Sexual Abuse, Exploitation and Trafficking in the Arab Region*, Child Maltreatment 13, https://doi.org/10.1007/978-3-030-66507-4_12

valley at the time of the Pharaohs.[2,3] Evidence from mummies has shown both Type I and Type III FGC present.[4]

Until the 1980s FGM was widely known as female circumcision, which implied equivalence in severity with male circumcision.[5] The Kenya Missionary Council began referring to it as the sexual mutilation of women in 1929, following the lead of Marion Scott Stevenson, a Church of Scotland missionary.[6]

References to the practice as mutilation increased throughout the 1970s.[7] In 1975 Rose Oldfield Hayes, an American anthropologist, called it female genital mutilation in the title of a paper,[8] and in 1979 Fran Hosken, an Austrian-American researcher and feminist, called it mutilation in her influential The Hosken Report: Genital and Sexual Mutilation of Females.[9]

The Inter-African Committee on Traditional Practices Affecting the Health of Women and Children and the World Health Organization (WHO) began referring to it as female genital mutilation in 1990 and 1991 respectively. In April 1997 the WHO,[10] United Nations Children's Fund (UNICEF) and United Nations Population Fund (UNFPA) issued a joint statement using that term.

Other terms in common use include female genital cutting (FGC) and female genital mutilation/cutting (FGM/C), preferred by those who work with practitioners.[11]

---

[2]Knight 2001, p. 331, citing G. Elliot Smith, A Contribution to the Study of Mummification in Egypt, Cairo: L'Institut Egyptien, 1906, p. 30, and Marc Armand Ruffer, Studies in the Paleopathology of Egypt, Chicago: University of Chicago Press, 1921, p. 171.

[3]F. G. Kenyon, Greek Papyri in the British Museum, British Museum, 1893, pp. 31–32.

[4]Female Genital Mutilation/Cutting: A Statistical Overview and Exploration of the Dynamics of Change, New York: United Nations Children's Fund, July 2013.

[5]Martha Nussbaum, Sex and Social Justice, New York: Oxford University Press, 1999, p. 119.

[6]James Karanja, The Missionary Movement in Colonial Kenya: The Foundation of Africa Inland Church, Göttingen: Cuvillier Verlag, 2009, p. 93, n. 63

[7]"Eliminating Female genital mutilation: An Interagency Statement", Geneva: World Health Organization, 2008.

[8]Rose Oldfield Hayes, "Female Genital Mutilation, Fertility Control, Women's Roles, and the Patrilineage in Modern Sudan: A Functional Analysis," American Ethnologist 2(4), November 1975, pp. 617–633. JSTOR 643328.

[9]Fran Hosken, The Hosken Report: Genital and Sexual Mutilation of Females, Lexington: Women's International Network, 1994 [1979].n2

[10]Female Genital Mutilation/Cutting: A Statistical Overview and Exploration of the Dynamics of Change, New York: United Nations Children's Fund, July 2013.

[11]"Eliminating Female genital mutilation: An Interagency Statement", Geneva: World Health Organization, 2008.

12.3 Female Genital Mutilation/Cutting/Female Circumcision (FGM): The Procedure

FGM is the ritual removal of some or all of the external female genitalia. UNICEF estimated in 2016 that 200 million women had undergone the procedures in 27 countries in Africa, as well as in Indonesia, Iraqi Kurdistan and Yemen, with a rate of 80–98 percent within the 15–49 age groups in Djibouti, Egypt, Eritrea, Guinea, Mali, Sierra Leone, Somalia and Sudan.[12]

Female genital cutting (FGC) is also known as female genital mutilation (FGM), female circumcision, or female genital mutilation/cutting (FGM/C); it is defined by the World Health Organization as "all procedures that involve partial or total removal of the external female genitalia, or other injury to the female genital organs for non-medical reasons." The term is exclusively used to describe traditional or religious procedures on a minor, which requires the parents' consent because of the age of the girl.

Typically carried out by a traditional circumciser using a blade, FGM is conducted from days after birth to puberty and beyond; in half the countries for which national figures are available, most girls are cut before the age of five.[13] Procedures differ according to the country or ethnic group. They include removal of the clitoral hood and clitoral glans; removal of the inner labia; and removal of the inner and outer labia and closure of the vulva. In this last procedure (known as infibulation), a small hole is left for the passage of urine and menstrual fluid; the vagina is opened for intercourse and opened further for childbirth.[14] Sunna circumcision usually refers to clitoridectomy, but is also used for more severe forms. Communities often refer to just two forms of FGM: pharaonic for infibulation and sunna for everything else.[15] Sunna means "path or way" in Arabic and refers to the tradition of Muhammad, although none of the procedures are required within Islam.[16]

The term infibulation derives from fibula, Latin for clasp; the Ancient Romans reportedly fastened clasps through the foreskins or labia of slaves to prevent sexual intercourse. The surgical infibulation of women came to be known as pharaonic

---

[12]"Female Genital Mutilation/Cutting: A Global Concern", New York: United Nations Children's Fund, February 2016.

[13]For the circumcisers, blade: UNICEF 2013, pp. 2, 44–46; for the ages: p. 50.

[14]Jasmine Abdulcadira, et al., "Care of women with female genital mutilation/cutting", Swiss Medical Weekly, 6(14), January 2011. doi:10.4414/smw.2011.13137 PMID 21213149.

[15]Ellen Gruenbaum, The Female Circumcision Controversy: An Anthropological Perspective, Philadelphia: University of Pennsylvania Press, 2001, pp. 2–3.

[16]Ibrahim Lethome Asmani, Maryam Sheikh Abdi, De-linking Female Genital Mutilation/Cutting from Islam, Washington: Frontiers in Reproductive Health, Population Council, 2008.

circumcision in Sudan, but as Sudanese circumcision in Egypt.[17] In Somalia it is known simply as qodob ("to sew up").[18]

The procedures are generally performed by a traditional circumciser (cutter or exciseuse) in the girls' homes, with or without anaesthesia. The cutter is usually an older woman, but in communities where the male barber has assumed the role of health worker he will perform FGM too.[19]

When traditional cutters are involved, non-sterile devices are likely to be used, including knives, razors, scissors, glass, sharpened rocks and fingernails.[20] A nurse in Uganda, quoted in 2007 in The Lancet, said that a cutter would use one knife on up to 30 girls at a time.[21]

Health professionals are often involved in Egypt, Kenya, Indonesia and Sudan. In Egypt 77 percent of FGM procedures, and in Indonesia over 50 percent, were performed by medical professionals as of 2008 and 2016.[22] Depending on the involvement of medical professionals, the procedures may include a local or general anesthetic, or neither. Women in Egypt reported in 1995 that a local anesthetic had been used on their daughters in 60 percent of cases, a general in 13 percent and neither in 25 percent.

The WHO, UNICEF and UNFPA issued a joint statement in April 1997 defining FGM as "all procedures involving partial or total removal of the external female genitalia or other injury to the female genital organs whether for cultural or other non-therapeutic reasons."[23]

The procedures vary considerably according to ethnicity and individual practitioners. During a 1998 survey in Niger, women responded with over 50 different terms when asked what was done to them.[24] Translation problems are compounded by the women's confusion over which type of FGM they experienced, or even

---

[17]Leonard J. Kouba, Judith Muasher, "Female Circumcision in Africa: An Overview," African Studies Review, 28(1), March 1985, pp. 95–110. JSTOR 524569.

[18]Raqiya D. Abdalla, "'My Grandmother Called it the Three Feminine Sorrows': The Struggle of Women Against Female Circumcision in Somalia", in Abusharaf 2007, p. 190.

[19]UNICEF 2013, pp. 42–44 and Table 5, p. 181 (for cutters), p. 46 (for home and anaesthesia).

[20]Elizabeth Kelly, Paula J. Adams Hillard, "Female genital mutilation", Current Opinion in Obstetrics & Gynecology, 17(5), October 2005, pp. 490–494. PMID 16141763

[21]Wairagala Wakabi, "Africa battles to make female genital mutilation history", The Lancet, 369 (9567), 31 March 2007, pp. 1069–1070. doi:10.1016/S0140-6736(07)60508-X PMID 17405200

[22]Female Genital Mutilation/Cutting: A Statistical Overview and Exploration of the Dynamics of Change, New York: United Nations Children's Fund, July 2013.43–45.

[23]"Eliminating Female genital mutilation: An Interagency Statement", Geneva: World Health Organization, 2008.

[24]Female Genital Mutilation/Cutting: A Statistical Overview and Exploration of the Dynamics of Change, New York: United Nations Children's Fund, July 2013.

whether they experienced it.[25] 190 Several studies have suggested that survey responses are unreliable.[26]

Standard questionnaires from United Nations bodies ask women whether they have undergone the following: cut, no flesh removed (pricking or symbolic circumcision); cut, some flesh removed; sewn closed; and type not determined/unsure/doesn't know.[27] The most common procedures fall within the "cut, some flesh removed" category and involve complete or partial removal of the clitoral glans.[28]

12.4 WHO Types I–IV

The World Health Organization has created a more detailed typology, Types I–II, based on how much tissue is removed. Type III is "sewn closed." Type IV describes symbolic circumcision and miscellaneous procedures.

12.4.1 Type I

It is subdivided into Ia, removal of the clitoral hood (rarely performed alone), [n 6] and the more common Ib (clitoridectomy), the complete or partial removal of the clitoral glans and clitoral hood.[29] 4 (When discussing FGM, the WHO uses clitoris to refer to the clitoral glans, the visible tip of the clitoris.)[30] "The clitoris is held between the thumb and index finger, pulled out and amputated with one stroke of a sharp object.

[25]Wairagala Wakabi, "Africa battles to make female genital mutilation history", The Lancet, 369 (9567) 31 March 2007, pp. 1069–1070. doi:10.1016/S0140-6736(07)60508-X PMID 17405200.

[26]P. Stanley Yoder, Shanxiao Wang, Elise Johansen, "Estimates of Female Genital Mutilation/Cutting in 27 African Countries and Yemen", Studies in Family Planning, 44(2), June 2013, pp. 189–204. doi:10.1111/j.1728-4465.2013.00352.x PMID 23720002.

[27]UNICEF 2013: "These categories do not fully match the WHO typology. Cut, no flesh removed describes a practice known as nicking or pricking, which currently is categorized as Type IV. Cut, some flesh removed corresponds to Type I (clitoridectomy) and Type II (excision) combined. And sewn closed corresponds to Type III, infibulation."[2]:48

[28]P. Stanley Yoder, Shanxiao Wang, Elise Johansen, "Estimates of Female Genital Mutilation/Cutting in 27 African Countries and Yemen", Studies in Family Planning, 44(2), June 2013, pp. 189–204. doi:10.1111/j.1728-4465.2013.00352.x PMID 23720002.

[29]Martha Nussbaum, Sex and Social Justice, New York: Oxford University Press, 1999, p. 119.

[30]"Eliminating Female genital mutilation: An Interagency Statement", Geneva: World Health Organization, 2008

12.4.2 Type II

It is an excision; this is the complete or partial removal of the inner labia, with or without removal of the clitoral glans and outer labia. Type IIa is removal of the inner labia; IIb, removal of the clitoral glans and inner labia; and IIc, removal of the clitoral glans, inner and outer labia. Excision in French can refer to any form of FGM.

12.4.3 Type III

It is called: infibulation or pharaonic circumcision; in such cases,

The "sewn closed" category, involves the removal of the external genitalia and fusion of the wound. The inner and/or outer labia are cut away, with or without removal of the clitoral glans.

Type IIIa is the removal and closure of the inner labia and IIIb the outer labia. The practice is found largely in Djibouti, Eritrea, Ethiopia, Somalia and Sudan (though not South Sudan) in northeast Africa. Estimates of numbers vary: according to one in 2008, over eight million women in Africa have experienced it. According to UNFPA in 2010, 20 percent of women with FGM have been infibulated.[31]

Type IIIb[32]: Comfort Momoh, a specialist midwife, writes of Type III: "[E]lderly women, relatives and friends secure the girl in the lithotomy position. A deep incision is made rapidly on either side from the root of the clitoris to the fourchette, and a single cut of the razor excises the clitoris and both the labia majora and labia minora."[33]: 12–14 In Somalia the clitoral glans is removed and shown to the girl's senior female relatives, who decide whether enough has been amputated. After this the labia are removed.[34,35]

A single hole of 2–3 mm is left for the passage of urine and menstrual fluid by inserting something, such as a twig, into the wound.[36] The vulva is closed with surgical thread, agave oracacia thorns, or covered with a poultice such as raw egg,

[31]"Frequently Asked Questions on Female Genital Mutilation/Cutting", United Nations Population Fund, April 2010.

[32]Jasmine Abdulcadira, et al., "Care of women with female genital mutilation/cutting", Swiss Medical Weekly, 6(14), January 2011. doi:10.4414/smw.2011.13137 PMID 21213149.

[33]Edna Adan Ismail, "Female genital mutilation survey in Somaliland", Edna Adan Maternity and Teaching Hospital, 2009.

[34]Comfort Momoh, "Female genital mutilation" in Comfort Momoh (ed.), Female Genital Mutilation, Oxford: Radcliffe Publishing, 2005, p. 7.

[35]Abusharaf 2007, p. 190.

[36]"67/146. Intensifying global efforts for the elimination of female genital mutilations", United Nations General Assembly, adopted 20 December 2012.

herbs and sugar.[37,38] The parts that have been removed might be placed in a pouch for the girl to wear. To help the tissue bond, the girl's legs are tied together, often from hip to ankle, for up to six weeks; the bindings are usually loosened after a week and may be removed after two. The entrance to the vagina is obliterated by a drum of skin extending across the orifice except for a small hole. Circumstances at the time may vary; the girl may struggle ferociously, in which case the incisions may become uncontrolled and haphazard. The girl may be pinned down so firmly that bones may fracture. If the remaining hole is too large in the view of the girl's family, the procedure is repeated. The vagina is opened for sexual intercourse, for the first time either by a midwife with a knife or by the woman's husband with his penis. In some areas, including Somaliland, female relatives of the bride and groom might watch the opening of the vagina to check that the girl is a virgin.

Psychologist Hanny Lightfoot-Klein interviewed hundreds of women and men in Sudan in the 1980s about sexual intercourse with Type III: The penetration of the bride's infibulation takes anywhere from 3 or 4 days to several months. Some men are unable to penetrate their wives at all (in my study over 15%), and the task is often accomplished by a midwife under conditions of great secrecy, since this reflects negatively on the man's potency. Some who are unable to penetrate their wives manage to get them pregnant in spite of the infibulation, and the woman's vaginal passage is then cut open to allow birth to take place.... Those men who do manage to penetrate their wives do so often, or perhaps always, with the help of the "little knife." This creates a tear which they gradually rip more and more until the opening is sufficient to admit the penis.[39] The woman is opened further for childbirth and closed afterwards, a process known as defibulation (or deinfibulation) and reinfibulation. Reinfibulation can involve cutting the vagina again to restore the pinhole size of the first infibulation. This might be performed before marriage, and after childbirth, divorce and widowhood.[40]

WHO defines Type IV as "[a]ll other harmful procedures to the female genitalia for non-medical purposes", including pricking, piercing, incising, scraping and cauterization. It includes nicking of the clitoris (symbolic circumcision), burning or scarring the genitals, and introducing substances into the vagina to tighten it.[41,42]

---

[37]Elizabeth Kelly, Paula J. Adams Hillard, "Female genital mutilation", Current Opinion in Obstetrics & Gynecology, 17(5), October 2005, pp. 490–494. PMID 16141763

[38]Edna Adan Ismail, "Female genital mutilation survey in Somaliland", Edna Adan Maternity and Teaching Hospital, 2009.

[39]Hanny Lightfoot-Klein, "The Sexual Experience and Marital Adjustment of Genitally Circumcised and Infibulated Females in The Sudan"], The Journal of Sex Research, 26(3), 1989, pp. 375–392. JSTOR 3812643.

[40]Eric K. Silverman, "Anthropology and Circumcision," Annual Review of Anthropology, 33, 2004, pp. 419–445. JSTOR 25064860

[41]"Eliminating Female genital mutilation: An Interagency Statement", Geneva: World Health Organization, 2008.

[42]Female Genital Mutilation/Cutting: A Statistical Overview and Exploration of the Dynamics of Change, New York: United Nations Children's Fund, July 2013.

Labia stretching is also categorized as Type IV. Common in southern and eastern Africa, the practice is supposed to enhance sexual pleasure for the man and add to the sense of a woman as a closed space. From the age of eight, girls are encouraged to stretch their inner labia using sticks and massage. Girls in Uganda are told they may have difficulty giving birth without stretched labia.[43]

A definition of FGM from the WHO in 1995 included gishiri cutting and angurya cutting, found in Nigeria and Niger. These were removed from the WHO's 2008 definition because of insufficient information about prevalence and consequences.[44] Gishiri cutting involves cutting the vagina's front or back wall with a blade or penknife, performed in response to infertility, obstructed labour and several other conditions. Over 30 percent of women with gishiri cuts in a study by Nigerian physician Mairo Usman Mandara had vesico-vaginal fistulae. Angurya cutting is excision of the hymen, usually performed seven days after birth.[45]

12.5 Regional Specificities

12.5.1 FGM in Indonesia[46]

FGM harms women's physical and emotional health throughout their lives.[47,48] It has no known health benefits.[49] The short-term and late complications depend on the type of FGM, whether the practitioner had medical training, and whether she used antibiotics and unsterilized or surgical single-use instruments. In the case of Type III, other factors include how small a hole was left for the passage of urine and menstrual blood, whether surgical thread was used instead of agave or acacia thorns, and whether the procedure was performed more than once (for example, to close an

---

[43]Eric K. Silverman, "Anthropology and Circumcision," Annual Review of Anthropology, 33, 2004, pp. 419–445. JSTOR 25064860

[44]"Eliminating Female genital mutilation: An Interagency Statement", Geneva: World Health Organization, 2008.

[45]Mairo Usman Mandara, "Female genital cutting in Nigeria: View of Nigerian Doctors on the Medicalization Debate", in Bettina Shell-Duncan and Ylva Hernlund (eds.), Female "Circumcision" in Africa: Culture Controversy and Change, Boulder: Lynne Rienner Publishers, 2000 (pp. 253–282), pp. 98, 100; for fistulae, p. 102.

[46]Preparations of the Girl before procedure; Nine-month-old afterwards — Stephanie Sinclair; The New York Times, 2006.

[47]Rigmor C. Berg, et al., "Effects of female genital cutting on physical health outcomes: a systematic review and meta-analysis", BMJ Open, 4(11), 2014: e006316. PMID 25416059 doi:10.1136/bmjopen-2014-006316

[48]Dan Reisel, Sarah M. Creighton, "Long term health consequences of Female Genital Mutilation (FGM)", Maturitas, 80(1), January 2015 (pp. 48–51), p. 49. PMID 25466303 doi:10.1016/j.maturitas.2014.10.009

[49]"Female genital mutilation", Geneva: World Health Organization, February 2016.

opening regarded as too wide or re-open one too small).[50] Common short-term complications include swelling, excessive bleeding, pain, urine retention and healing problems/wound infection. A 2015 systematic review of 56 studies that recorded immediate complications suggested that each of these occurred in more than one in ten girls and women undergoing any form of FGM, including symbolic nicking of the clitoris (Type IV), although the risks increased with Type III. The review also suggested that there was under-reporting.[51] Other short-term complications include fatal bleeding, anemia, urinary infection, septicemia, tetanus, gangrene, necrotizing fasciitis (flesh-eating disease) and endometritis. It is not known how many girls and women die as a result of the practice, because complications may not be recognized or reported. The practitioners' use of shared instruments is thought to aid the transmission of hepatitis B, hepatitis C and HIV, although no epidemiological studies have shown this.[52,53]

12.5.2 FGM in Africa: Population Awareness and Education

Late complications of FGM vary depending on the type of FGM.[54] They include the formation of scars and keloids that lead to strictures and obstruction, epidermoid cysts that may become infected, and neuroma formation (growth of nerve tissue) involving nerves that supplied the clitoris.[55,56]

An infibulated girl may be left with an opening as small as 2–3 mm, which can cause prolonged, drop-by-drop urination, pain while urinating, and a feeling of needing to urinate all the time. Urine may collect underneath the scar, leaving the area under the skin constantly wet, which can lead to infection and the formation of

[50]Jasmine Abdulcadira, et al., "Care of women with female genital mutilation/cutting", Swiss Medical Weekly, 6(14), January 2011. doi:10.4414/smw.2011.13137 PMID 21213149

[51]Rigmor C Berg, Vigdis Underland, "Immediate health consequences of female genital mutilation/cutting (FGM/C)", Kunnskapssenteret (Norwegian Knowledge Centre for the Health Services), systematic review no. 8, 2014, pp. 4–5 (full text). ISBN 978-82-8121-856-7

[52]Dan Reisel, Sarah M. Creighton, "Long term health consequences of Female Genital Mutilation (FGM)", Maturitas, 80(1), January 2015 (pp. 48–51), p. 49. PMID 25466303 doi:10.1016/j.maturitas.2014.10.009

[53]Christos Iavazzo, Thalia A. Sardi, Ioannis D. Gkegkes, "Female genital mutilation and infections: a systematic review of the clinical evidence", Archives of Gynecology and Obstetrics, 287(6), June 2013, pp. 1137–1149. PMID 23315098 doi:10.1007/s00404-012-2708-5

[54]Elizabeth Kelly, Paula J. Adams Hillard, "Female genital mutilation", Current Opinion in Obstetrics & Gynecology, 17(5), October 2005, pp. 490–494. PMID 161417

[55]Elizabeth Kelly, Paula J. Adams Hillard, "Female genital mutilation", Current Opinion in Obstetrics & Gynecology, 17(5), October 2005, pp. 490–494. PMID 161417

[56]El Dareer 1982, p. 37. Also see Asma El Dareer, "Preliminary report on a study on prevalence and epidemiology of female circumcision in Sudan today", WHO seminar, Khartoum, 10–15 February 1979; Asma el Dareer, "Female circumcision and its consequences for mother and child", Yaounde, 12–15 December 1979, cited in Rushwan 2013.

small stones. The opening is larger in women who are sexually active or have given birth by vaginal delivery, but the urethra opening may still be obstructed by scar tissue. Vesicovaginal or rectovaginal fistulae can develop (holes that allow urine or faeces to seep into the vagina).[57] This and other damage to the urethra and bladder can lead to infections and incontinence, pain during sexual intercourseand infertility. Painful periods are common because of the obstruction to the menstrual flow, and blood can stagnate in the vagina and uterus. Complete obstruction of the vagina can result in hematocolpos and hematometra (where the vagina and uterus fill with menstrual blood).[58] The swelling of the abdomen that results from the collection of fluid, together with the lack of menstruation, can lead to suspicion of pregnancy. Asma El Dareer, a Sudanese physician, reported in 1979 that a girl in Sudan with this condition was killed by her family.[59]

FGM may place women at higher risk of problems during pregnancy and childbirth, which are more common with the more extensive FGM procedures. Infibulated women may try to make childbirth easier by eating less during pregnancy to reduce the baby's size.[60] In women with vesico-vaginal or rectovaginal fistulae, it is difficult to obtain clear urine samples as part of prenatal care, making the diagnosis of conditions such as pre-eclampsia harder.[61]

Cervical evaluation during labor may be impeded and labor prolonged or obstructed. Third-degree laceration (tears), anal-sphincter damage and emergency caesarean section are more common in infibulated women.[62]

Neonatal mortality is increased. The WHO estimated in 2006 that an additional 10–20 babies die per 1000 deliveries as a result of FGM. The estimate was based on a study conducted on 28,393 women attending delivery wards at 28 obstetric centres in Burkina Faso, Ghana, Kenya, Nigeria, Senegal and Sudan. In those settings all types of FGM were found to pose an increased risk of death to the baby: 15% higher for Type I, 32% for Type II and 55% for Type III.

The reasons for this were unclear, but may be connected to genital and urinary tract infections and the presence of scar tissue. The researchers wrote that FGM was

---

[57]Hamid Rushwan, "Female genital mutilation: A tragedy for women's reproductive health", African Journal of Urology, 19(3), September 2013, pp. 130–133. doi:10.1016/j.afju.2013.03.002

[58]Jasmine Abdulcadira, et al., "Care of women with female genital mutilation/cutting", Swiss Medical Weekly, 6(14), January 2011. doi:10.4414/smw.2011.13137 PMID 21213149

[59]El Dareer 1982, p. 37. Also see Asma El Dareer, "Preliminary report on a study on prevalence and epidemiology of female circumcision in Sudan today", WHO seminar, Khartoum, 10–15 February 1979; Asma el Dareer, "Female circumcision and its consequences for mother and child", Yaounde, 12–15 December 1979, cited in Rushwan 2013

[60]Mumtaz Rashid, Mohammed H. Rashid, "Obstetric management of women with female genital mutilation", The Obstetrician and Gynaecologist, 9(2), April 2007, pp. 95–101. doi:

[61]Elizabeth Kelly, Paula J. Adams Hillard, "Female genital mutilation", Current Opinion in Obstetrics & Gynecology, 17(5), October 2005, pp. 490–494. PMID 16141763

[62]Mumtaz Rashid, Mohammed H. Rashid, "Obstetric management of women with female genital mutilation", The Obstetrician and Gynaecologist, 9(2), April 2007, pp. 95–101. doi:10.1576/toag.9.2.095.27310

associated with an increased risk to the mother of damage to the perineum and excessive blood loss, as well as a need to resuscitate the baby, and stillbirth, perhaps because of a long second stage of labor.[63]

12.6 FGM in the Arab Region

12.6.1 Data on FGM

Female Genital Mutilation (FGM) is still practiced in some countries in the region. A report by the Population Council of Egypt in 1997 showed that 86 per cent of adolescent girls had undergone FGM. The fact that it is increasingly dealt with as a medical issue points to its becoming legitimized. In Sudan, in contrast, FGM has been illegal since 1991, but is still commonly practiced by elderly women in the community at the request of parents. FGM is also still prevalent in Djibouti.

This cultural phenomenon is not reported in Tunisia, Algeria, Syria, Qatar, Morocco, Lebanon, Jordan; on the other side, there is no law preventing female genital mutilation in Sudan, Egypt, Yemen; other countries did not provide information on FGM.[64]

In the Arab region, The many variants of FGM are reflected in dozens of local terms in countries where it is common.[65] These often refer to purification. A common Arabic term for purification has the root t-h-r, used for male and female circumcision (tahur and tahara).[66] It is also known in Arabic as khafḍ or khifaḍ.[67,68] In the Bambara language, spoken mostly in Mali, FGM is known as bolokoli ("washing your hands")[69] and in the Igbo language in eastern Nigeria as isa aru or

[63]Emily Banks, et al, "Female genital mutilation and obstetric outcome: WHO collaborative prospective study in six African countries", The Lancet, 367(9525), 3 June 2006, pp. 1835–1841. PMID 16753486 doi:10.1016/S0140-6736(06)68805-3

[64]"FGM still largely an unknown quantity in Arab world", IRIN, http://www.irinnews.org/InDepthMain aspx?InDepthId=15&ReportId=62474&Country=Yes

[65]Female Genital Mutilation/Cutting: A Statistical Overview and Exploration of the Dynamics of Change, New York: United Nations Children's Fund, July 2013:48

[66]Fadwa El Guindi, "Had This Been Your Face, Would You Leave It as Is?" in Rogaia Mustafa Abusharaf (ed.), Female Circumcision: Multicultural Perspectives, Philadelphia: University of Pennsylvania Press, 2007, p. 30.

[67]Clarence-Smith, William G. "Islam and Female Genital Cutting in Southeast Asia: The Weight of the Past", Finnish Journal of Ethnicity and Migration, 3(2), 2008, p. 14.

[68]Ibrahim Lethome Asmani, Maryam Sheikh Abdi, De-linking Female Genital Mutilation/Cutting from Islam, Washington: Frontiers in Reproductive Health, Population Council, 2008.

[69]Chantal Zabus, "The Excised Body in African Texts and Contexts," in Merete Falck Borch (ed.), Bodies and Voices: The Force-field of Representation and Discourse in Colonial and Postcolonial Studies, New York: Rodopi, 2008, p. 47.

iwu aru ("having your bath," as in "a young woman must 'have her bath' before she has a baby").[70]

FGM is found mostly in what Gerry Mackie called an "intriguingly contiguous"[71,72] zone in Africa—east to west from Somalia to Senegal, and north to south from Egypt[73] to Tanzania.[74] Nationally representative figures available as of 2016 suggest that the practice is concentrated in 27 countries in Africa, as well as in Indonesia, Iraqi Kurdistan and Yemen. Over 200 million women and girls are thought to be living with FGM in those 30 countries.[75] As of 2013, 27.2 million women had undergone FGM in Egypt, 23.8 million in Ethiopia, and 19.9 million in Nigeria.[76]:2

The highest concentrations among the 15–49 age group are in Somalia (98%), Guinea (97%), Djibouti (93%), Egypt (91%) and Sierra Leone (90%).There is also a high concentration in Indonesia; national figures for adults are not available, but the prevalence rate for the 0–11 age group there is 49%, mostly Types I and IV.:2

Smaller studies or anecdotal reports suggest that FGM is also practised in Colombia, the Congo, Malaysia, Oman, Peru, Saudi Arabia, Sri Lanka, and the United Arab Emirates, as well as among the Bedouin in Israel; in Rahmah, Jordan; and among the Dawoodi Bohra in India.[77] It is also found within immigrant communities in Australasia, Europe, North America and Scandinavia.[78]:4

---

[70]Chantal Zabus, "'Writing with an Accent': From Early Decolonization to Contemporary Gender Issues in the African Novel in French, English, and Arabic," in Simona Bertacco (ed.), Language and Translation in Postcolonial Literatures, New York: Routledge, 2013, p. 40.

[71]Gerry Mackie, 1996: "FGM is pre-Islamic but was exaggerated by its intersection with the Islamic modesty code of family honor, female purity, virginity, chastity, fidelity, and seclusion."[85]:1008

[72]Gerry Mackie, 1996: "The Koran is silent on FGM, but several hadith (sayings attributed to Mohammed) recommend attenuating the practice for the woman's sake, praise it as noble but not commanded, or advise that female converts refrain from mutilation because even if pleasing to the husband it is painful to the wife."[85]:1004–1005

[73]Mohammed A. Tag-Eldin (World Health Organization, 2008): "The most common forms of FGC still widely practised throughout Egypt are type I (commonly referred to as clitoridectomy) and type II (commonly referred to as excision)."[76]

[74]Gerry Mackie, John LeJeune, "Social Dynamics of Abandonment of Harmful Practices: A New Look at the Theory", Innocenti Working Paper No. 2008-XXX, UNICEF Innocenti Research Centre, 2008, p. 5.

[75]"Female Genital Mutilation/Cutting: A Global Concern", New York: United Nations Children's Fund, February 2016.

[76]Female Genital Mutilation/Cutting: A Statistical Overview and Exploration of the Dynamics of Change, New York: United Nations Children's Fund, July 2013

[77]For the Dawoodi Bohra: Diane Cole, "UNICEF Estimate Of Female Genital Mutilation Up By 70 Million", NPR, 8 February 2016.

For Rahmah, Jordan: Dana Charkasi, "Female circumcision still haunts Jordanian tribe in southern Jordan", ArabNews West, 2012; Rana Sabbagh-Gargour, "The Jordanian town that still circumcises women", The Daily Star (Lebanon), 13 November 2003.

[78]Michael Miller and Francesca Moneti, Changing a harmful social convention: Female genital cutting/mutilation, Florence: UNICEF Innocenti Research Centre, 2005.

Algeria (no Data) Female genital cutting—mutilation is present in Algeria.[79]

Djibouti (90–98% prevalence, Type II and III)

FGC was outlawed in the country's revised Penal Code that went into effect in April 1995. Article 333 of the Penal Code provides that persons found guilty of this practice will face a five year prison term and a fine of one million Djibouti francs (approximately US$5,600). Djibouti ratified the Maputo Protocol in 2005.[80]

Egypt (78–97% prevalence, Type I, II and III)

In Egypt, the decision of Egyptian Health Minister No. 261 of 1996 prohibits female circumcision in public hospitals and private clinics, except in medical cases only, approved by the Department of Obstetrics and Gynecology.

Although this decision has been a significant development in the Department's position on the issue of female genital mutilation, it still contains a loophole for those who want to practice female circumcision. The National Council for Childhood and Motherhood organized a national project to combat female genital mutilation, which aims to mobilization of society at large, changing behaviors and renouncing the habit.

The project builds on empowerment of girls at risk of female genital mutilation and information on their rights; the project aims to reach 120 villages free of female genital mutilation within a three years period.

Statistics show that in 2003, the size of this phenomenon in Egypt was high, with a rate of FGM of 97% among married women between 15–45 years old, and 82% for girls below the age of 15 years. There was a disparity in the practice of circumcision between rural and urban areas, with higher proportions in rural areas. The study performed by the National Council for Motherhood and Childhood with UNDP in 2004 to change the trend towards the practice of female genital mutilation reported that about 50% of young people—male and female—manifested their opposition to this phenomenon.

Egypt's Ministry of Health and Population has banned all forms of female genital cutting since 2007.[81] The ministry's order declared it is 'prohibited for any doctors, nurses, or any other person to carry out any cut of, flattening or modification of any natural part of the female reproductive system'. Islamic authorities in the nation also stressed that Islam opposes female circumcision. The Grand Mufti of Egypt, Ali Gomaa, said that it is "Prohibited, prohibited, prohibited."[82] The June 2007 Ministry ban eliminated a loophole that allowed girls to undergo the procedure for health

[79]Fuambai Ahmadu, "Rites and Wrongs: An Insider/Outsider Reflects on Power and Excision," in Shell-Duncan and Hernlund 2000, pp. 284–285.

[80]Rogaia Mustafa Abusharaf, "Introduction: The Custom in Question," in Abusharaf 2007, p. 8; El Guindi 2007, pp. 36–37

[81]Rogaia Mustafa Abusharaf, "Introduction: The Custom in Question," in Abusharaf 2007, p. 8; El Guindi 2007, pp. 36–37

[82]Asma El Dareer, "Attitudes of Sudanese People to the Practice of Female Circumcision", International Journal of Epidemiology, 12(2), 1983 (pp. 138–144), p. 140. doi:10.1093/ije/12.2.138 PMID 6874206

reasons.[83] There had previously been provisions under the Penal Code involving "wounding" and "intentional infliction of harm leading to death", as well as a ministerial decree prohibiting FGC. In December 1997, the Court of Cassation (Egypt's highest appeals court) upheld a government banning of the practice providing that those who did not comply would be subjected to criminal and administrative punishments. This law had proved ineffective and in a survey in 2000, a study found that 97% of the country's population still practiced FGC. In light of the widespread practice of FGC, even after the ban in 1997, some Egyptian villages decided to voluntarily give up the practice, as was the case with Abou Shawareb, which vowed in July 2005 to end the practice. However, it remains a culturally accepted practice, and a 2005 study found that over 95% of Egyptian women have undergone some form of FGC.[84]

Therefore, in Egypt, the decision of Egyptian Health Minister No. 261 of 1996 prohibits female circumcision in public hospitals and private clinics, except in medical cases only, approved by the Department of Obstetrics and Gynecology. Although this decision has been a significant development in the Department's position on the issue of female genital mutilation, it still contains a loophole for those who want to practice female circumcision. The National Council for Childhood and Motherhood organized a national project to combat female genital mutilation, which aims to mobilization of society at large, changing behaviors and renouncing the habit. The project builds on empowerment of girls at risk of female genital mutilation and information on their rights; the project aims to reach 120 villages free of female genital mutilation within a three years period.

Libya (No Data) Female genital cutting—mutilation is practiced in Libya.[85]

Sudan (91% prevalence, Type I, II and III)

Sudan was among the countries trying early to tackle the process; however, the Penal Code of 1993 does not contain any reference to criminalize the practice, which is still widespread among a large proportion of married women 15–49 years old, up to about 89%. The ratio varies between areas, where less cases are reported in the Darfur region, to reach 87% in the eastern region, and different ratios are also noted based on religion, where Muslim women FGM incidence reaches 90%, as compared to 47% for Christians.

Currently there is no law forbidding FGC, although Sudan was the first country to outlaw it in 1946, under the British. Type III was prohibited under the 1925 Penal Code, with less severe forms allowed. Outreach groups have been trying to eradicate the practice for 50 years, working with NGOs, religious groups, the government, the

---

[83]UNICEF 2013, p. 52: "The highest levels of support can be found in Mali, Guinea, Sierra Leone, Somalia, Gambia and Egypt, where more than half the female population think the practice should continue." Also see Figure 6.1, p. 54 and Figures 8.1A – 8.1D, pp. 90–91.

[84]Nafissatou J. Diop, Amadou Moreau, Hélène Benga, "Evaluation of the Long-term Impact of the TOSTAN Programme on the Abandonment of FGM/C and Early Marriage: Results from a qualitative study in Senega", UNICEF, January 2008.

[85]"Fresh progress toward the elimination of female genital mutilation and cutting in Egypt", UNICEF, 2 July 2007.

media and medical practitioners. Arrests have been made but no further action seems to have taken place. [86]Sudan signed the Maputo Protocol in June, 2008 but no ratification has yet been deposited with the African Union.

Afghanistan (no data available, however, Female genital cutting—mutilation is present in Afghanistan.[87]

Iran; No national prevalence figures available ; however, Female genital cutting—mutilation exists in Western and Southern Iran, primarily in Iranian Kurdistan where it is reported to be widespread, but also in regions such as Khuzestan.[88]

Iraq, Iraqi Kurdistan (72.7% prevalence (excluding Dohuk), Type I and II

There is no law against FGM in Iraqi Kurdistan, but in 2007 a draft legislation condemning the practice was submitted to the Regional Parliament, but was not passed.

Jordan: No national prevalence figures available; however, Female genital cutting—mutilation is prevalent in Jordan.

Oman: No national prevalence figures available; however, the practice is prevalent in Oman.

Pakistan No national prevalence figures available; however, the practice is present in certain ethnic groups in Pakistan i.e. (Dawoodi Bohra Muslims).

Palestinian territories : No national prevalence figures available; however, Female genital cutting—mutilation is prevalent in Palestinian territories.

Saudi-Arabia: No national prevalence figures available; however, Female gender cutting—mutilation is prevalent in Northern Saudi-Arabia.

Syria : No national prevalence figures available; however, circumstantial evidence suggests that Female genital cutting—mutilation exists in Syria. There is no available war data on changes in FGM in Syria

Turkey: No national prevalence figures available; however, Circumstantial evidence suggests that Female genital cutting—mutilation exists in Turkey.

United Arab Emirates: No national prevalence figures available; however, WHO mentions a study that documents Female genital cutting in United Arab Emirates, but does not provide data. A report at a conference in 2003 about the findings by the authors suggests that the practice is prevalent in rural and urban UAE, but is declining.

Yemen (23% prevalence in women 15 to 49); there is no available data on per-conflict FGM in Yemen

[86]Rogaia Mustafa Abusharaf, "Introduction: The Custom in Question," in Abusharaf 2007, p. 8; El Guindi 2007, pp. 36–37.

[87]"48/104. Declaration on the Elimination of Violence against Women", United Nations General Assembly, 20 December 1993.

[88]Sarah W. Rodriguez, "Rethinking the History of Female Circumcision and Clitoridectomy: American Medicine and Female Sexuality in the Late Nineteenth Century", Journal of the History of Medicine and Allied Sciences. 63(3), July 2008, pp. 323–347. doi:10.1093/jhmas/jrm044 PMID 18065832

In addition to the adult prevalence,[89] UNICEF reports that 20% of women aged 15–49 have a daughter who had the procedure.

In Yemen, the national level of female genital mutilation is 25%, with variations by region, where up to 96% in coastal areas, up to 38% in the mountains, and up to 38–40% in desert areas. Some studies suggest that circumcision in Yemen is prevalent in coastal areas because of the multiple waves of migration from East Africa, and that most cases of genital mutilation are done in the first weeks after birth, and that practice is mostly based on conviction of religious heritage. The Minister of Health issued in this regard a decision No. 1/3 of 2001, which prohibits carrying out female genital mutilation for all workers in public and private health services. Yemen also addressed the subject of female circumcision in a number of provinces in the framework of female genital mutilation. As a response to the catastrophic, although non-islamic, consequences of FGM, Al-Azhar Supreme Council of Islamic Research, the highest religious authority in Egypt, issued a statement saying FGM/C has no basis in core Islamic law or any of its partial provisions and that it is harmful and should not be practiced."[90] Coptic Pope Shenouda, the leader of Egypt's minority Christian community, said that neither the Qur'an nor the Bible demand or mention female circumcision.

In conclusion, FGC is predominantly practiced in Northeast Africa and parts of the Near East and Southeast Asia, although it has also been reported to occur in individual tribes in South America and Australia. Opposition is motivated by concerns regarding the consent (or lack thereof, in most cases) of the patient, and subsequently the safety and long-term consequences of the procedures. In the past several decades, there have been many concerted efforts by the World Health Organization (WHO) to end the practice of FGC. The United Nations has also declared February 6 as "International Day of Zero Tolerance to Female Genital Mutilation".[91]

The World Health Organization estimates that between 125 and 150 million women and girls alive today have experience female genital mutilation (FGM), which involves the partial or complete removal and, in some cases, reshaping of external female genitalia. This practice has no proven health benefits and puts women at risk for hemorrhaging, infection (including HIV), infertility, and complications of childbirth, cysts, as well as various other physical and psychological problems.

---

[89]Shorter 2008, p. 82; Uriel Elchalal, et al., "Ritualistic Female Genital Mutilation: Current Status and Future Outlook", Obstetrical & Gynecological Survey, 52(10), October 1997, pp. 643–651. PMID 9326757

[90]Abusharaf 2007, p. 190

[91]Martha Nussbaum, Sex and Social Justice, New York: Oxford University Press, 1999, p. 119

12.6.2 *Social Perspectives on FGM in the Arab Region*

12.6.2.1 The Culture

Cultures that practice FGM believe it is necessary for social acceptance, hygiene, and controlling female sexual desire. FGM is performed in 28 countries across Africa, as well as in parts of the Middle East and Southeast Asia. The reasons behind the continuation of this practice are related to cultural heritage and aims at ensuring the girl's marriage, social status. Despite the existence of legislation in a number of Arab countries to curb the practice of this habit, it is still widespread in some of them due to weak legislation and lack of implementation. It is worth noting the position of the OIC edited in Cairo in December 2009 as recommendations to countries against FGM.[92]

12.6.2.2 The Response

In 1959 the UN asked the WHO to investigate FGM, but the latter responded that it was not a medical matter.[93] Feminists took up the issue throughout the 1970s.[94] *Women and Sex* (1972), a book by the Egyptian physician and feminist Nawal El Saadawi, criticized FGM; the book was banned in Egypt and El Saadawi lost her job as director general of public health.[95] She followed up with a chapter, "The Circumcision of Girls," in *The Hidden Face of Eve: Women in the Arab World* (1980), which described her own clitoridectomy when she was six years old[96]

Throughout the 1990s and 2000s governments in Africa and the Middle East passed legislation banning or restricting FGM. In 2003 the African Union ratified the Maputo Protocol on the rights of women, which supported the elimination of FGM.[97] By 2015 laws restricting FGM had been passed in at least 23 of the 27 African countries in which it is concentrated, although several fell short of a ban.

Nawal El Saadawi criticized FGM in 1972, one of the first African feminists to do so publicly.

---

[92]For the Dawoodi Bohra: Diane Cole, "UNICEF Estimate Of Female Genital Mutilation Up By 70 Million", NPR, 8 February 2016. For Rahmah, Jordan: Dana Charkasi, "Female circumcision still haunts Jordanian tribe in southern Jordan", ArabNews West, 2012; Rana Sabbagh-Gargour, "The Jordanian town that still circumcises women", The Daily Star (Lebanon), 13 November 2003.

[93]Boyle 2002, p. 41.

[94]Bagnol and Mariano 2011, p. 281.

[95]Gruenbaum 2001, p. 22.

[96]Nawal El Saadawi, The Hidden Face of Eve, London: Zed Books, 2007 [1980], p. 14.

[97]Emma Bonino, "A brutal custom: Join forces to banish the mutilation of women", The New York Times, 15 September 2004; Ma UNFPA-UNICEF Joint Evaluation of the UNFPA-UNICEF Joint Programme on Female Genital Mutilation/Cutting (FGM/C): Accelerating Change, New York: United Nations Population Fundputo Protocol, pp. 7–8.

The International Response

In December 1993 the United Nations General Assembly included FGM in resolution 48/104, the Declaration on the Elimination of Violence against Women. From 2003 the UN began sponsoring an International Day of Zero Tolerance to Female Genital Mutilation, which is held every 6 February.[98]

UNICEF began in 2003 to promote an evidence-based social norms approach to the evaluation of intervention, using ideas from game theory about how communities reach decisions about FGM, and building on the work of Gerry Mackie on the ending of footbinding in China.[99] In 2005 the UNICEF Innocent Research Centre in Florence published its first report on FGM[100] UNFPA and UNICEF launched a joint program in Africa in 2007 to reduce FGM by 40% within the 0–15 age group and eliminate it entirely from at least one country by 2012, goals that were not met. [101] In 2008 several United Nations bodies, including the Office of the High Commissioner for Human Rights, published a statement recognizing FGM as a human-rights violation. In December 2012 the General Assembly passed resolution 67/146, "Intensifying global efforts for the elimination of female genital mutilations."[102] In July 2014 UNICEF and the UK government co-hosted the first Girl Summit, aimed at ending FGM and child marriage.[103] As of 2013 legislation banning FGM had been passed by 33 countries outside Africa and the Middle East[104]: As a result of immigration the practice spread to Australia, New Zealand, Europe, North America and Scandinavia, all of which outlawed it entirely or restricted it to consenting adults. Sweden outlawed it in 1982, the first Western country to do so.[105] Several former colonial powers, including Belgium, Britain, France and the Netherlands,

---

[98] "48/104. Declaration on the Elimination of Violence against Women", United Nations General Assembly, 20 December 1993.

Charlotte Feldman-Jacobs, "Commemorating International Day of Zero Tolerance to Female Genital Mutilation", Population Reference Bureau, February 2009.

[99] Francesca Moneti, David Parker, The Dynamics of Social Change, Florence: UNICEF Innocenti Research Centre, October 2010, p. 6.

[100] Michael Miller and Francesca Moneti, Changing a harmful social convention: Female genital cutting/mutilation, Florence: UNICEF Innocenti Research Centre, 2005.

[101] UNFPA-UNICEF Joint Evaluation of the UNFPA-UNICEF Joint Programme on Female Genital Mutilation/Cutting (FGM/C): Accelerating Change, New York: United Nations Population Fund, 2013 (for goals not met: "Executive Summary", p. 2).

[102] "67/146. Intensifying global efforts for the elimination of female genital mutilations", United Nations General Assembly, adopted 20 December 2012.

[103] "No time to lose: New UNICEF data show need for urgent action on female genital mutilation and child marriage", UNICEF, 22 July 2014; "Girl Summit", The Guardian.

[104] Female Genital Mutilation/Cutting: A Statistical Overview and Exploration of the Dynamics of Change, New York: United Nations Children's Fund, July 2013.

[105] Birgitta Essén, Sara Johnsdotter, "Female Genital Mutilation in the West: Traditional Circumcision versus Genital Cosmetic Surgery", Acta Obstetricia Gynecologica Scandinavica, 83(7), July 2004, pp. 611–613. PMID 15225183

followed suit, either with new laws or by making clear that it was covered by existing legislation.[106]

Canada recognized FGM as a form of persecution in July 1994, when it granted refugee status to Khadra Hassan Farah, who had fled Somalia to avoid her daughter being cut.[107] In 1997 section 268 of its Criminal Code was amended to ban FGM, except where "the person is at least eighteen years of age and there is no resulting bodily harm." As of May 2016 there had been no prosecutions.[108] In the United States the Centers for Disease Control (CDC) estimated in 2015 that 513,000 women and girls living there had experienced FGM or were at risk, as of 2012;[109] their previous estimate was 168,000 as of 1990.[110] A Nigerian woman successfully contested deportation in March 1994 on the grounds that her daughters might be cut,[111] and in 1996 Fauziya Kasinga from Togo became the first to be granted asylum to escape FGM.[112] In 1996 the Federal Prohibition of Female Genital Mutilation Act made it illegal to perform FGM on minors for non-medical reasons, and in 2013 the Transport for Female Genital Mutilation Act prohibited transporting a minor out of the country for the purpose of FGM. In addition, 24 states have legislation banning FGM.[113] The American Academy of Pediatrics opposes all forms of the practice; in 2010 it suggested that "pricking or incising the clitoral skin" was a harmless procedure that might satisfy parents, but it withdrew the statement after complaints.[114,115] The first FGM conviction in the US was in 2006, when Khalid Adem, who had emigrated from Ethiopia, was sentenced to ten years

---

[106]Boyle 2002 p. 97.

[107]Clyde H. Farnsworth, "Canada Gives Somali Mother Refugee Status", The New York Times, 21 July 1994.

[108]Corinne Packer, et al., "Canada's response to female genital mutilation: Are we failing our girls?", Canadian Medical Association Journal, 187(6), 17 February 2015, E188–189. doi:10.1503/cmaj.141215 PMC 4387059

[109]"Female Genital Mutilation/Cutting in the United States: Updated Estimates of Women and Girls at Risk, 2012", Centers for Disease Control and Prevention, Public Health Reports, 131, March–April 2016.

[110]Wanda K. Jones, et al., "Female Genital Mutilation/Female Circumcision: Who Is at Risk in the U.S.?", Public Health Reports, 112(5), September-October 1997 (pp. 368–377), p. 372. PMID 9323387

[111]Patricia Dysart Rudloff, "In Re: Oluloro: Risk of female genital mutilation as 'extreme hardship' in immigration proceedings", 26 Saint Mary's Law Journal, 877, 1995.

[112]Celia W. Dugger, "June 9–15; Asylum From Mutilation",The New York Times, 16 June 1996.

[113]"Female Genital Mutilation/Cutting in the United States: Updated Estimates of Women and Girls at Risk, 2012", Centers for Disease Control and Prevention, Public Health Reports, 131, March–April 2016.

[114]Current policy: "Female Genital Mutilation", Pediatrics, 102(1), 1 July 1998, pp. 153–156. PMID 9651425

[115]Pam Belluck, "Group Backs Ritual 'Nick' as Female Circumcision Option", The New York Times, 6 May 2010.

after severing his two-year-old daughter's clitoris with a pair of scissors.[116] According to the European Parliament, 500,000 women in Europe had undergone FGM as of March 2009.[117] France is known for its tough stance against FGM.[118] Up to 30,000 women there were thought to have experienced FGM as of 1995. Colette Gallard, a family-planning counselor, writes that when FGM was first encountered in France, the reaction was that Westerners ought not to intervene, and it took the deaths of two girls in 1982, one of them three months old, for that attitude to change.[119] The practice is outlawed by a provision of France's penal code dealing with violence against children.[120] All children under six who were born in France undergo medical examinations that include inspection of the genitals, and doctors are obliged to report FGM.[121] The first civil suit was in 1982 and the first criminal prosecution in 1993.[122] In 1999 a woman was given an eight-year sentence for having performed FGM on 48 girls.[123] By 2014 over 100 parents and two practitioners had been prosecuted in over 40 criminal cases.[124] Around 137,000 women and girls living in England and Wales were born in countries where FGM is practised (as of 2011).[125] Performing FGM on children or adults was outlawed under the Prohibition of Female Circumcision Act 1985.[126] This was replaced by the Female Genital Mutilation Act 2003 and Prohibition of Female Genital Mutilation (Scotland) Act 2005, which added a prohibition on arranging FGM outside the

---

[116]"Man gets 10-year sentence for circumcision of 2-year-old daughter", Associated Press, 1 November 2006.

[117]P. Stanley Yoder, Shanxiao Wang, Elise Johansen, "Estimates of Female Genital Mutilation/ Cutting in 27 African Countries and Yemen", Studies in Family Planning, 44(2), June 2013, pp. 189–204. doi:10.1111/j.

[118]Renée Kool and Sohail Wahedi, "Criminal Enforcement in the Area of Female Genital Mutilation in France, England and the Netherlands: A Comparative Law Perspective", International Law Research, 3(1), 2014, pp. 3–5.

[119]Colette Gallard, "Female genital mutilation in France", British Medical Journal, 310, 17 June 1995, p. 1592. PMID 7787655 PMC

[120]Megan Rowling "France reduces genital cutting with prevention, prosecutions – lawyer", Thomson Reuters Foundation, 27 September 2012.

[121]Renée Kool and Sohail Wahedi, "Criminal Enforcement in the Area of Female Genital Mutilation in France, England and the Netherlands: A Comparative Law Perspective", International Law Research, 3(1), 2014, pp. 3–5. doi:10.5539/ilr.v3n1p1

[122]Gallard 1995, p. 1593; for 1993, Farnsworth (New York Times) 1994.

[123]David Gollaher, Circumcision: A History of the World's Most Controversial Surgery, New York: Basic Books, 2000, p. 189

[124]Renée Kool and Sohail Wahedi, "Criminal Enforcement in the Area of Female Genital Mutilation in France, England and the Netherlands: A Comparative Law Perspective", International Law Research, 3(1), 2014, pp. 3–5. doi:10.5539/ilr.v3n1p1

[125]J. A. Black, G. D. Debelle, "Female genital mutilation in Britain", British Medical Journal, 310, 17 June 1995. PMID 7787654 PMC 2549951 doi:10.1136/bmj.310.6994.1590

[126]Kool and Wahedi 2014, pp. 5–7; "Prohibition of Female Circumcision Act 1985", legislation. gov.uk.

country for British citizens or permanent residents.[127] The United Nations Committee on the Elimination of Discrimination against Women asked the government in 2013 to "ensure the full implementation of its legislation on FGM."[128] The first charges were brought the following year against a physician and another man, after the physician stitched an infibulated woman after opening her for childbirth. Both men were acquitted in 2015

The Regional Response

Recent research conducted on female genital mutilation shows that the continuation of this practice is linked to "cultural heritage", specifically the notion that its practice will help ensure that girls get married and attain a respectable social status. Despite the existence of legislation in a number of Arab countries to help reduce FGM practices, it is still widely practiced due to weak enforcement of the legislation.

Sudan was among the first countries that tried to combat FGM practices, but the country's Penal Code of 1993 makes no reference whatsoever to the criminalization of such practices, which are still prevalent among a large proportion of married women in the age group of 15–49 years. Prevalence rates stood at 68.4% in 2006 with disparities between regions; while the Darfur region experienced the lowest prevalence rate, it was as high as 87% in the Eastern region. The FGM/C rates also vary by religion, with 90% of Muslim women being affected compared to 47% of Christian women. Sudan is implementing a national strategy to eliminate female genital mutilation within the generation of women (2008–2018) under the Program for Elimination of FGM/C, which is being implemented by National Council for Child Welfare

In Egypt, the state has given special attention to the issue of FGM/C, prioritizing it on the national agenda for child issues in Egypt. In this context, the National Council for Childhood and Motherhood, which was first established in 2003, created a national program to combat FGM/C practices in the country. This socio-cultural practice was considered as a violation to the fundamental rights of females in Egypt and is not proscribed by religion and does not promote health, two rationales the practice was linked with previously. A comprehensive program has been designed to handle this aspect of FGM.

In Yemen, female circumcision rates are as high as 25% nationally, but with wide regional variations; prevalence rates stand at 96% in coastal areas, 38% in the mountains and 38–40% in desert areas. According to some studies conducted in Yemen, female circumcision is more prevalent in coastal areas because of multiple

[127] "Female Genital Mutilation Act 2003" and "Prohibition of Female Genital Mutilation (Scotland) Act 2005", legislation.gov.uk.

[128] "Concluding observations on the seventh periodic report of the United Kingdom of Great Britain and Northern Ireland", United Nations Convention on the Elimination of All Forms of Discrimination against Women, 26 July 2013, p. 6, paras 36, 37.

waves of migration from Eastern Africa. Most circumcisions are performed in the first weeks after birth, and the practice is based mostly on a legacy of religious heritage. In this regard, a decision by the Minister of Health (No. 01 /03 of 2001) bans the practice of FGM/C by all health service providers in both the public and private sectors. The subject of female circumcision is also being addressed in a number of provinces within the framework of a project to combat FGM/C.

Whilst FGM is widely practiced out in the open by many communities of varied faiths in its locus of concentration in Northeastern Africa,[129] it is practiced in different parts of the Middle East. In the Arab peninsula, Types I and II FGM are usually performed, often referred to as Sunna circumcision. The practice occurs particularly in northern Saudi Arabia, southern Jordan, and northern Iraq (Kurdistan)[130.131] In the Iraqi village of Hasira, a recent study found that 60% of the women and girls reported having undergone FGM.[132] Before the study, there had been no solid proof of the prevalence of the practice. There is also circumstantial evidence to suggest that Female genital cutting is practiced in the Kurdish regions of Syria, Turkey and Iran. In Oman, a few communities still practice Female genital cutting; however, experts believe that the number of such cases is small and declining annually. In the United Arab Emirates and Saudi Arabia, it is practiced mainly among foreign workers from East Africa and the Nile Valley. A 2009 study suggested that FGM had virtually disappeared among the Negev Bedouin due to modernization process under Israeli rule. Female genital Cutting—mutilation is practiced in Palestinian territories. The countries where FGC is commonly practiced were identified by the US State Department.[133,134] The practice is rooted in gender inequality, attempts to control women's sexuality, and ideas about purity, modesty and aesthetics. It is usually initiated and carried out by women, who see it as a source of honor, and who fear that failing to have their daughters and granddaughters cut will expose the girls to social exclusion.[135] The health effects depend on the

[129]Salah M. Rasheedemail, Ahmed H. Abd-Ellah, Fouad M. Yousef, "Female genital mutilation in Upper Egypt in the new millennium", International Journal of Gynecology and Obstetrics, 114(1), July 2011, pp. 47–50. doi:10.1016/j.ijgo.2011.02.003 PMID 21513937

[130]UNICEF 2013. For eight percent in Iraq: p. 27, box 4.4, group 5); for the regions in Iraq: p. 31, map 4.6).

Berivan A. Yasin, et al, "Female genital mutilation among Iraqi Kurdish women: a cross-sectional study from Erbil city", BMC Public Health, 13, September 2013. PMID 24010850 PMC 3844478 doi:10.1186/1471-2458-13-809

[131]Chad: UNICEF 2013, pp. 35–36.

[132]"Guinea" (2012), UNICEF statistical profile, July 2014, p. 2/4.

[133]Rogaia Mustafa Abusharaf, "Introduction: The Custom in Question," in Abusharaf 2007, p. 8; El Guindi 2007, pp. 36–37

[134]"Female Genital Mutilation/Cutting in the United States: Updated Estimates of Women and Girls at Risk, 2012", Centers for Disease Control and Prevention, Public Health Reports, 131, March–April 2016.

[135]UNICEF 2013: "There is a social obligation to conform to the practice and a widespread belief that if they [families] do not, they are likely to pay a price that could include social exclusion, criticism, ridicule, stigma or the inability to find their daughters suitable marriage partners."[2]:15

procedure; they can include recurrent infections, difficulty urinating and passing menstrual flow, chronic pain, the development of cysts, an inability to get pregnant, complications during childbirth, and fatal bleeding.[136] There are no known health benefits.[137]

Over 80% (of those cut) are cut before the age of five in Nigeria, Mali, Eritrea, Ghana and Mauritania. The 1997 Demographic and Health Survey in Yemen found that 76 percent of girls had been cut within two weeks of birth.[138] The percentage is reversed in Somalia, Egypt, Chad and the Central African Republic, where over 80 percent (of those cut) are cut between five and 14.[139] Just as the type of FGM is often linked to ethnicity, so is the mean age. In Kenya, for example, the Kisi cut around age 10 and the Kamba at 16.[140]

UNICEF has noted that the Arab world has yet to make decisive moves in the eradication of the practice of female genital mutilation (FGM), a practice that jeopardizes the health, safety and development of girls.[141] A recent survey showed that 97 per cent of Egyptian women of reproductive age have been subjected to the practice, while 8 out of 10 mothers had either circumcised their daughters or intended to have a daughter circumcised in the future.[142]

Prevalence rates are estimated to be 23 per cent in Yemen, and there are also reports, but no clear evidence, of this practice in southern Jordan, Gaza, Oman and Iraq.[143] A 2005 survey by WADI, a German NGO, had found that 60 per cent of women and girls aged older than 10 had undergone the operation in Kurdish areas of Iraq.[144]

FGM has been outlawed or restricted in most of the countries in which it occurs, but the laws are poorly enforced. There have been international efforts since the 1970s to persuade practitioners to abandon it, and in 2012 the United Nations General Assembly, recognizing FGM as a human-rights violation, voted

[136]Jasmine Abdulcadira, et al., “Care of women with female genital mutilation/cutting”, Swiss Medical Weekly, 6(14), January 2011. doi:10.4414/smw.2011.13137 PMID 21213149

[137]“Female genital mutilation”, Geneva: World Health Organization, February 2016.

[138]Michael Miller and Francesca Moneti, Changing a harmful social convention: Female genital cutting/mutilation, Florence: UNICEF Innocenti Research Centre, 2005.

[139]Female Genital Mutilation/Cutting: A Statistical Overview and Exploration of the Dynamics of Change, New York: United Nations Children’s Fund, July 2013.

[140]Female Genital Mutilation/Cutting: A Statistical Overview and Exploration of the Dynamics of Change, New York: United Nations Children’s Fund, July 2013.

[141]UNICEF 2014:

[142]“Female genital mutilation: issues and impact”, UNICEF, http://www.unicef.org/egypt/protection_148.html

[143]State of the World’s Children 2007 – Middle East and North Africa edition”, UNICEF, 2007

[144]Iraqi Kurdistan: Draft for a Law Prohibiting Female Genital Mutilation is submitted to the Kurdish Regional Parliament”, Stop FGM in Kurdistan, 23 November 2007, Suleymaniya/Berlin, http://www.stopfgmkurdistan.org/en/press2.htm

unanimously to intensify those efforts.[145] The opposition is not without its critics, particularly among anthropologists. Eric Silverman writes that FGM has become one of anthropology's central moral topics, raising difficult questions about cultural relativism, tolerance and the universality of human rights.[146]

Advocacy efforts to criminalize FGM are being led by women's organizations in the region.

Women's organizations in Kurdish Regional Government have been advocating for legislation that will criminalize FGM and a draft Law prohibiting FGM has been submitted to the Kurdish Regional Parliament. In Egypt, the amendments to 1996 Child Law condemn this practice, which has persisted despite Decrees by the Ministry of Health, while in Yemen, a January 2001 Ministerial Decree banning FGM, combined with awareness efforts by civil society groups, have reportedly reduced incidences of FGM.

Tolerance Versus Human Rights

Anthropologist Eric Silverman wrote in 2004 that FGM had "emerged as one of the central moral topics of contemporary anthropology." Anthropologists have accused FGM eradicationists of cultural colonialism. In turn, anthropologists have been criticized for their moral relativism and failure to defend the idea of universal human rights.[147] According to the opposition's critics, the biological reductionism of the opposition to FGM, and the failure to appreciate FGM's cultural context, serves to "other" the people who practice it and undermines their agency—in particular when African parents are referred to as "mutilators."[148] Africans who object to the tone of the opposition to FGM risk appearing to defend the practice[149,150,151]—including dry sex, polygyny, bride price and levirate marriage.[152,153]

---

[145]Intensifying global efforts for the elimination of female genital mutilations", United Nations General Assembly, adopted 20 December 2012. Emma Bonino, "Banning Female Genital Mutilation", The New York Times, 19 December 2012.

[146]Eric K. Silverman, "Anthropology and Circumcision," Annual Review of Anthropology, 33, 2004, pp. 419–445. JSTOR 25064860

[147]Eric K. Silverman, "Anthropology and Circumcision," Annual Review of Anthropology, 33, 2004, pp. 419–445. JSTOR 25064860

[148]Vicky Kirby, "Out of Africa: 'Our Bodies Ourselves?'" in Obioma Nnaemeka (ed.), Female Circumcision and the Politics of Knowledge: African Women in Imperialist Discourses, Westport: Praeger, 2005, p. 83.

[149]Obioma Nnaemeka, "African Women, Colonial Discourses, and Imperialist Interventions: Female Circumcision as Impetus," in Nnaemeka 2005, p. 33.

[150]Nnaemeka 2005, p. 34.

[151]Tamale 2011, pp. 19–20.

[152]Tamale 2011, pp. 19–20.

[153]Tamale 2011, pp. 19–20.

The debate has highlighted a tension between anthropology and feminism, with the former's focus on tolerance and the latter's on equal rights for all women, presenting African women as victims of false consciousness participating in their own oppression, a position promoted by several feminists in the 1970s and 1980s. It prompted the French Association of Anthropologists to issue a statement in 1981, at the height of the early debates, that "a certain feminism resuscitates (today) the moralistic arrogance of yesterday's colonialism.[154] As an example of the disrespect arguably shown toward women who have undergone FGM, commentators highlight the appropriation of the women's bodies as exhibits, such asthe publication in 1996 of the Pulitzer-prize-winning photographs of a 16-year-old Kenyan girl undergoing FGM. The photographs were published by 12 American newspapers, but according to Korieh the girl had not given permission for the images to be taken, much less published.[155]

Comparison with Other Procedures

The crucial question, broader than FGM, is why the female body is subjected to so much "abuse and indignity" around the world, including a parallel between FGM and cosmetic procedures.[156] Some cosmetic genital procedures drive the advance of female genital mutilation by encouraging women to see natural variations as defects,[157] like comparing FGM to breast enhancement, in which the maternal function of the breast becomes secondary to men's sexual pleasure[158] or citing FGM and cosmetic surgery as sexist and patriarchal[159] , although some maintain that FGM may be conducive to women's well-being within their communities in the same way that rhinoplasty and male circumcision may help people elsewhere.[160] In Egypt, despite the 2007 ban, women wanting FGM for their daughters discuss the need for *amalyet tajmeel* (cosmetic surgery) to remove what is viewed as excess genital tissue for a more acceptable appearance.[161]

---

[154] Christine J. Walley, "Searching for 'Voices': Feminism, Anthropology, and the Global Over Female Genital Operations" in James and Robertson 2002, pp. 18, 34 (for false consciousness), 43.

[155] Chima Korieh, "'Other' Bodies: Western Feminism, Race and Representation in Female Circumcision Discourse," in Nnaemeka 2005, pp. 121–122.

[156] Marge Berer, "It's female genital mutilation and should be prosecuted", British Medical Journal, 334(7608), 30 June 2007, p. 1335. PMID 17599983 PMC 1906631 doi:10.1136/bmj.39252.646042.3A

[157] Ronán M. Conroy, "Female genital mutilation: whose problem, whose solution?", British Medical Journal, 333(7559), 15 July 2006. PMID 16840444 PMC 1502236

[158] El Guindi 2007, p. 33.

[159] Lora Wildenthal, The Language of Human Rights in West Germany, Philadelphia: University of Pennsylvania Press, 2012, p. 148.

[160] Obermeyer 1999, p. 94.

[161] Rahim (Tahrir Institute) 2014.

The WHO does not cite procedures such as labiaplasty and clitoral hood reduction as examples of FGM, but its definition aims to avoid loopholes, so several elective practices on adults do fall within its categories.[162] Some of the laws banning FGM, including in Canada and the US, focus only on minors. Several countries, including Sweden and the UK, have banned it regardless of consent, and the legislation would seem to cover cosmetic procedures. Sweden, for example, has banned "operations on the external female genital organs which are designed to mutilate them or produce other permanent changes in them . . . regardless of whether consent to this operation has or has not been given. It seems the law distinguishes between Western and African genitals, and deems only African women (such as those seeking reinfibulation after childbirth) unfit to make their own decisions.[163]

Arguing against suggested similarities between FGM and dieting or body shaping, a key difference is that FGM is mostly conducted on children using physical force. She argues that the distinction between social pressure and physical force is morally and legally salient, comparable to the distinction between seduction and rape. She argues further that the literacy of women in practicing countries is generally poorer than in developed nations, and that this reduces their ability to make informed choices.[164]

Several commentators maintain that children's rights are violated with the genital alteration of intersex children, who are born with anomalies that physicians choose to correct; thousands of these procedures take place every year in the United States, and say that they are medically unnecessary, more extensive than FGM, and have more serious physical and mental consequences. They attribute the silence of anti-FGM campaigners about intersex procedures to white privilege and a refusal to acknowledge that "similar unnecessary and harmful genital cutting occurs in their own backyards."[165]

12.6.3 Example of National Strategy to Reduce FGM: Egypt

Some countries that prohibited FGC still experience the practice in secrecy. In many cases, enforcement of this prohibition is a low priority for governments. Other countries have tried to educate practitioners to make it easier and safer instead of outlawing the practice entirely. However, with pressure from the WHO and other

---

[162] "Eliminating Female genital mutilation: An Interagency Statement", Geneva: World Health Organization, 2008.

[163] Sara Johnsdotter and Birgitta Essén, "Genitals and ethnicity: the politics of genital modifications", Reproductive Health Matters, 18(35), 2010, pp. 29–37. PMID 20541081 doi:10.1016/S0968-8080(10)35495-4

[164] Nussbaum 1999, pp. 123–124.

[165] Nancy Ehrenreich, Mark Barr, "Intersex Surgery, Female Genital Cutting, and the Selective Condemnation of 'Cultural Practices'", Harvard Civil Rights-Civil Liberties Law Review, 40(1), 2005 (pp. 71–140), pp. 74–75.

groups, laws are being passed in regards to FGC. The first known non-colonial campaign against FGM began in Egypt in the 1920s, when the Egyptian Doctors' Society called for a ban.[166] There was a parallel campaign in Sudan, run by religious leaders and British women. Infibulation was banned there in 1946, but the law was unpopular and barely enforced.[167] The Egyptian government banned infibulation in state-run hospitals in 1959, but allowed partial clitoridectomy if parents requested it.[168]

On June 28, 2007 Egypt banned female genital cutting after the death of 12-year-old Badour Shaker during a genital circumcision. The Guardian of Britain reported that her death "sparked widespread condemnation" of the practice.[169]

Egypt has launched the FGM/C National Program to fight this socio-cultural practice that violates the fundamental rights of the Egyptian child (a practice that has no health or religious precedents). These efforts are part of an integrated program covering the following key themes aimed at:

- Building a resource test-base against FGM/C in Egyptian villages, relying on partnerships with NGOs (21 NGOs) and local leaders; adopting initiatives to deliver health, educational, cultural and social services. Such initiatives would help inform public opinion against FGM/C within each village. The (model) program has been implemented in 120 villages, targets the girl child and can be replicated at the national level. It allocates 40% of its total funding to the national program for support to NGOs through institutional capacity building and implementation of community based initiatives at the sites where the program is executed.
- Developing a public opinion against FGM/C practices through a strategy involving media campaigns. An extensive media response to the concerns of the community has been developed and is, perceived and viewed as an integrated medical, religious, social and legal campaign; all media outlets, including the press, radio and television and the Internet, in addition to advertising in public places and on roads,, contributed to this effort.
- Tackling the phenomenon of practicing FGM/C by doctors, this can be achieved through support to doctors in rural health units by supplying them with scientific and medical information on FGM/C. It can also be achieved through training of doctors to provide appropriate advice to Egyptian families with a view to preventing FGM/C, and activating ministerial decisions on the prohibition of

[166]UNICEF 2013, p. 10, calls the Egyptian Doctors' Society opposition the "first known campaign" against FGM; for independence, Boddy 2007, p. 147.

[167]FGM is still practised in Sudan. Some states banned it in 2008–2009, but as of 2013, there was no national legislation.

[168]Elizabeth Heger Boyle, Female Genital Cutting: Cultural Conflict in the Global Community, Baltimore: Johns Hopkins University Press, 2002, pp. 92, 103. (Egypt banned FGM entirely in 2007.)

[169]El Guindi 2007, p. 4

FGM/C practices through medical health service providers, and enforce the law incriminating perpetrators of FGM/C.

- Issuing a new legislation to criminalize FGM/C practices by raising awareness amongst the judiciary (judges and prosecutors) and the members of the People's Assembly about FGM/C-related health issues and the various related social, religious and legal aspects. The purpose is to render meaningful and instrumental the involvement of all these stakeholders in a proposed bill to incriminate the FGM/C practice.
- Encouraging male and female youth volunteerism, and form youth groups within educational and cultural institutions; the aim is to change prevailing misconceptions/beliefs about FGM/C amongst future parents, extending "child-to-child" education.
- Coordinating national efforts with line ministries, civil society and the media to incorporate FGM/C prevention in the strategies of the institutions concerned with this phenomenon.
- Educating the public about the issues to increase reporting on planned FGM/C incidences from across Egypt via a dedicated 24-hour toll-free line (Child Helpline 16000). These calls were received confidentially, and FGM/C-specific questions and counseling communications were also received via the Child Rescue Helpline, accounting for 65% of the total calls.
- Having FGM/C criminalization approved by the People's Assembly and Shura Council, and punish those who perform this practice, which violates the rights and dignity of girls in Egypt. The provisions of the law criminalizing FGM/C, Article 242 bis, punish: "FGM/C practitioners without prejudice, to any severe penalty provided for under the law by a minimum three-month to a maximum two-year imprisonment, or a minimum of one-thousand to a maximum of five-thousand Egyptians-Pound fine for all wounds punishable under Articles 241 and 242 of the Penal Code". i. A Circular was issued to the Attorney General, illustrating the general philosophy behind the amendments to the Children's Rights Act; the letter includes a separate section explaining steps for the implementation and investigation of FGM/C cases.

Chapter 13
Honor Killings and Crimes; Familial and Tribal Homicide

13.1 Abstract

Honor killings are directed mostly against women and girls.[1] Although rarely, men can also be the victims of honor killings by members of the family of a woman with whom they are perceived to have an inappropriate relationship.[2] The loose term "honor killing" applies to killing of both men and women in cultures that practice it.[3] There is a strong positive correlation between violence against women—as well as LGBT—and women's lack of social power and equality on the one hand, and a baseline of development, associated with access to basic resources, health care, and human capital, such as literacy on the other.[4] In a male-dominated society, there is more inequality between men, and women lose out not just physically and economically, but crucially because men who feel subordinated will often try to regain a sense of their authority in turn by excessive subordination of those below them, i.e. women, although both men and women in such societies suffer more violence and worse health. Some women who bridge social divides, publicly engage other communities, or adopt some of the customs or the religion of an outside group may be attacked. In countries that receive immigrants, some otherwise low-status immigrant men and boys have asserted their dominant patriarchal status by inflicting

---

[1] "Violence Against Women and "Honor" Crimes". Human Rights Watch. Retrieved 6 April 2001.

[2] Afghan couple stoned to death – Central & South Asia. Al Jazeera English (16 August 2010). Retrieved on 1 October 2011.

[3] Ouis, P. and Myhrman, T., editors. Gender-Based Sexual Violence against Teenage Girls in the Middle East: A Comparative Situation Analysis of Honour Violence, Early Marriages and Sexual Abuse in Lebanon, the Occupied Palestinian Territories and Yemen. Save the Children Sweden, Regional Office for the Middle East and North Africa, 2007.

[4] "Ethics: Honour Crimes". BBC. 1 January 1970. Retrieved 23 December 2013.

B. Gerbaka et al., *Child Sexual Abuse, Exploitation and Trafficking in the Arab Region*, Child Maltreatment 13, https://doi.org/10.1007/978-3-030-66507-4_13

honor killings on female family members who have participated in public life, for example, in feminist and integration politics.[5]

13.2 What Is It? Who Are the Victims?

An honor killing or honor killing[6] is the killing of a member of a family or social group by other members, due to the belief of the perpetrators (and potentially the wider community) that the victim has brought dishonor upon the family or community. or has violated the principles of a community or a religion, usually for reasons such as refusing to enter an arranged marriage, being in a relationship that is disapproved by their family, having sex outside marriage, becoming the victim of rape, dressing in ways which are deemed inappropriate,[7] engaging in non-heterosexual relations[8] or renouncing a faith.[9,10]

Furthermore, Honor killings are acts of vengeance, usually death, committed by male family members against female family members, who are held to have brought dishonor upon the family. A woman can be targeted by (individuals within) her family for a variety of reasons, including: refusing to enter into an arranged marriage, being the victim of a sexual assault, seeking a divorce—even from an abusive husband—or (allegedly) committing adultery. The mere perception that a woman has behaved in a way that "dishonors" her family is sufficient to trigger an attack on her life.[11] In some honor-based societies individuals are punished by death for violating cultural and religious norms.

Women and LGBT[12] identified people are disproportionately affected by this custom, as this punishment is carried out for individuals who have been raped, refuse suitors, have extra-marital sexual relations, seek divorce, or engage in homosexual acts. These killings are often carried out through stoning, shooting, burning, and live burial. Husbands and male family members who commit these killings often escape punishment or face reduced sentences because these crimes are viewed as socially acceptable in certain areas.

[5]Teen Lovers killed in India Honor Killing. LiveLeak.com

[6]"SECRETARY-GENERAL, IN ADDRESS TO "WOMEN 2000" SPECIAL SESSION, SAYS FUTURE OF PLANET DEPENDS UPON WOMEN". United Nations.

[7]"Honor killing definition". dictionary.reference.com. Retrieved 23 December 2013.

[8]"Shocking gay honor killing inspires movie – CNN.com". Edition.cnn.com. Retrieved 16 August 2013.

[9]"Ethics: Honour Crimes". BBC. 1 January 1970. Retrieved 23 December 2013

[10]"Honor killing: Definition and More from the Free Merriam-Webster Dictionary". merriam-webster.com. 31 August 2012. Retrieved 23 December 2013.

[11]"Violence Against Women and "Honor" Crimes". Human Rights Watch. Retrieved 6 April 2001.

[12] *"Shocking gay honor killing inspires movie – CNN.com". Edition.cnn.com*

13.3 Honor Killings in International Human Rights

In its annual report, Amnesty International confirmed that 'Honor killings persisted in Jordan, occupied Palestinian territories, Iraq, Syria and other states in which the perpetrators benefited from laws that belittled their crimes'.[13,14]According to UNICEF, available data indicate that honor killings also occur in Egypt, Lebanon, Morocco, and Yemen—in 1999, Jordan's Family Protection Department dealt with 507 cases of family violence, of which 38% were crimes of honor; in the Occupied Palestinian Territory, 20 honor killings and 15 attempts were recorded between March 2004 and March 2005.[15]

Perpetrators of honor killings are often unpunished, and when cases are brought to court, tend to receive lenient sentences. In Jordan, civil society organizations have raised concerns about Article 97 of the Penal Code, which allows the guardian of an abused child to drop charges against perpetrators, and articles 340, 98 and 99, which accords lenience to "honor" crimes, with sentences not severe enough to have a deterring effect.[16] UNICEF reports that in Syria, women themselves were found to be responsible for the defendants' actions in 55% of cases where husbands killed their wives for adultery.[17] Civil society groups across the region are advocating for legislative environment that better protects women and girls.

The cultural features which lead to honor killings are complex. Honor killings involve violence and fear as a tool of maintaining control. Honor killings are argued to have their origin among nomadic peoples and herdsmen: such populations carry all their valuables with them and risk having them stolen, and do not have proper recourse to law. As a result, inspiring fear, using aggression, and cultivating a reputation for violent revenge in order to protect property is preferred to other behaviors. In societies where there is a weak rule of law, people must build fierce reputations.[18]

[13]Amnesty International Report 2007 – The State of the World' Human Rights', Amnesty International.

[14]"*Broken bodies, shattered minds: Torture and ill-treatment of women". Amnesty International.*

[15]UNICEF, 2007, Op. Cit

[16]"Making Children's Rights Work: Country Profile on Jordan", International Bureau for Children's Rights, 2007.

[17]UNICEF, 2007, Op. Cit.

[18]"Historical Context – Origins of Honour Killing/Honour Killing – Worldwide/Honour Killing – In Countries with Islamic Law – Preliminary Examination of so-called Honour Killings in Canada". Justice.gc.ca. Retrieved 2015-02-15.

13.4 Honor Crimes and Violence

Honor crimes represent the most severe type of criminal acts and domestic violence against females. This type of crime is driven by dominant beliefs concerning honor within the family unit, in many cases pertaining to relationships conducted outside of wedlock by female members of family. Generally, information about this type of violence is rare. Honor crimes are indeed the most severe types of domestic violence against girls, and are led by prevailing beliefs about shame and honor. In general, little information is available on this kind of violence.[19] The distinctive nature of honor killings is the collective nature of the crime—many members of an extended family plan the act together, sometimes through a formal "family council". Another significant feature is the connection of honor killings to the control of women's behavior, in particular in regard to sexuality/male interaction/marriage, by the family as a collective. Another key aspect is the importance of the reputation of the family in the community, and the stigma associated with losing social status, particularly in tight-knit communities.[20] Another characteristic of honor killings is that the perpetrators often don't face negative stigma within their communities, because their behavior is seen as justified.[21,22]

13.5 Societal Approaches

The incidence of honor killings is very difficult to determine and estimates vary widely.[23,24] Most of such crimes are described in Arab countries, but also in Asian and African countries, as well as, increasingly, in western countries.[25] Algeria, Oman, Morocco do not report the existence of the phenomenon, as well as Jordan,[26] Syria and Lebanon, where there are laws to prevent crimes of honor; in Libya, a law

[19]"Iraqi immigrant convicted in Arizona 'honor killing' awaits sentence – CNN.com". Edition.cnn.com. 23 February 2011. Retrieved 16 August 2013.

[20]"FAQ". Hbv-awareness.com. Retrieved 2015-02-15.

[21]"Introduction – Preliminary Examination of so-called Honour Killings in Canada". Justice.gc.ca. Retrieved 2015-02-15.

[22]Holt, Gerry (2014-05-29). "BBC News – Why do families kill their daughters?". Bbc.com. Retrieved 2015-02-15.

[23]http://www.unl.edu/rhames/courses/212/readings/honor-kil-ng.pdf

[24]"Honor Killings: Amnesty USA". webcache.googleusercontent.com. Retrieved 23 December 2013.

[25]""Honor killing" under growing scrutiny in the U.S. – Crimesider". CBS News. Retrieved 16 August 2013.

[26]Maher, Ahmed (20 June 2013). "Many Jordan teenagers 'support honour killings'". bbc.co.uk. Retrieved 23 December 2013.

bans and punishes crimes of honor. Other countries did not provide information on the subject.[27]

The OIC edited recommendations in December 2009 to stop crimes of honor. In most countries data on honor killings is not collected systematically, and many of these killings are reported by the families as suicides or accidents and registered as such. A forced suicide may be a substitute for an honor killing. In this case, the family members do not directly kill the victim themselves, but force him or her to commit suicide, in order to avoid punishment. Such suicides are reported to be common in southeastern Turkey,[28] Iraq and Iran.[29] It was reported that in 2001, 565 women lost their lives in honor-related crimes in Iran, of which 375 were reportedly staged as self-immolation.[30] In 2008, self-immolation, "occurred in all the areas of Kurdish settlement (in Iran), where it was more common than in other parts of Iran". It is claimed that in Iraqi Kurdistan, many deaths are reported as "female suicides" in order to conceal honor-related crimes.[31]

Although honor killings are often associated with the Asian continent, especially the Middle East Arab and non-Arab countries like Turkey,[32,33] including different cultures and Kurdish areas,[34,35]Pakistan,[36] Iran, Afghanistan[37,38]and South Asia, they occur all over the world, including immigrant populations.[39] In 2000, the United Nations estimated that 5000 women were victims of honor killings each

---

[27]"UNICEF Turkey: Protective Environment for Children; Honour Crimes and Forced Suicides". unicef.org.tr. Retrieved 23 December 2013.

[28]"UN probes Turkey 'forced suicide'". BBC News. 24 May 2006. Retrieved 23 December 2013.

[29]"UNICEF Turkey: Protective Environment for Children; Honour Crimes and Forced Suicides". unicef.org.tr. Retrieved 23 December 2013.

[30]Amnesty International (2008, July). Human Rights Abuses against the Kurdish Minority. London: Amnesty International.

[31]Kurdish Human Rights Project European Parliament Project: The Increase in Kurdish Women Committing Suicide Final Report

[32]"UNICEF Turkey: Protective Environment for Children; Honor Crimes and Forced Suicides". unicef.org.tr. Retrieved 23 December 2013.

[33]AYSAN SEV'ER. "Feminist Analysis of Honor Killings in Rural Turkey" (PDF). 'University of Toronto'. Retrieved 2 January 2015.

[34]Ahmet Kaya, Ahmet Yildiz's cousin, said Mr. Yildiz was the only son of a deeply religious and wealthy Kurdish family from Sanliurfa, in the predominantly Kurdish southeast.

[35]Hilal Onur Ince, Aysun Yarali and Dogancan Ozsel. "Customary Killings in Turkey and Turkish Modernization". Middle Eastern Studies. Middle Eastern Studies. 45: 537–551. Retrieved 2 December 2011.

[36]"PAKISTAN Honour killings of girls and women". Amnesty International. Archived from the original on 5 June 2008. Retrieved 15 April 2008.

[37]Afghan couple stoned to death – Central & South Asia. Al Jazeera English (16 August 2010). Retrieved on 1 October 2011.

[38]"PAKISTAN Honour killings of girls and women". Amnesty International. Archived from the original on 5 June 2008. Retrieved 15 April 2008.

[39]"Iraqi immigrant convicted in Arizona 'honor killing' awaits sentence – CNN.com". Edition.cnn.com. 23 February 2011. Retrieved 16 August 2013.

year.[40] According to BBC, "Women's advocacy groups, however, suspect that more than 20,000 women are killed worldwide each year."[41] Murder is not the only form of honor crime, other crimes such as acid attacks, abduction, mutilations, beatings occur; in 2010 the UK police recorded at least 2823 such crimes.[42] An honor killing or honor killing is the killing of a member of a family or social group by other members, due to the belief of the perpetrators (and potentially the wider community) that the victim has brought dishonor upon the family or community. Honor killings are directed mostly against women and girls. In some honor-based societies individuals are punished by death for violating cultural and religious norms. Women and LGBT identified people are disproportionately affected by this custom, as this punishment is carried out for individuals who have been raped, refuse suitors, have extra-marital sexual relations, seek divorce, or engage in homosexual acts. These killings are often carried out through stoning, shooting, burning, and live burial. Husbands and male family members who commit these killings often escape punishment or face reduced sentences because these crimes are viewed as socially acceptable in certain areas.

13.6 How Does the Concept of Honor Lead to Violence?

In, what we can refer to as, honor-cultures children are threatened by or exposed to violence in issues related to their sexual morality and general behavior. In each country concerned here, a number of teenage girls are being killed annually. It should be noted that honor violence is not a sexual-violent act in itself, but is violence based on controlling the sexuality of females. The perceived dishonor is normally the result of one of the following behaviors, or the suspicion of such behaviors:

- Dressing in a manner unacceptable to the family or community,
- Wanting to terminate or prevent an arranged marriage or desiring to marry by own choice,
- Engaging in heterosexual sexual acts outside marriage, or even due to a non-sexual relationship perceived as inappropriate, and
- Engaging in homosexual acts. Women and girls are killed at a much higher rate than men.

---

[40]""Honor killing" under growing scrutiny in the U.S. – Crimesider". CBS News. Retrieved 16 August 2013.

[41]Holt, Gerry (2014-05-29). "BBC News – Why do families kill their daughters?". Bbc.com. Retrieved 2015-02-15.

[42]"'Honor' attack numbers revealed by UK police forces". bbc.co.uk. 3 December 2011. Retrieved 23 December 2013.

The United Nations Population Fund (UNFPA) estimates that perhaps as many as 5000 women and girls a year are killed by members of their own families. Many women's groups in the Middle East and Southwest Asia suspect the victims are at least four times more.

Methods of killing include stoning, stabbing, beating, burning, beheading, hanging, throat slashing, lethal acid attacks, shooting and strangulation.[43] The murders are sometimes performed in public to warn the other women within the community of possible consequences of engaging in what is seen as illicit behavior.[44]

Often, minor girls and boys are selected by the family to act as the killers, so that the killer may benefit of the most favorable legal outcome. Boys and sometimes women in the family are often asked to closely control and monitor the behavior of their sisters or other females in the family (there are also few cases of men or boys being killed in the name of 'honor', to ensure that the females do not do anything to tarnish the 'honor' and 'reputation' of the family. The boys are often asked to carry out the murder, and if they refuse, they may face serious repercussions from the family and community for failing to perform their "duty".[45,46]

13.7 The Role of Religion

Human Rights Watch said that the practice "goes across cultures and across religions".[47] Worldwide, 91% of perpetrators were Muslims.[48] Resolution 1327 (2003) of the Council of Europe states that[49]: "The Assembly notes that whilst so-called 'honor crimes' emanate from cultural and not religious roots and are perpetrated worldwide (mainly in patriarchal societies or communities), the majority of reported cases in Europe have been amongst Muslim or migrant Muslim communities (although Islam itself does not support the death penalty for honor-related misconduct)."

Killing one's wife or sister for tarnishing her honor or that of her family has not received approval from any Islamic scholar of any note, in either medieval or modern era.[50] Many Muslim commentators and organizations condemn honor killings as an

[43] http://www.genevadeclaration.org/fileadmin/docs/CoPublications/Femicide

[44] http://www.genevadeclaration.org/fileadmin/docs/Co-publications/Femicide_A

[45] http://www.genevadeclaration.org/fileadmin/docs/Co-publications/Femicide

[46] http://www.humanrights.ch/upload/pdf/070419_Kvinnoforum_HRV.pdf

[47] "Thousands of Women Killed for Family "Honor"". news.nationalgeographic.com. Retrieved 2016-07-19.

[48] Worldwide Trends in Honor Killings by Phyllis Chesler http://www.meforum.org/2646/worldwide-trends-in-honor-killings

[49] "Council of Europe Parliamentary Assembly". Retrieved 10 June 2016.

[50] A.C. Brown, Jonathan (2014). Misquoting Muhammad: The Challenge and Choices of Interpreting the Prophet's Legacy. Oneworld Publications. p. 180. ISBN 978–1,780,744,209.

un-Islamic cultural practice.[51] Aga Khan University says that there is nothing in the Qur'an that permits or sanctions honor killings. Khan instead blames it on attitudes (across different classes, ethnic, and religious groups) that view women as property with no rights of their own as the motivation for honor killings.[52] Salafi scholar Muhammad Al-Munajjid asserts that the punishment of any crime is reserved for the Islamic ruler only. Ali Gomaa, Egypt's ex-Grand Mufti, has also spoken out forcefully against honor killings.[53]

In history, honor killings were encouraged in ancient Rome, where male family members who did not take actions against the female adulterers in their family were "actively persecuted".[54] The origin of honor killings and the control of women are evidenced throughout history in the culture and tradition of many regions. The Roman law of pater familias gave complete control to the men of the family over both their children and wives. Under these laws, the lives of children and wives were at the discretion of the men in their family. Ancient Roman Law also justified honor killings by stating that women found guilty of adultery could be killed by their husbands. Among the Ching dynasty in China, fathers and husbands had the right to kill females deemed to have dishonored them. Among the Amerindian Aztecs and Incas, adultery was punishable by death. During John Calvin's control over Geneva, women found guilty of adultery were punished by being drowned in the Rhone river.[55] Honor killings have a long tradition in Mediterranean Europe.[56,57] According to the *Honor Related Violence—European Resource Book and Good Practice*: "Honor in the Mediterranean world is a code of conduct, a way of life and an ideal of the social order, which defines the lives, the customs and the values of many of the peoples in the Mediterranean moral".

13.8 The Social Background of HK

The relation between social views on female sexuality and honor killings is complex. The way through which women in honor-based societies are considered to bring dishonor to men is often through their sexual behavior. Indeed, violence related to

---

[51] John Esposito (2011), What Everyone Needs to Know About Islam, p. 177. Oxford University Press. ISBN 978–0–19-979,413-3.

[52] Mayell, Hillary (12 February 2002). "Thousands of women killed for family "honor"". National Geographic News. National Geographic Society.pdf.

[53] John Esposito (2011), What Everyone Needs to Know About Islam, p. 177. Oxford University Press. ISBN 978–0–19-979,413-3.

[54] Matthew A. Goldstein (September 2002). "The biological roots of heat-of-passion crimes and honor killings" (PDF). Politics and the Life Sciences. p. 29. Retrieved 21 July 2012.

[55] http://hbv-awareness.com/history/

[56] "How the West should treat 'honor' killings". Reuters. Retrieved 20 April 2015.

[57] "http://www.medinstgenderstudies.org/wp-content/uploads/hrvresourcebook.pdfExplainer: Why Is It So Hard To Stop 'Honor Killings'?". RadioFreeEurope/RadioLiberty. Retrieved 20 April 2015.

female sexual expression has been documented since Ancient Rome,[58] when the pater familias had the right to kill an unmarried sexually active daughter or an adulterous wife. In medieval Europe, early Jewish law mandated stoning for an adulterous wife and her partner.[59]

Carolyn Fluehr-Lobban, an anthropology professor at Rhode Island College, writes that an act, or even alleged act, of any female sexual misconduct, upsets the moral order of the culture, and bloodshed is the only way to remove any shame brought by the actions and restore social equilibrium.[60] However, the relation between honor and female sexuality is a complicated one, and some authors argue that it is not women's sexuality per se that is the 'problem', but rather women's self-determination in regard to it, as well as fertility. Sharif Kanaana, professor of anthropology at Birzeit University, says that honor killing is a complicated issue that cuts deep into the history of Islamic society... What the men of the family, clan, or tribe seek control of in a patrilineal society is reproductive power. Women for the tribe were considered a factory for making men. The honor killing is not a means to control sexual power or behavior. What's behind it is the issue of fertility, or reproductive power.[61] In some cultures, honor killings are considered less serious than other murders simply because they arise from long-standing cultural traditions and are thus deemed appropriate or justifiable.[62] Additionally, according to a poll done by the BBC's Asian network, 1 in 10 of the 500 young Asians surveyed said they would condone any murder of someone who threatened their family's honor.[63] The women's resource center in Lahore, Pakistan says: "It is an unholy alliance that works against women: the killers take pride in what they have done, the tribal leaders condone the act and protect the killers and the police connive the cover-up."[64] The lawyer and human rights activist Hina Jilani says, "The right to life of women in Pakistan is conditional on their obeying social norms and traditions."[65]

A July 2008 Turkish study on honor killings has so far shown that little if any social stigma is attached to honor killing. It also comments that the practice is not related to a feudal societal structure, "There are also perpetrators who are well-

---

[58]Greg Woolf (2007). *Ancient civilizations: the illustrated guide to belief, mythology, and art.* Barnes & Noble. p. 386. ISBN 978-1-4351-0121-0

[59]"Historical Context – Origins of Honour Killing/Honour Killing – Worldwide/Honour Killing – In Countries with Islamic Law – Preliminary Examination of so-called Honour Killings in Canada". Justice.gc.ca. Retrieved 2015-02-15.

[60]Carolyn Fluehr-Lobban. "Cultural Relativism and Universal Rights" (PDF). Retrieved 2 December 2011

[61]Suzanne Ruggi. "Commodifying Honor in Female Sexuality: Honor Killings in Palestine". Middle East Research and Information Project. Retrieved 8 February 2008.

[62]*Maher, Ahmed (20 June 2013). "Many Jordan teenagers 'support honour killings'". bbc.co.uk*

[63]"One in 10 'backs honor killings'". BBC News. Retrieved 8 December 2001.

[64]Culture of Discrimination: A Fact Sheet on "Honor" Killings. Amnestyusa.org. Retrieved on 1 October 2011.

[65]"PAKISTAN Honour killings of girls and women". Amnesty International. Archived from the original on 5 June 2008. Retrieved 15 April 2008.

educated university graduates. Of all those surveyed, 60% are either high school or university graduates or at the very least, literate."[66]

In contemporary times, the changing cultural and economic status of women has also been used to explain the occurrences of honor killings.[67] Women in largely patriarchal cultures who have gained economic independence from their families go against their male-dominated culture.[68] Some researchers argue that the shift towards greater responsibility for women and less for their fathers may cause their male family members to act in oppressive and sometimes violent manners in order to regain authority.[69] This change of culture can also be seen to have an effect in Western cultures such as Britain where honor killings often arise from women seeking greater independence and adopting seemingly Western values. For women who trace their ancestry back to the Middle East or South Asia, wearing clothes that are considered Western, having a boyfriend, or refusing to accept an arranged marriage are all offenses that can and have led to an honor killing.[70] Honor killings which arise in Western cultures such as Britain are a tactic for immigrant families to cope with the alienating consequences of urbanization; immigrants remain close to the home culture and their relatives because it provides a safety net; it is thus the attempt to regain control and the feelings of alienation that ultimately leads to an honor killing.[71]

13.9 Cultures of Honor and Shame

The concept of family honor is extremely important in many communities.[72] The family is viewed as the main source of honor and the community highly values the relationship between honor and the family. Acts by family members which may be considered inappropriate are seen as bringing shame to the family in the eyes of the

---

[66]Murat Gezer. "Honor killing perpetrators welcomed by society, study reveals". Today's Zaman. Archived from the original on 19 July 2008. Retrieved 15 July 2008.

[67] *"UNICEF Turkey: Protective Environment for Children; Honour Crimes and Forced Suicides". unicef.org.tr*

[68]*Krishan Bir Singh (1 January 1970). "Honour Killing – A Study of the Causes and Remedies in its Socio Legal Aspect". academia.edu*

[69]Hilal Onur Ince, Aysun Yarali and Dogancan Ozsel. "Customary Killings in Turkey and Turkish Modernization". Middle Eastern Studies. Middle Eastern Studies. 45: 537–551. doi:https://doi.org/10.1080/00263200903009593. Retrieved 2 December 2011.

[70]Hilal Onur Ince, Aysun Yarali and Dogancan Ozsel. "Customary Killings in Turkey and Turkish Modernization". Middle Eastern Studies. Middle Eastern Studies. 45: 537–551.

[71]Fareena Alam (6 July 2004). "Take the Honor Out of Killing". London: The Guardian. Retrieved 2 December 2011.

[72]*Mayell, Hillary (12 February 2002). "Thousands of Women Killed for Family "Honor"". National Geographic News. National Geographic Society.*

community.[73] Such acts often include female behaviors that are related to sex outside marriage or way of dressing, but may also include male homosexuality (like the emo killings in Iraq). The family loses face in the community, and may be shunned by relatives. The only way the shame can be erased is through a killing.[74] The cultures in which honor killings take place are usually considered "high-context", where the family is more important than the individual, and individualistic autonomy is seen as a threat to the collective family and its honor.[75] In many cultures where honor is of central value, men are sources, or active generators/agents of that honor, while the only effect that women can have on honor is to destroy it.[76] Once the family's or clan's honor is considered to have been destroyed by a woman, there is a need for immediate revenge to restore it, in order for the family to avoid losing face in the community. Amnesty International statement notes that the regime of honor is unforgiving[77]: women on whom suspicion has fallen are not given an opportunity to defend themselves, and family members have no socially acceptable alternative but to remove the stain on their honor by attacking the woman.[78]

13.10 Specific Triggers of Honor Killings

There are multiple causes and triggers for which honor killings occur, and numerous factors interact with each other.

[73]*Foblets, Marie-Claire; Renteln, Alison Dundes (16 January 2009). Multicultural Jurisprudence: Comparative Perspectives on the Cultural Defense. Bloomsbury Publishing. ISBN 978-1-84731-481-9*

[74]Krishan Bir Singh (1 January 1970). "Honour Killing – A Study of the Causes and Remedies in its SocioLegal Aspect". academia.edu. Retrieved 23 December 2013.

[75]"FAQ". Hbv-awareness.com. Retrieved 2015-02-15.

[76]"Historical Context – Origins of Honour Killing/Honour Killing – Worldwide/Honour Killing – In Countries with Islamic Law – Preliminary Examination of so-called Honour Killings in Canada". Justice.gc.ca. Retrieved 2015-02-15.

[77]Male Asylum Applicants Who Fear Becoming the Victims of Honor Killings: The Case for Gender Equality

[78]"Broken bodies, shattered minds: Torture and ill-treatment of women". Amnesty International. Retrieved 6 March 2001.

13.10.1 Refusal of an Arranged Marriage: Forced Marriage[79]

Refusal of an arranged marriage is often a cause of an honor killing.[80] The family which has prearranged the marriage risks disgrace if the marriage does not proceed.[81] Yet, another way of restoring honor is through a forced marriage. In the case of an unmarried girl associating herself with a man, losing virginity, or being raped, the family may attempt to restore its 'honor' with a 'shotgun wedding'. The groom will usually be the man who has 'dishonored' the girl, but if this is not possible the family may try to arrange a marriage with another man, often a man who is part of the extended family of the one who has committed the acts with the girl. This being an alternative to an honor killing, the girl has no choice but to accept the marriage. The family of the man is expected to cooperate and provide a groom for the girl.[82]

13.10.2 Seeking a Divorce[83]

A woman attempting to obtain a divorce or separation without the consent of the husband/extended family can also be a trigger for honor killings. In cultures where marriages are arranged and goods are often exchanged between families, a woman's desire to seek a divorce is often viewed as an insult to the men who negotiated the deal. By making their marital problems known outside the family, the women are seen as exposing the family to public dishonor.[84]

---

[79]http://www.honordiaries.com/wp-content/uploads/2013/06/HD-FactSheet-HonorViolenceEast.pdf

[80]"Ethics: Honour crimes". BBC. 1 January 1970. Retrieved 23 December 2013.

[81]https://tspace.library.utoronto.ca/bitstream/1807/17543/1/cultureofhonour.pdf

[82]"United Nations Population Fund | Publications" (PDF). UNFPA. Retrieved 2015-02-15.

[83]"Thousands of Women Killed for Family "Honor"". News.nationalgeographic.com. 2010-10-28. Retrieved 2015-02-15.

[84]"Introduction – Preliminary Examination of so-called Honour Killings in Canada". Justice.gc.ca. Retrieved 2015-02-15.

13.10.3 Allegations and Rumors About a Family Member[85,86]

In certain cultures, an *allegation* against a woman can be enough to tarnish her family's reputation, and to trigger an honor killing: the family's fear of being ostracized by the community is enormous.[87]

13.10.4 Victims of Rape: Victim Blaming

In many cultures, victims of rape face severe violence, including honor killings, from their families and relatives. In many parts of the world, women who have been raped are considered to have brought 'dishonor' or 'disgrace' to their families. This is especially the case if the victim becomes pregnant.[88] Central to the code of honor, in many societies, is a woman's virginity, which must be preserved until marriage. A woman's virginity is perceived as the property of the men around her, first her father, later a gift for her husband; a virtual dowry as she graduates to marriage."[89]

13.10.5 Homosexuality[90]: Violence Against LGBT People[91]

There is evidence that homosexuality can also be perceived as grounds for honor killing by relatives.[92] It is not only same-sex sexual acts that trigger violence—behaviors that are regarded as inappropriate gender expression (e.g. a male acting or dressing in a "feminine way") can also raise suspicion and lead to honor violence.[93]

---

[85]Bhaskar Dasgupta (21 February 2004). "No Honour In Honour Killings". countercurrents.org. Retrieved 23 December 2013.

[86]"Ethics: Honour crimes". BBC. 1 January 1970. Retrieved 23 December 2013.

[87]http://www.octevaw-cocvff.ca/sites/all/files/pdf/factsheets/Honour_Killing.pdf

[88]Harter, Pascale (14 June 2011). "BBC News – Libya rape victims 'face honour killings'". Bbc.co.uk. Retrieved 16 August 2013.

[89]Susan Ruggi; "Dafka". Dafka. Retrieved 2015-02-15.

[90]UNHCR Guidance Note on Refugee Claims Relating to Sexual Orientation and Gender Identity, II, B. para 14. Unhcr.org

[91]"Father confesses to killing his own son in landmark homosexual murder case – LOCAL". Hurriyetdailynews.com. 2011-09-13. Retrieved 2015-02-15.

[92]*Razzall, Katie; Khan, Yasminara (11 April 2017). "Male 'honour' cases 'underreported*

[93]http://www.humanrights.ch/upload/pdf/070419_Kvinnoforum_HRV.pdf

Gay people may be shot by father or siblings[94] or in a café.[95]Sociologists have called this Turkey‘s[96] first publicized gay honor killing.[97,98,99]

United Nations High Commissioner for Refugees state that "claims made by LGBT persons often reveal exposure to physical and sexual violence, extended periods of detention, medical abuse, threat of execution and honor killing."[100]

13.11 International Approach

13.11.1 The UN Report on HK

The report of the Special Rapporteur... concerning cultural practices in the family that are violent towards women (E/CN.4/2002/83), indicated that honor killings had been reported in Egypt, Jordan, Lebanon, Morocco, Pakistan, the Syrian Arab Republic, Turkey, Yemen, and other Mediterranean and Persian Gulf countries, and that they had also taken place in western countries such as France, Germany and the United Kingdom, within migrant communities.
A June 2008 report by the Turkish Prime Ministry's Human Rights Directorate said that in Istanbul alone there was one honor killing every week, and reported over 1000 during the previous five years. It added that metropolitan cities were the location of many of these, due to growing Kurdish immigration to these cities from the East. In 2009 a Turkish news agency reported that a 2-day-old boy who was born out of wedlock had been killed for honor. The maternal grandmother of the infant, along with six other persons, including a doctor who had reportedly accepted a bribe in order to not report the birth, were arrested. The grandmother is suspected

[94]Marina Jimenez. "Gay Jordanian now 'gloriously free' in Canada". Toronto: The Globe and Mail. Retrieved 20 May 2004.[dead link]

[95] *"Father gets life imprisonment for murdering gay son in Turkey – LGBTQ Nation". Lgbtqnation. com*

[96]The German Democratic Turkey Forum (DTF) has prepared a report with details on the killing and the subsequent court case; accessed on 31 March 2011.

[97]http://www.nytimes.com/2009/11/26/world/europe/26turkey.html?_r=0 Ahmet Kaya, Ahmet Yildiz's cousin, said Mr. Yildiz was the only son of a deeply religious and wealthy Kurdish family from Sanliurfa, in the predominantly Kurdish southeast.

[98]Nicholas Birch (19 July 2008). "Was Ahmet Yildiz the victim of Turkey's first gay honor killing?". London: The Independent. Retrieved 27 September 2008

[99]"Father gets life imprisonment for murdering gay son in Turkey – LGBTQ Nation". Lgbtqnation. com. 2012-07-02. Retrieved 2015-02-15.

[100]UNHCR Guidance Note on Refugee Claims Relating to Sexual Orientation and Gender Identity, II, B. para 14. Unhcr.org (21 November 2008). Retrieved on 1 October 2011.

of fatally suffocating the infant.[101] The child's mother, 25, was also arrested; she stated that her family had made the decision to kill the child.[102]

A girl in Turkey was killed after her family heard a song and thought she had a boyfriend. In 2010 a 16-year-old girl was buried alive by relatives for befriending boys in Southeast Turkey; her corpse was found 40 days after she went missing. Ahmet Yilciz, 26, a Turkish physics student who represented his country at an international gay conference in the United States in 2008, was shot leaving a cafe in Istanbul. It is believed Yildiz was the victim of the country's first gay honor killing.[103]

There are no exact official numbers about honor killings of women in Lebanon; many honor killings are arranged to look like accidents, but the figure is believed to be 40 to 50 per year. A 2007 report by Amnesty International said that the Lebanese media in 2001 reported 2–3 honor killings per month in Lebanon, although the number is believed by lawyers to be higher. Most killings in the Gaza Strip and the West Bank are carried out by villagers; honor killing is extremely rare in Palestinian cities and larger towns. The Palestinian authority uses Jordanian law, which gives men reduced punishment for killing a female relative if she has brought dishonor to the family. Due to Palestinian protests, Mahmoud Abbas, President of the Palestinian Authority, promised to change the discriminatory law by the year 2010, but As of November 2010 this has not happened.

According to UNICEF, in 2000 two-thirds of all killings in the Palestinian territories were honor killings.[104] As many as 133 women were killed in the Iraqi city of Basra alone in 2006—79 for violation of "Islamic teachings" and 47 for honor killings, according to IRIN, the news branch of the U.N.'s Office for the Coordination of Humanitarian Affairs. Amnesty International says that armed groups, not the government, also kill politically active women and those who did not follow a strict dress code, as well as women who are perceived as human rights defenders.[105]

Jordan, considered one of the most liberal countries in the Middle East, still has instances of honor killings. In Jordan there is minimal sex discrimination, and women are permitted to vote, but men receive reduced sentences for killing their wives or female family members if they have brought dishonor to their family. Families often get sons under the age of 18—legally minors—to commit honor killings; the juvenile law allows convicted minors to serve time in a juvenile detention center and be released with a clean criminal record at the age of 18.

---

[101] *Holt, Gerry (29 May 2014). "BBC News – Why do families kill their daughters?". BBC News. Bbc.com*

[102] Hilal Onur Ince, Aysun Yarali and Dogancan Ozsel. "Customary Killings in Turkey and Turkish Modernization". Middle Eastern Studies. Middle Eastern Studies. 45: 537–551.

[103] AYSAN SEV'ER. "Feminist Analysis of Honor Killings in Rural Turkey" (PDF). 'University of Toronto'. Retrieved 2 January 2015.

[104] Suzanne Ruggi. "Commodifying Honor in Female Sexuality: Honor Killings in Palestine". Middle East Research and Information Project. Retrieved 8 February 2008.

[105] "Thousands of Women Killed for Family "Honor"". News.nationalgeographic.com. 2010-10-28. Retrieved 2015-02-15.

Rana Husseini, a leading journalist on the topic of honor killings, states that "under the existing law, people found guilty of committing honor killings often receive sentences as light as six months in prison".[106]

There has been public support in Jordan to amend Articles 340 and 98. In 1999 King Abdullah created a council to review the sex inequalities in the country. The Council returned with a recommendation to repeal Article 340. "The cabinet approved the recommendation, the measure was presented to parliament twice in November 1999 and January 2000 and in both cases, though approved by the upper house, it failed to pass the elected lower house".[107] In 2001, after parliament was suspended, a number of temporary laws were created which were subject to parliamentary ratification. One of the amendments was that "husbands would no longer be exonerated for killing unfaithful wives, but instead the circumstances would be considered as evidence for mitigating punishments". In the interest of sex equality, women were given the same reduction in punishment if found guilty of the crime. But parliament returned to session in 2003 and the new amendments were rejected by the lower house after two successful readings in the upper house.

According to the report of the Special Rapporteur submitted to the 58th session of the United Nations Commission on Human Rights in 2002 concerning cultural practices in the family that reflect violence against women (E/CN.4/2002/83)[108]: The Special Rapporteur indicated that legislative provisions allowing for partial or complete defense could be found in the penal codes of Egypt, Iran, Israel, Jordan, Syria and the Palestinian National Authority. The report of the Special Rapporteur... concerning cultural practices in the family that are violent towards women (E/CN.4/2002/83), indicated that honor killings had been reported in Egypt, Jordan, Lebanon (the Lebanese Parliament abolished the Honor killing in August 2011), Morocco, Pakistan, the Syrian Arab Republic, Turkey, Yemen, and other Mediterranean and Persian Gulf countries, and that they had also taken place in western countries such as France, Germany and the United Kingdom, within migrant communities.[109]

In addition, the United Nations Commission on Human Rights gathered reports from several countries and considering only the countries that submitted reports it was shown that honor killings have occurred in Bangladesh, Great Britain, Brazil, Ecuador, Egypt, India, Israel, Italy, Jordan, Pakistan, Morocco, Sweden, Turkey, and Uganda.[110,111] According to Human Rights Watch, the practice of honor killing "goes across cultures and across religions."

[106]"Ethics: Honour crimes". BBC. 1 January 1970. Retrieved 23 December 2013.

[107]"Ethics: Honour crimes". BBC. 1 January 1970. Retrieved 23 December 2013.

[108]"One in 10 'backs honor killings'". BBC News. Retrieved 8 December 2001.

[109]"Working towards the elimination of crimes against women committed in the name of honour" (PDF). Office of the United Nations High Commissioner for Human Rights. Retrieved 8 February 2008.

[110]"International Domestic Violence Issues". Sanctuary For Families. Retrieved 5 December 2011.

[111]"Thousands of Women Killed for Family "Honor"". National Geographic News. 12 February 2002. Retrieved 6 August 2013

13.11.2 International Response

Honor killings are condemned as a serious human rights violation and are addressed by several international instruments. The Council of Europe Convention on preventing and combating violence against women and domestic violence addresses this issue. Article 42 reads:

Article 42—Unacceptable justifications for crimes, including crimes committed in the name of so-called "honour".

1. Parties shall take the necessary legislative or other measures to ensure that, in criminal proceedings initiated following the commission of any of the acts of violence covered by the scope of this Convention, culture, custom, religion, tradition or so-called "honor" shall not be regarded as justification for such acts. This covers, in particular, claims that the victim has transgressed cultural, religious, social or traditional norms or customs of appropriate behavior.
2. Parties shall take the necessary legislative or other measures to ensure that incitement by any person of a child to commit any of the acts referred to in paragraph 1 shall not diminish the criminal liability of that person for the acts committed.

The World Health Organization (WHO) addressed the issue of honor killings and stated: "Murders of women to 'save the family honor' are among the most tragic consequences and explicit illustrations of embedded, culturally accepted discrimination against women and girls." According to the UNODC: "Honor crimes, including killing, are one of history's oldest forms of gender-based violence. It assumes that a woman's behavior casts a reflection on the family and the community.... In some communities, a father, brother or cousin will publicly take pride in a murder committed in order to preserve the 'honor' of a family. In some such cases, local justice officials may side with the family and take no formal action to prevent similar deaths."

13.11.3 National Legal Codes

Legislation on this issues varies, but today the vast majority of countries no longer allow a husband to legally kill a wife for adultery (although adultery itself continues to be punishable by death in some countries) or to commit other forms of honor killings. However, in many places, adultery and other "immoral" sexual behaviors by female family members can be considered mitigating circumstances in case when they are killed, leading to significantly shorter sentences.

In the Western world, a country that is often associated with "crimes of passion" and adultery related violence is France, and indeed, recent surveys have shown French public to be more accepting of these practices than the public in other countries. One 2008 Gallup survey compared the views of the French, German and British public and those of French, German and British Muslims on several social issues: 4% of French public said "honor killings" were "morally acceptable" and 8% of French public said "crimes of passion" were "morally acceptable"; honor killings were seen as acceptable by 1% of German public and also 1% of British public; crimes of passion were seen as acceptable by 1% of German public and 2% of British public. Among Muslims 5% in Paris, 3% in Berlin and 3% in London saw honor killings as acceptable, and 4% in Paris (less than French public), 1% in Berlin and 3% in London saw crimes of passion as acceptable.

According to the report of the United Nations Special Rapporteur submitted to the 58th session of the United Nations Commission on Human Rights in 2002 concerning cultural practices in the family that reflect violence against women (E/CN.4/2002/83):

The Special Rapporteur indicated that there had been contradictory decisions with regard to the honor defense in Brazil, and that legislative provisions allowing for partial or complete defense in that context could be found in the penal codes of Argentina, Ecuador, Egypt, Guatemala, Iran, Israel, Jordan, Peru, Syria, Venezuela and the Palestinian National Authority.

The legal aspects of honor killings in different countries are discussed below:

- Jordan: In recent years, Jordan has amended its Code to modify its laws which used to offer a complete defense for honor killings.[112]
- Many former French colonies offer the possibility of reduced sentences in regard to adultery related violent crimes (inspired by the French Napoleonic Code).
- In Brazil, an explicit defense to murder in case of adultery has never been part of the criminal code, but a defense of "honor" (not part of the criminal code) has been widely used by lawyers in such cases to obtain acquittals. Although this defense has been generally rejected in modern parts of the country (such as big cities) since the 1950s, it has been very successful in the interior of the country. In 1991 Brazil's Supreme Court explicitly rejected the "honor" defense as having no basis in Brazilian law.
- Haiti: In 2005, the laws were changed, abolishing the right of a husband to be excused for murdering his wife due to adultery. Adultery was also decriminalized
- Syria: In 2009, Article 548 of the Syrian Law code was amended. Beforehand, the article waived any punishment for males who committed murder on a female family member for inappropriate sex acts. Article 548 states that "He who catches his wife or one of his ascendants, descendants or sister committing adultery (flagrante delicto) or illegitimate sexual acts with another and he killed or injured one or both of them benefits from a reduced penalty, that should not be less than 2 years in prison in case of a killing." Article 192 states that a judge may opt for reduced punishments (such as short-term imprisonment) if the killing was done with an honorable intent. In addition to this, Article 242 says that a judge may

[112] *"'Historic Day for Jordanian Women': Joy as Marriage Loophole for Rapists Removed". Al Bawaba. 2 August 2017*

reduce a sentence for murders that were done in rage and caused by an illegal act committed by the victim.

- Turkey: In Turkey, persons found guilty of this crime are sentenced to life in prison. There are well documented cases, where Turkish courts have sentenced whole families to life imprisonment for an honor killing. The most recent was on 13 January 2009, where a Turkish Court sentenced five members of the same Kurdish family to life imprisonment for the honor killing of Naile Erdas, 16, who got pregnant as a result of rape.
- Pakistan: Honor killings are known as karo kari (Sindhi: ڪارو ڪاري) (Urdu: کاروکاری). The practice is supposed to be prosecuted under ordinary killing, but in practice police and prosecutors often ignore it. Cases that do result in a conviction may end with the killers being freed as Pakistani law allows a victim's family to forgive their killer. As a woman's killers usually are her family, the law allows them to nominate family members to do the murder which they then forgive.[293] Often a man must simply claim the killing was for his honor and he will go free. Nilofar Bakhtiar, advisor to Prime Minister Shaukat Aziz, stated that in 2003, as many as 1261 women were killed in honor killings. The Hudood Ordinances of Pakistan, enacted in 1979 by then ruler General Zia-ul-Haq, created laws that realigned Pakistani rule with Islamic law. The law had the effect of reducing the legal protections for women, especially regarding sex outside of the marriage. Women who made accusations of rape, after this law, were required to provide four male witnesses. If unable to do this, the alleged rape could not be prosecuted in the courts. Because the woman had admitted to sex outside of marriage, however, she could be punished for having sex outside of the marriage, a punishment that ranged from stoning to public lashing. This law made it that much more risky for women to come forward with accusations of rape. In 2006, the Women's Protection Bill amended these Hudood Ordinances by removing four male witnesses as a requirement for rape allegations. On 8 December 2004, under international and domestic pressure, Pakistan enacted a law that made honor killings punishable by a prison term of seven years, or by the death penalty in the most extreme cases. Women's rights organizations were, however, wary of this law as it stops short of outlawing the practice of allowing killers to buy their freedom by paying compensation to the victim's relatives. Women's rights groups claimed that in most cases it is the victim's immediate relatives who are the killers, so inherently the new law is just whitewash. It did not alter the provisions whereby the accused could negotiate pardon with the victim's family under the Islamic provisions. In March 2005, the Pakistani parliament rejected a bill which sought to strengthen the law against the practice of honor killing. However, the bill was brought up again, and in November 2006, it passed. It is doubtful whether or not the law would actually help women.
- Egypt: A number of studies on honor crimes by The Centre of Islamic and Middle Eastern Law, at the School of Oriental and African Studies in London, includes one which reports on Egypt's legal system, noting a gender bias in favor of men in general, and notably article 17 of the Penal Code: judicial discretion to allow reduced punishment in certain circumstance, often used in honor killings case.

13.12 Laws in the Arab Region

13.12.1 Legal Frames Through History

Legal frameworks can encourage honor killings. Such laws include on one side leniency towards such killings, and on the other side criminalization of various behaviors, such as extramarital sex, 'indecent' dressing in public places, or homosexual sexual acts, with these laws acting as a way of reassuring perpetrators of honor killings that people engaging in these behaviors deserve punishment.[113,114]

In the Roman Empire the Roman law Lex Julia de adulteriis coercendis implemented by Augustus Caesar permitted the murder of daughters and their lovers who committed adultery at the hands of their fathers and also permitted the murder of the adulterous wife's lover at the hand of her husband.[115]

The Napoleonic Code did not allow women to murder unfaithful husbands, while it permitted the murder of unfaithful women by their husbands.[116] The Napoleonic Code Article 324 which was passed in 1810 permitted the murders of an unfaithful wife and her lover at the hand of her husband.[117] It was abolished only in 1975. On November 7, 1975, Law no. 617/75 Article 17 repealed the 1810 French Penal Code Article 324. The 1810 penal code Article 324 passed by Napoleon was copied by Middle Eastern Arab countries. It inspired Jordan's Article 340 which permits murder of a wife and her lover if caught in the act at the hands of her husband.[118] France's 1810 Penal Code Article 324 also inspired the 1858 Ottoman Penal Code's Article 188, both the French Article 324 and Ottoman article 188 were drawn on to create Jordan's Article 340 which was retained even after a 1944 revision of Jordan's laws[119] which did not touch public conduct and family law so Article 324 still applies to this day.[120] France's Mandate over Lebanon resulted in its penal code being imposed there in 1943–1944, with the French inspired Lebanese law for adultery allowing the mere accusation of adultery against women resulting in a maximum punishment of two years in prison while men have to be caught in the act and not merely accused, and are punished with only one year in prison.

Jordan's Article 98 says *he who commits a crime in a fit of fury caused by an unrightful and dangerous act on the part of the victim benefits from a reduction in*

---

[113] Women of the Jordan: Islam, Labor, and the Law. Retrieved 23 December 2013.

[114] 'Honour': Crimes, Paradigms and Violence Against Women. Retrieved 23 December 2013.

[115] Greg Woolf (2007). Ancient civilizations: the illustrated guide to belief, mythology, and art. Barnes & Noble. p. 386. ISBN 978–1–4351-0121-0.

[116] http://www.napoleon-series.org/research/government/code/c_code2.html

[117] http://www.napoleon-series.org/research/government/france/penalcode/c_penalcode3b.html

[118] Women of the Jordan: Islam, Labor, and the Law. Retrieved 23 December 2013.

[119] http://www.centerforinquiry.net/isis/articles_and_books/intrafamily_femicide_in_defence_of_honour_the_case_of_jordan/

[120] http://digitalcollections.sit.edu/cgi/viewcontent.cgi?article=1427&context=isp_collection

penalty.[121] In Jordan six months is the usual penalty for murderers in honor killings, the murderer in honor killings are allowed to get off by Article 97 while the "fit of fury" in Article 98 is used to justify the defense for committing an honor killing, while the murderer can also justify the honor killing with Article 340.[122]

France's Article 324 inspired laws in other Arab countries such as:

- Algeria's 1991 Penal Code Article 279
- Egypt's 1937 Penal Code no. 58 Article 237
- Iraq's 1966 Penal Code Article 409
- Jordan's 1960 Penal Code no. 16 Article 340
- Kuwait's Penal Code Article 153
- Lebanon's Penal Code Articles 193, 252, 253 and 562
  - These were amended in 1983, 1994, 1995, 1996 and 1999 and were eventually repealed by the Lebanese Parliament on August 4, 2011
- Libya's Penal Code Article 375
- Morocco's 1963 amended Penal Code Article 418
- Oman's Penal Code Article 252
- Palestine, which had two codes
- Jordan's 1960 Penal Code 1960 in the West Bank and British Mandate Criminal Code Article 18 in the Gaza Strip[123]
  - These were respectively repealed by Article 1 and Article 2 and both by Article 3 of the 2011 Law no. 71 which was signed on May 5, 2011 by President Mahmoud Abbas into the October 10, 2011 Official Gazette no. 91 applying in the Criminal Code of Palestine's Northern Governorates and Southern Governorates
- Syria's 1953 amended 1949 Penal Code Article 548
- Tunisia's 1991 Penal Code Article 207 (which was repealed)
- United Arab Emirate's law no.3/1978 Article 334
- Yemen's law no. 12/1994 Article 232

[121]Stefanie Eileen Nanes, "Fighting Honor Crimes: Evidence of Civil Society in Jordan," Middle East Journal, vol. 57, no.1 (Winter 2003), p. 6.

[122]Ellen R. Sheeley (2007). Reclaiming Honor in Jordan: A National Public Opinion Survey on "honor" Killings. Author. ISBN 978–9957-8607-0-7.

[123]Women of the Jordan: Islam, Labor, and the Law. Retrieved 23 December 2013.

13.12.2 Reports of Cases

A court in the UK dropped murder charges and instead only filed manslaughter[124] for the murder of Paul Wilkins and Kay Morton after Kay's boyfriend William Cranston killed them in his fury.[125] "Loss of control" in the murder of unfaithful women by their male partners was considered acceptable as a reason to kill by Lord Chief Justice Lord Judge of England, the murder of the wife of Jon Clinton by Jon was examined by Lord Judge who ordered a retrial, overturning the original life sentence and allowing the infidelity of his wife to be entered as evidence.[126]

The murderer of Tonya Lynn, who committed infidelity, her husband James Lynn Jr., was given a retrial with evidence of his wife's cheating included while his original murder conviction was thrown out by the Georgia Supreme Court[127] In the murder case of Fumiko Ogawa, a plea deal which agreed that the murder was committed due to a "sudden quarrel in the heat of passion" saw her husband Anthony Simoneau's sentence reduced from murder to 11 years for voluntary manslaughter.[128]

13.12.3 Responsive Legislations

Countries where the law is interpreted to allow men to kill female relatives in a premeditated effort as well as for crimes of passions, in flagrante delicto in the act of committing adultery, include:

[124]http://www.telegraph.co.uk/news/uknews/law-and-order/9020905/Murder-can-be-crime-of-passion-says-top-judge.html

[125]http://news.bbc.co.uk/2/hi/uk_news/england/beds/bucks/herts/8126350.stm

[126]http://www.dailymail.co.uk/news/article-2087868/Men-murder-cheating-partners-CAN-use-loss-control-defence.html

[127]http://www.dailymail.co.uk/news/article-2819819/Husband-wins-retrial-court-wasn-t-told-wife-killed-dropped-taunted-affairs.html

[128]http://www.dailymail.co.uk/news/article-2994159/Man-admits-killing-wife-moment-passion-dumping-body-desert-fleeing-Hawaii-eight-years-ago.html

- Jordan: Part of article 340 of the Penal Code states that "he who discovers his wife or one of his female relatives committing adultery and kills, wounds, or injures one of them, is exempted from any penalty."[71] This has twice been put forward for cancellation by the government, but was retained by the Lower House of the Parliament, in 2003: a year in which at least seven honor killings took place. [72] Article 98 of the Penal Code is often cited alongside Article 340 in cases of honor killings. "Article 98 stipulates that a reduced sentence is applied to a person who kills another person in a 'fit of fury'".

Countries that allow men to kill female relatives in flagrante delicto (but without premeditation) include:

- Syria: Article 548 states that "He who catches his wife or one of his ascendants, descendants or sister committing adultery (flagrante delicto) or illegitimate sexual acts with another and he killed or injured one or both of them benefits from a reduced penalty, that should not be less than 2 years in prison in case of a killing."

Countries that allow husbands to kill only their wives in flagrante delicto (based upon the Napoleonic code) include:

- Morocco: Revisions to Morocco's criminal code in 2003 helped improve women's legal status by eliminating unequal sentencing in adultery cases. Article 418 of the penal code granted extenuating circumstances to a husband who kills, injures, or beats his wife and/or her partner, when catching them in flagrante delicto while committing adultery. While this article has not been repealed, the penalty for committing this crime is at least now the same for both genders.

Countries where honor killing is not legal but is known to occur include:

- Turkey: In Turkey, persons found guilty of this crime are sentenced to life in prison.[74] There are well documented cases, where Turkish courts have sentenced whole families to life imprisonment for an honor killing. The most recent was on January 13, 2009, where a Turkish Court sentenced five members of the same Kurdish family to life imprisonment for the "honor killing" of Naile Erdas, 16, who got pregnant as a result of rape.
- Pakistan: Honor killings are known as karo kari (Sindhi: ڪارو ڪاري) (Urdu: کاروکاری). The practice is supposed to be prosecuted under ordinary killing, but in practice police and prosecutors often ignore it. Often a man must simply claim the killing was for his honor and he will go free. Nilofar Bakhtiar, advisor to Prime Minister Shaukat Aziz, stated that in 2003, as many as 1261 women were killed in honor killings. On December 8, 2004, under international and domestic pressure, Pakistan enacted a law that made honor killings punishable by a prison term of seven years, or by the death penalty in the most extreme cases. Women's rights organizations were, however, wary of this law as it stops short of outlawing the practice of allowing killers to buy their freedom by paying compensation to the victim's relatives. Women's rights groups claimed that in most cases it is the victim's immediate relatives who are the killers, so inherently the new law is just eyewash. It did not alter the provisions whereby the accused could negotiate

pardon with the victim's family under the Islamic provisions. In March 2005 the Pakistani parliament rejected a bill which sought to strengthen the law against the practice of honor killing. However, the bill was brought up again, and in November 2006, it passed. It is doubtful whether or not the law would actually help women.

- Egypt: A number of studies on honor crimes by The Centre of Islamic and Middle Eastern Law, at the School of Oriental and African Studies in London, includes one which reports on Egypt's legal system, noting a gender bias in favor of men in general, and notably article 17 of the Penal Code: judicial discretion to allow reduced punishment in certain circumstance, often used in honor killings case.

Honor crimes represent the most severe types of domestic violence against girls, and are led by prevailing beliefs about shame and honor. In general, little information is available on this kind of violence.

13.13 Data in the Arab and Middle-East Region

13.13.1 Limitations of Data

In 2010 inquiry, Algeria, Oman, Morocco did not report HK, as well as Jordan, Syria and Lebanon, where there are laws to prevent crimes of honor; in Libya, a law bans and punishes crimes of honor. In this state inquiry, other countries did not provide information on the subject. OIC edited recommendations in December 2009 to stop crimes of honor.

In Jordan, the phenomenon of so-called 'honor crimes' does not exist officially, despite criminal occurrences of a similar description that involve women occurring on a yearly basis. These incidences are legally justified in some cases, and are labeled as honor crimes. Jordan has amended the Penal Code to impose harsher punishments on perpetrators and abolish impunity in cases of honor crimes.

Bahrain, Tunisia, Algeria, Oman, Egypt and Morocco, did not report any cases of honor crimes.

In Syria and Lebanon, legislation prohibits honor crimes. In Libya, the law prohibits and punishes crimes of honor. In Syria, a law which made an exception for the perpetrator in cases of honor crimes has been amended and punishment was gradually extended to 5–7 years of imprisonment. Other countries did not provide information about laws against honor crimes to the LAS.

13.13.2 Egypt

Honor killings in Egypt occur due to reasons such as a woman meeting an unrelated man, even if this is only an allegation; or adultery (real or suspected). The exact number of honor killings is not known, but a report in 1995 estimated about 52 honor killings that year.[129] In 2013, a woman and her two daughters were murdered by 10 male relatives, who strangled and beat them, and then threw their bodies in the Nile. Honor killings are illegal in Egypt and five of the ten men were arrested.

13.13.3 Iran

In Iran, honor killings occur primarily among tribal minority groups, such as Kurdish, Arab, Lori, Baluchi, and Turkish-speaking tribes, while honor-related crimes are not a tradition among Persians who are generally less socially conservative. Discriminatory family laws, articles in the Criminal Code that show leniency towards honor killings, and a strongly male dominated society have been cited as causes of honor killings in Iran. Honor killings are particularly prevalent in the provinces of Kordistan and Ilam.

Discriminatory family laws, articles in the Criminal Code that show leniency towards honor killings, and a strongly male dominated society have been cited as causes of honor killings in Iran.[130] It was reported that in 2001, 565 women lost their lives in honor-related crimes in Ilam, Iran, of which 375 were reportedly staged as self-immolation. In 2008, self-immolation, "occurred in all the areas of Kurdish settlement (in Iran), where it was more common than in other parts of Iran".

13.13.4 Iraq

In 2008, the United Nations Assistance Mission for Iraq (UNAMI) has stated that honor killings are a serious concern in Iraq, particularly in Iraqi Kurdistan[131] and including Iraki citizen outside Irak.[132] The Free Women's Organization of Kurdistan (FWOK) released a statement on International Women's Day 2015 noting that "6082 women were killed or forced to commit suicide during the past year in Iraqi Kurdistan, which is almost equal to the number of the Peshmerga martyred fighting Islamic State (IS)," and that a large number of women were victims of honor killings or enforced suicide—mostly self-immolation or hanging. About 500 honor killings per year are reported in hospitals in Iraqi Kurdistan, although real numbers are likely much higher. It is speculated that alone in Erbil there is one honor killing per day.

---

[129] http://www.un.org/womenwatch/daw/egm/vaw-gp-2005/docs/experts/khafagy.honorcrimes.pdf

[130] http://www.landinfo.no/asset/960/1/960_1.pdf

[131] https://www.hrw.org/report/2011/02/21/crossroads/human-rights-iraq-eight-years-after-us-led-invasion

[132] *"Iraqi immigrant convicted in Arizona 'honor killing' awaits sentence – CNN.com". Edition. cnn.com*

The UNAMI reported that at least 534 honor killings occurred between January and April 2006 in the Kurdish Governorates. It is claimed that many deaths are reported as "female suicides" in order to conceal honor-related crimes. Aso Kamal of the Doaa Network Against Violence claimed that they have estimated that there were more than 12,000 honor killings in Iraqi Kurdistan from 1991 to 2007. He also said that the government figures are much lower, and show a decline in recent years, and Kurdish law has mandated since 2008 that an honor killing be treated like any other murder. Honor killings and other forms of violence against women have increased since the creation of Iraqi Kurdistan, and "both the KDP and PUK claimed that women's oppression, including 'honor killings', are part of Kurdish 'tribal and Islamic culture'". The honor killing and self-immolation condoned or tolerated by the Kurdish administration in Iraqi Kurdistan has been labeled as "gendercide" by Mojab (2003).[133]

As many as 133 women were killed in the Iraqi city of Basra alone in 2006. 79 were killed for violation of "Islamic teachings" and 47 for honor, according to IRIN, the news branch of the U.N.'s Office for the Coordination of Humanitarian Affairs. Amnesty International says that armed groups, not the government, also kill politically active women and those who did not follow a strict dress code, as well as women who are perceived as human rights defenders. 17-year-old Du'a Khalil Aswad, an Iraqi girl of the Yazidi faith, was stoned to death in front of a mob of about 2000 men in 2007, possibly because she was allegedly planning to convert to Islam.[134]

13.13.5 Jordan

There are still "honor" killings in Jordan.[135] A 2008 report of the National Council of Family Affairs in Jordan, an NGO affiliated with the Queen of Jordan, indicated that the National Forensic Medicine Center recorded 120 murdered women in 2006, with 18 cases classified officially as crimes of honor

In 2013, the BBC cited estimates by the National Council of Family Affairs in Jordan, an NGO, that as many as 50 Jordanian women and girls had been killed in the preceding 13 years. But the BBC indicated "the real figure" was probably "far higher," because "most honor killings go unreported."

Men receive reduced sentences for killing their wives or female family members if they are

[133]Shahrzad Mojab. (2003). Kurdish Women in the Zone of Genocide and Gendercide. Al-Raida 21 (103): 20–25.

[134]"Iraq: Amnesty International appalled by stoning to death of Yezidi girl and subsequent killings" Amnesty International. *27 April 2007.*

[135]*Jordan: Special Report on Honour Killings*

deemed to have brought dishonor to their family. Families often get sons under the age of 16—legally minors—to commit honor killings; the juvenile law allows convicted minors to serve time in a juvenile detention center and be released with a clean criminal record at the age of 16. Rana Husseini, a leading journalist on the topic of honor killings, states that "under the existing law, people found guilty of committing honor killings often receive sentences as light as six months in prison".

According to UNICEF, there is an average of 23 honor killings per year in Jordan.[136]

There has been public support in Jordan to amend Articles 340 and 98. In 1999 King Abdullah created a council to review the sex inequalities in the country. The Council returned with a recommendation to repeal Article 340. "The cabinet approved the recommendation, the measure was presented to parliament twice in November 1999 and January 2000 and in both cases, though approved by the upper house, it failed to pass the elected lower house".[137] In 2001, after parliament was suspended, a number of temporary laws were created which were subject to parliamentary ratification. One of the amendments was that "husbands would no longer be exonerated for killing unfaithful wives, but instead the circumstances would be considered as evidence for mitigating punishments". In the interest of sex equality, women were given the same reduction in punishment if found guilty of the crime. But parliament returned to session in 2003 and the new amendments were rejected by the lower house after two successful readings in the upper house.

A 2013 survey of "856 ninth graders—average age of 15—from a range of secondary schools across Amman—including private and state, mixed-sex and single gender" showed that attitudes favoring honor killings are present in the "next generation" Jordanians: "In total, 33.4% of all respondents either "agreed" or "strongly agreed" with situations depicting honor killings. Boys were more than twice as likely to support honor killings: 46.1% of boys and 22.1% of girls agreed with at least two honor killing situations in the questionnaire." The parents' education was found to be a significant correlation: "61% of teenagers from the lowest level of educational background showed supportive attitudes towards honor killing, as opposed to only 21.1% where at least one family member has a university degree.[138]

13.13.6 Kuwait

Kuwait is relatively liberal (by Middle East standards), and honor killings are rare, but not unheard of—in 2006 a young woman died in an honor killing committed by

[136]UNICEF Executive Director targets violence against women. UNICEF. 7 March 2000

[137]"*Jordan: Special Report on Honour Killings". Retrieved 8 February 2009.*

[138]*Belief that honour killings are 'justified' still prevalent among Jordan's next generation, study shows | University of Cambridge".* Cam.ac.uk. *20 June 2013.*

her brothers. In 2008, a girl was given police protection after reporting that her family intended to kill her for having an affair with a man.

13.13.7 Lebanon

There are no exact official numbers about honor killings of women in Lebanon; many honor killings are arranged to look like accidents, but the figure is believed to be 40 to 50 per year. A 2007 report by Amnesty International said that the Lebanese media in 2001 reported 2 or 3 honor killings per month in Lebanon, although the number is believed to be higher by other independent sources.

On 4 August 2011, however, the Lebanese Parliament agreed by a majority to abolish Article 562, which for the past years had worked as an excuse to commute the sentence given for honor killing.[139,140]

13.13.8 Palestinian Authority

The Palestinian Authority, using a clause in the Jordanian penal code still in effect in the West Bank, exempts men from punishment for killing a female relative if she has brought dishonor to the family.[141] Mahmoud Abbas, President of the Palestinian Authority, issued a decree in May 2014 under which the exemption of men was abolished in cases of honor killings. According to UNICEF estimates in 1999, two-thirds of all murders in the Palestinian territories were likely honor killings.

The Palestinian Independent Commission for Human Rights has reported 29 women were killed 2007–2010, whereas 13 women were killed in 2011 and 12 in the first seven months of 2012. According to a PA Ministry of Women's Affairs report the rate of 'Honor Killings' went up by 100% in 2013, "reporting the number of 'honor killing' victims for 2013 at 27".[142]

[139] *"Lebanon at last removes honor crime article from its penal code". Retrieved 2011.*

[140] *"Hedersmord". Amnesty. Retrieved 2007.*

[141] *Suzanne Ruggi. "Commodifying Honor in Female Sexuality: Honor Killings in Palestine". Middle East Research and Information Project.*

[142] *Yashar, Ari. "PA 'Honor Killings' Up 100% in 2013". Arutz Sheva. Retrieved 26 February 2014.*

13.13.9 Saudi Arabia

In 2008 a woman was killed in Saudi Arabia by her father for "chatting" with a man on Facebook. The killing became public only when a Saudi cleric referred to the case, to criticize Facebook for the strife it caused.[143]

13.13.10 Syria

Some estimates suggest that more than 200 honor killings occur every year in Syria. The Syrian Civil War has been reported as leading to an increase in honor killings in the country, mainly due to the common occurrence of war rape, which led to the stigmatization of victims by their relatives and communities, and in turn to honor killings.[144,145]

13.13.11 Turkey

A report compiled by the Council of Europe estimated that over 200 women were killed in honor killings in Turkey in 2007.[146] A June 2008 report by the Turkish Prime Ministry's Human Rights Directorate said that in Istanbul alone there was one honor killing every week, and reported over 1000 during the previous five years. It added that metropolitan cities were the location of many of these, due to growing immigration to these cities from the East.[147] The mass migration during the past decades of rural population from Southeastern Turkey to big cities in Western Turkey has resulted in "modern" cities such as Istanbul, Ankara, Izmir, and Bursa having the highest numbers of reported honor killings.[148]

A report by UNFPA identified the following situations as being common triggers for honor killings: a married woman having an extra-marital relationship; a married woman running away with a man; a married woman getting separated or divorced; a divorced woman having a relationship with another man; a young unmarried girl

---

[143] *Damien McElroy (31 March 2008). "Saudi woman killed for chatting on Facebook". London: The Daily Telegraph. Retrieved 27 September 2008.*

[144] *Sinjab, Lina (12 October 2007). "Honour crime fear of Syria women". BBC News.*

[145] *Thomson Reuters Foundation. "Syrian war causing 'honour killings', child marriages – doctor". Retrieved 20 April 2015.*

[146] *"Number of Honor Killings in Europe Higher Than Thought".* voanews.com. *Retrieved 23 December 2013.*

[147] *AYSAN SEV'ER. "Feminist Analysis of Honor Killings in Rural Turkey" (PDF). 'University of Toronto'*

[148] http://middlab.middlebury.edu/files/2111/04/Honor-Killings-essay1.pdf

having a relationship; a young unmarried girl running away with a man; a woman (married or unmarried) being kidnapped and/or raped.

In Turkey, young boys are often ordered by other family members to commit the honor killing, so that they can get a shorter jail sentence (because they are minors). Forced suicides—where the victim who is deemed to have 'dishonored' the family is ordered to commit suicide in an attempt by the perpetrator to avoid legal consequences—also take place in Turkey, especially in Batman in southeastern Turkey, which has been nicknamed "Suicide City".

In 2009 a Turkish news agency reported that a 2-day-old boy who was born out of wedlock had been killed for honor in Istanbul. The maternal grandmother of the infant, along with six other persons, including a doctor who had reportedly accepted a bribe to not report the birth, were arrested. The grandmother is suspected of fatally suffocating the infant. The child's mother, 25, was also arrested; she stated that her family had made the decision to kill the child.[149]

In 2010 a 16-year-old girl was buried alive by relatives for befriending boys in Southeast Turkey; her corpse was found 40 days after she went missing. Ahmet Yildiz, 26, a Turkish-Kurdish physics student who represented his country at an international gay conference in the United States in 2008, was shot dead leaving a cafe in Istanbul. Ahmet Yildiz was who was from deeply religious family was believed to be the victim of the country's first gay honor killing.

Honor killings continue have some support in the conservative parts of Turkey. In 2005, a small survey in Diyarbakir in southeastern Turkey found that, when asked the appropriate punishment for a woman who has committed adultery, 37% of respondents said she should be killed, while 21% said her nose or ears should be cut off.[150]

A July 2008 Turkish study by a team from Dicle University on honor killings in the Southeastern Anatolia Region, the predominantly Kurdish area of Turkey, has so far shown that little if any social stigma is attached to honor killing. It also comments that the practice is not related to a feudal societal structure, "There are also perpetrators who are well-educated university graduates. Of all those surveyed, 60 percent are either high school or university graduates or at the very least, literate." There are well documented cases, where Turkish courts have sentenced whole families to life imprisonment for an honor killing. The most recent was on 13 January 2009, where a Turkish Court sentenced five members of the same Kurdish family to life imprisonment for the honor killing of Naile Erdas, a 16-year-old girl who got pregnant as a result of rape.

[149]*Le Monde* (France), Un bébé de 2 jours victime d'un "crime d'honneur" en Turquie. LEMONDE.FR with Reuters. 16 April 2010. Accessed 17 April 2010.

[150]*Rainsford, Sarah (19 October 2005). "'Honour' crime defiance in Turkey". BBC News. Retrieved 23 December 2013.*

13.13.12 Yemen

Honor killings are common in Yemen. In some parts of the country, traditional tribal customs forbid contact between men and women before marriage.[151] Yemeni society is strongly male dominated, Yemen being ranked last of 135 countries in the 2012 Global Gender Gap Report. It was estimated that about 400 women and girls died in honor killings in 1997 in Yemen. In 2013, a 15-year-old girl was killed by her father, who burned her to death, because she talked to her fiancé before the wedding.[152]

13.13.13 Maghreb

Honor killings in Maghreb are not as common as in the Asian countries of the Middle East and South Asia, but they do occur.[153] In Libya, they are targeted particularly against rape victims.

13.14 International Data

13.14.1 Europe

The issue of honor killings has risen to prominence in Europe in recent years, prompting the need to address the occurrence of honor killings. The 2009 European Parliamentary Assembly noted this in their Resolution 1681 which noted the dire need to address honor crimes. The resolution stated that: "On so-called 'honor crimes,' the Parliamentary Assembly notes that the problem, far from diminishing, has worsened, including in Europe. It mainly affects women, who are its most frequent victims, both in Europe and the rest of the world, especially in patriarchal and fundamentalist communities and societies. For this reason, it asked the Council of Europe member states to 'draw up and put into effect national action plans to combat violence against women, including violence committed in the name of so-called 'honor,' if they have not already done so."[154]

The Honor Based Violence Awareness Network (HBVA) writes[155]:

---

[151] *Yemeni 'burns daughter to death for contacting fiance'"*. bbc.co.uk. *23 October 2013. Retrieved 23 December 2013.*

[152] *Yemeni girl, 15, 'burned to death by father'"*. edition.cnn.com. *24 October 2013. Retrieved 23 December 2013.*

[153] *Five dead in Algeria 'honour' killings". News24. Retrieved 20 April 2015.*

[154] "Council of Europe Parliamentary Assembly". assembly.coe.int. 26 June 2009. Retrieved 23 December 2013.

[155] http://hbv-awareness.com/regions/

"Certain Eastern European countries have recorded cases of HBV [honor based violence] within the indigenous populations, such as Albania and Chechnya, and there have been acts of 'honor' killings within living memory within Mediterranean countries such as Italy and Greece".

13.14.1.1 Albania

Honor based violence has a long tradition in Albania, and although much rarer today than in the past, it still exists.[156] The Kanun is a set of traditional Albanian laws and customs. Honor (in Albanian: Nderi) is one of the four pillars on which the Kanun is based. Honor crimes happen especially in northern Albania. In Albania (and in other parts of the Balkans) the phenomenon of blood feuds between males was more common historically than honor killings of females; but honor violence against women and girls also has a tradition.[157]

13.14.1.2 Belgium

In 2011, Belgium held its first honor killing trial, in which four Pakistani family members were found guilty of killing their daughter and sibling, Sadia Sheikh.[158] As a legacy of the very influential Napoleonic Code, before 1997, Belgian law provided for mitigating circumstances in the case of a killing or assault against a spouse caught in the act of adultery.[159] (Adultery itself was decriminalized in Belgium in 1987.)[160]

13.14.1.3 Denmark

Ghazala Khan was shot and killed in Denmark in September 2005, by her brother, after she had married against the will of the family. She was of Pakistani origin. Her murder was ordered by her father to save the family 'honor', and several relatives were involved.

---

[156] http://www.mcser.org/images/stories/2_journal/mjss_september_2012/miranda%20rira.pdf

[157] http://www.etd.ceu.hu/2011/xhaho_armela.pdf

[158] "Pakistani family guilty of Belgian honour killing: media". AFP. 12 December 2011. Retrieved 16 December 2011.

[159] http://orbi.ulg.ac.be/bitstream/2268/36305/1/ULg-Liber%20amicorum%20Bosly%20-%20Masset.pdf

[160] http://www.senate.be/www/?MIval=/publications/viewPub.html&COLL=S&LEG=4&NR=162&VOLGNR=1&LANG=fr

13.14.1.4 France

France has a large immigrant community from North Africa (especially from Algeria, Morocco and Tunisia) and honor violence occurs in this community.[161] A 2009 report by the Council of Europe cited the United Kingdom, Germany, Belgium, France, and Norway as countries where honor crimes and honor killings occur.[162] France traditionally provided for leniency in regard to honor crimes, particularly against women who had committed adultery. The Napoleonic Code of 1804, established under Napoleon Bonaparte, is one of the origins of the legal leniency in regard to adultery-related killings in a variety of legal systems in several countries around the world. Under this code, a man who killed his wife whom he caught in the act of adultery could not be charged with premeditated murder—although he could be charged with other lesser offenses. This defense was available only for a husband, not for a wife. The Napoleonic Code has been very influential, and many countries, inspired by it, provided for lesser penalties or even acquittal for such crimes. This can be seen in the criminal codes of many former French colonies.[163][164]

13.14.1.5 Germany

In 2005 Der Spiegel reported: "In the past four months, six Muslim women living in Berlin have been killed by family members". The article went on to cover the case of Hatun Sürücü, a Turkish-Kurdish woman who was killed by her brother for not staying with the husband she was forced to marry, and of "living like a German". Precise statistics on how many women die every year in such honor killings are hard to come by, as many crimes are never reported, said Myria Boehmecke of the Tuebingen-based women's group Terre des Femmes. The group tries to protect Muslim girls and women from oppressive families. The Turkish women's organization Papatya has documented 40 instances of honor killings in Austria and Germany since 1996.[165] Hatun Sürücü's brother was convicted of murder and jailed for nine years and three months by a German court in 2006.[166] In March 2009, a Kurdish immigrant from Turkey, Gülsüm S., was killed for a relationship not in keeping with her religious family's plan for an arranged marriage.[167] In a well-known case, a Kurdish man killed his pregnant girlfriend in Berlin in January 2015

[161] Geesy, Patricia "North African Immigrants in France: Integration and Change" 1995 Substance 77(76) p137.

[162] "Number of Honor Killings in Europe Higher Than Thought". VOA. Retrieved 20 April 2015.

[163] "Honour Killings By Region". Hbv-awareness.com. 18 March 2012. Retrieved 16 August 2013.

[164] Lethal Imagination: Violence and Brutality in American History. Retrieved 16 August 2013

[165] "The Whore Lived Like a German". Der Spiegel, Germany.

[166] "Turkish man in Berlin jailed for 'honour killing' of sister".

[167] "Erschlagen, weil sie schwanger war? – Killed, because she was pregnant?". Der Bild

and burned her alive.[168] In 2016 a Kurdish woman was shot dead at her wedding in Hannover for refusing to marry her cousin in a forced marriage.[169]

13.14.1.6 Italy

Similar to other Southern/Mediterranean European areas, "honor" was traditionally important in Italy. Indeed, until 1981, the Criminal Code provided for mitigating circumstances for such killings; until 1981 the law read: Art. 587: He who causes the death of a spouse, daughter, or sister upon discovering her in illegitimate carnal relations and in the heat of passion caused by the offence to his honor or that of his family will be sentenced to three to seven years. The same sentence shall apply to whom, in the above circumstances, causes the death of the person involved in illegitimate carnal relations with his spouse, daughter, or sister. Traditionally, honor crimes used to be more prevalent in Southern Italy. In 1546, Isabella di Morra, a young poet from Valsinni, Matera, was stabbed to death by her brothers for a suspected affair with a married nobleman, whom they also murdered.

In 2006, 20-year-old Hina Saleem, a Pakistani woman who lived in Brescia, Italy, was murdered by her father who claimed he was "saving the family's honor". She had refused an arranged marriage, and was living with her Italian boyfriend. In 2009, in Pordenone, Italy, Sanaa Dafani, an 18-year-old girl of Moroccan origin, was murdered by her father because she had a relationship with an Italian man.

In 2011, in Cerignola, Italy, a man stabbed his brother 19 times because his homosexuality was a "dishonor to the family".

13.14.1.7 Norway

Anooshe Sediq Ghulam was a 22-year-old Afghan refugee in Norway, who was killed by her husband in an honor killing. She had reported her husband to the police for domestic violence and was seeking a divorce.

---

[168] Von Jörg Burger und Johannes Dudziak; 20. Februar 2016, 16:25 Uhr / 89 Kommentare; http://www.zeit.de/gesellschaft/zeitgeschehen/2016-02/prozess-mord-junge-frau-migrantenmilieus/komplettansicht

[169] http://www.telegraph.co.uk/women/life/kurdish-woman-shot-dead-at-wedding-for-refusing-to-marry-her-cou/

13.14.1.8 Sweden

In Sweden the 26-year-old Iraqi Kurdish woman Fadime Şahindal was killed by her father in 2002.[170] Pela Atroshi was a Kurdish girl who was shot by her uncle who was radical Muslim in a brutal honor killing in Sweden.

13.14.1.9 Switzerland

In 2010, a 16-year-old Pakistani girl was killed near Zurich, Switzerland, by her father who was dissatisfied with her lifestyle and her Christian boyfriend.

13.14.1.10 United Kingdom

Every year in the United Kingdom (UK), officials estimate that at least a dozen women are victims of honor killings, almost exclusively within Asian and Middle Eastern families.[171] Often, cases cannot be resolved due to the unwillingness of family, relatives and communities to testify.[172] A 2006 BBC poll for the Asian network in the UK found that one in ten of the 500 young Asians polled said that they could condone the killing of someone who dishonored their family.[173] In the UK, in December 2005, Nazir Afzal, Director, west London, of Britain's Crown Prosecution Service, stated that the United Kingdom has seen "at least a dozen honor killings" between 2004 and 2005.

In 2010, Britain saw a 47% rise of honor-related crimes. Data from police agencies in the UK report 2283 cases in 2010, and an estimated 500 more from jurisdictions that did not provide reports. These "honor-related crimes" also include house arrests and other parental punishments. Most of the attacks were conducted in cities that had high immigrant populations.[174]

Banaz Mahmod, a 20-year-old Iraqi Kurd woman from Mitcham, south London, was killed in 2006, in a murder orchestrated by her father, uncle and cousins. Her life and murder were presented in a documentary called Banaz a Love Story, directed and produced by Deeyah Khan. Another well-known case was Heshu Yones, stabbed to death by her Kurdish father in London in 2002 when her family heard a love song dedicated to her and suspected she had a boyfriend. Other examples

---

[170]Hellgren, Zenia; Hobson, Barbara (1 September 2008). "Cultural dialogues in the good society: The case of honour killings in Sweden". Ethnicities. 8 (3): 385–404. doi:https://doi.org/10.1177/1468796808092449

[171]*"BBC: Honour killings in the UK". BBC. Archived from the original on 6 January 2009. Retrieved 27 September 2008.*

[172]*" 'Honour' attack numbers revealed by UK police forces". bbc.co.uk*

[173]*One in 10 'backs honour killings'". BBC. 4 September 2006. Retrieved 27 September 2008.*

[174]*Ashis Ray (4 December 2011). "Honor Killing Cases Among South Asians in the UK Rising". The Indian Times. Retrieved 8 December 2011.*

include the killing of Tulay Goren, a Kurdish Shia Muslim girl who immigrated with her family from Turkey,and Samaira Nazir (Pakistani Muslim). A highly publicized case was that of Shafilea Iftikhar Ahmed, a 17-year-old British Pakistani girl from Great Sankey, Warrington, Cheshire, who was murdered in 2003 by her parents. However, a lesser-known case is that of Gurmeet Singh Ubhi, a Sikh man who, in February 2011, was found guilty of the murder of his 24-year-old daughter, Amrit Kaur Ubhi in 2010. Ubhi was found to have murdered his daughter because he disapproved of her being 'too westernised'. Likewise he also disapproved of the fact that she was dating a non-Sikh man. In 2012, the UK had the first white victim of an honor killing: 17 year old Laura Wilson was killed by her Asian boyfriend, Ashtiaq Ashgar, because she revealed details of their relationship to his family, challenging traditional cultural values of the Asian family. Laura Wilson's mother told Daily Mail, "I honestly think it was an honor killing for putting shame on the family. They needed to shut Laura up and they did". Wilson was repeatedly knifed to death as she walked along a canal in Rotherham city. In 2013, Mohammed Inayat was jailed for killing his wife and injuring three daughters by setting his house on fire in Birmingham. Inayat wanted to stop his daughter from flying to Dubai to marry her boyfriend, because he believed the marriage would dishonor his family.[175] In 2014, the husband of a Syrian 25-year-old Rania Alayed, as well as three brothers of the husband, were jailed for killing her.

According to the prosecution, the motive for the murder was that she had become "too westernised" and was "establishing an independent life".

Honor killings also affect LGBT. In 2008 a man had to flee from Turkey after his Kurdish boyfriend was killed by his own father.

13.14.2 South Asia

13.14.2.1 Afghanistan

In 2012, Afghanistan recorded 240 cases of honor killings, but the total number is believed to be much higher.[176] Of the reported honor killings, 21% were committed by the victims' husbands, 7% by their brothers, 4% by their fathers, and the rest by other relatives.[177]

---

[175] *Tyseley 'honour killing' father jailed for blaze murder". BBC News. Retrieved 20 April 2015.*

[176] Afghan couple stoned to death – Central & South Asia. Al Jazeera English

[177] *"AIHRC: 400 rape, honor killings registered in Afghanistan in 2 years".* latinbusinesstoday.com. *10 June 2013. Retrieved 23 December 2013.*

13.14.2.2 India

Honor killings have been reported in northern regions of India, mainly in the Indian states of Punjab, Rajasthan, Haryana and Uttar Pradesh, as a result of people marrying without their family's acceptance, and sometimes for marrying outside their caste or religion. In contrast, honor killings are prevalent to a lesser extent but are not completely non-existent[178] in South India and the western Indian states of Maharashtra and Gujarat. In some other parts of India, notably West Bengal, honor killings completely ceased about a century ago, largely due to the activism and influence of reformists such as Vivekananda, Ramakrishna, Vidyasagar and Raja Ram Mohan Roy. Haryana is notorious for incidents of honor killings, mainly in the upper caste of society, among Rajputs and Jats. Honor killings have been described as "chillingly common in villages of Haryana dominated by the lawless 'khap panchayats' (caste councils of village elders)".[179] In a landmark judgment in March 2010, Karnal district court ordered the execution of five perpetrators of an honor killing in Kaithal, and imprisoning for life the khap (local caste-based council) chief who ordered the killings of Manoj Banwala and Babli a man and woman of the same clan who eloped and married in June 2007. Despite having been given police protection on court orders, they were kidnapped; their mutilated bodies were found a week later in an irrigation canal. In 2013, a young couple who were planning to marry were murdered in Garnauthi village, Haryana, due to having a love affair. The woman, Nidhi, was beaten to death and the man, Dharmender, was dismembered alive. People in the village and neighboring villages approved of the killings.

The Indian state of Punjab also has a large number of honor killings. According to data compiled by the Punjab Police, 34 honor killings were reported in the state between 2008 and 2010: 10 in 2008, 20 in 2009, and four in 2010. Bhagalpur in the eastern Indian state of Bihar has also been notorious for honor killings.[180] Recent cases include a 16-year-old girl, Imrana, from Bhojpur who was set on fire inside her house in a case of what the police called 'moral vigilantism'. The victim had screamed for help for about 20 minutes before neighbors arrived, only to find her smoldering body. She was admitted to a local hospital, where she later died from her injuries. In May 2008, Jayvirsingh Bhadodiya shot his daughter Vandana Bhadodiya and struck her on the head with an axe. Honor killings occur even in Delhi.

Honor killings take place in Rajasthan, too. In June 2012, a man chopped off his 20-year-old daughter's head with a sword in Rajasthan after learning that she was dating men. According to police officer, "Omkar Singh told the police that his daughter Manju had relations with several men. He had asked her to mend her

---

[178] *"Suspected Honor killing in South Indian state*

[179] http://www.bbc.com/news/world-asia-india-24170937

[180] Eight beheaded in Indian 'honor killing'. United Press International. 12 February 2009.

ways several times in the past. However, she did not pay heed. Out of pure rage, he chopped off her head with the sword".[181]

In 1990 the National Commission for Women set up a statutory body in order to address the issues of honor killings among some ethnic groups in North India. This body reviewed constitutional, legal and other provisions as well as challenges women face. The NCW's activism has contributed significantly towards the reduction of honor killings in rural areas of North India. According to Pakistani activists Hina Jilani and Eman M Ahmed, Indian women are considerably better protected against honor killings by Indian law and government than Pakistani women, and they have suggested that governments of countries affected by honor killings use Indian law as a model in order to prevent honor killings in their respective societies.[182] In June 2010, scrutinizing the increasing number of honor killings, the Supreme Court of India demanded responses about honor killing prevention from the federal government and the state governments of Punjab, Haryana, Bihar, Uttar Pradesh, Rajasthan, Jharkhand, Himachal Pradesh and Madhya Pradesh.

Alarmed by the rise of honor killings, the Government planned to bring a bill in the Monsoon Session of Parliament July 2010 to provide for deterrent punishment for 'honor' killings. According to the survey done by AIDWA, over 30% of the total honor killings in the country take place in Western Uttar Pradesh.[183]

13.14.2.3 Pakistan

In Pakistan honor killings are known locally as karo-kari.[184] An Amnesty International report noted "the failure of the authorities to prevent these killings by investigating and punishing the perpetrators." Recent cases include that of three teenage girls who were buried alive after refusing arranged marriages.[185] Another case was that of Taslim Khatoon Solangi, 17, of Hajna Shah village in Khairpur district, which was widely reported after her father, 57-year-old Gul Sher Solangi, publicized the case. He alleged his eight-months-pregnant daughter was tortured and killed on 7 March on the orders of her father-in-law, who accused her of carrying a child conceived out of wedlock. Statistically, honor killings have a high level of support in Pakistan's rural society, despite widespread condemnation from human rights groups. In 2002 alone over 382 people, about 245 women and 137 men, became victims of honor killings in the Sindh province of Pakistan. Over the course of six years, more than 4000 women have died as victims of honor killings in

---

[181]*Man beheads daughter in gory Rajasthan".* Zeenews.india.com. *17 June 2012. Retrieved 1 October 2012.*

[182]*Goonesekere, Savitri (2004). Violence, Law and Women's Rights in South Asia. SAGE Publications. p. 149. ISBN 0-7619-9796-2*

[183]*AIDWA survey "News 18. 29 October 2015.*

[184]*PAKISTAN Honour killings of girls and women". Amnesty International.*

[185]*Three teenagers buried alive in Pakistan 'honour killing'". Irish Time. 9 September 2008.*

Pakistan from 1999 to 2004. In 2005 the average annual number of honor killings for the whole nation was stated to be more than 1000 per year.[186]

A 2009 study by Muazzam Nasrullah et al. reported a total of 1957 honor crime victims reported in Pakistan's newspapers from 2004 to 2007. Of those killed, 18% were below the age of 18 years, and 88% were married. Husbands, brothers and close relatives were direct perpetrators of 79% of the honor crimes reported by mainstream media. The method used for honor crime included firearms (most common), stabbing, axe and strangulation.[187]

According to women's rights advocates, the concepts of women as property, and of honor, are so deeply entrenched in the social, political and economic fabric of Pakistan that the government mostly ignores the regular occurrences of women being killed and maimed by their families." Frequently, women killed in honor killings are recorded as having committed suicide or died in accidents. Savitri Goonesekere states that Islamic leaders in Pakistan use religious justifications for sanctioning honor killings. On 27 May 2014, a pregnant woman was stoned to death by her own family in front of a Pakistani high court for marrying the man she loved. "I killed my daughter as she had insulted all of our family by marrying a man without our consent, and I have no regret over it," Mujahid, the police investigator, quoted the father as saying. Prime Minister Nawaz Sharif described the stoning as "totally unacceptable," and ordered the chief minister of Punjab province to provide an immediate report. He demanded to know why police did nothing, despite the killing taking place outside one of the country's top courts, in the presence of police.[188]

Honor killings are tried by the 1990 Qisas and Diyat Ordinance of Pakistan, which permits the individual and his or her family to retain control over a crime, including the right to determine whether to report the crime, prosecute the offender, or demand *diyat* (or compensation). Since most honor killings are committed by a close relative, if and when the case reaches a court of law, the victim's family may 'pardon' the murderer, or be pressured to accept diyat (financial compensation). The murderer then goes free.[189] Once such a pardon has been secured, the state has no further writ on the matter although often the killers are relatives of the victim. Scholars suggest that the Islamic law doctrine of Qisas and Diyya encourages honor killings, particularly against females, as well as allows the murderer to go unpunished.

---

[186]Sohail Warraich, "'Honour Killings' and the Law in Pakistan", in Sara Hossain and Lynn Welchman, *Honour, Crimes, Paradigms, and Violence against Women*, Zed Books (10 November 2005),

[187]Muazzam Nasrullah et al. (March 2009), The epidemiological patterns of honour killing of women in Pakistan, The European Journal of Public Health, Oxford University Press, pp. 1–5

[188]*Nawaz Sharif orders action on stoning of pregnant Pakistani woman". Pakistan Telegraph. Retrieved 29 May 2014.*

[189]Beena Sarwar. Pakistan: No compromise on murder. 17 October 2004.

13.14.3 The Americas

13.14.3.1 Brazil

Throughout the twentieth century, husbands have used in court cases the "legitimate defense of their honor" (*legitima defesa da honra*) as justification for adultery-related killings. Although this defense was not explicitly stipulated in the twentieth century Criminal Code, it has been successfully pleaded by lawyers throughout the twentieth century, in particular in the interior of the country, though less so in the coastal big cities. In 1991 Brazil's Supreme Court explicitly rejected the "honor defense" as having no basis in Brazilian law.[190]

13.14.3.2 Canada

A 2007 study by Dr. Amin Muhammad and Dr. Sujay Patel of Memorial University, Canada, investigated how the practice of honor killings has been brought to Canada. The report explained that "When people come and settle in Canada they can bring their traditions and forcefully follow them. In some cultures, people feel some boundaries are never to be crossed, and if someone would violate those practices or go against it, then killing is justified to them." The report noted that "In different cultures, they can get away without being punished—the courts actually sanction them under religious contexts". The report also said that the people who commit these crimes are usually mentally ill, and that the mental health aspect is often ignored by Western observers because of a lack of understanding of the insufficiently developed state of mental healthcare in developing countries in which honor killings are prevalent.[191]

Canada has been host to a number of high-profile killings[192],[193] including the murder of Kaur Sidhu, the murder of Amandeep Atwal, the double murder of Khatera Sadiqi and her fiance, and the Shafia family murders. Honor killings have become such a pressing issue in Canada that the Canadian citizenship study guide mentions it specifically, saying, "Canada's openness and generosity do not extend to barbaric cultural practices that tolerate spousal abuse, 'honor killings', female genital mutilation, forced marriage or other gender-based violence."[194]

---

[190]http://www.nytimes.com/1991/03/29/us/honor-killing-of-wives-is-outlawed-in-brazil.html

[191]*Jamie Baker. "Cultural 'honour' killing brought to Canada". The Telegram. Retrieved 27 September 2008.*

[192]*Introduction – Preliminary Examination of so-called Honour Killings in Canada". Justice.gc.ca*

[193]*Historical Context – Origins of Honour Killing / Honour Killing – Worldwide / Honour Killing – In Countries with Islamic Law – Preliminary Examination of so-called Honour Killings in Canada". Justice.gc.ca*

[194]*"The History of Honor Killings". CBC News. Retrieved 2 December 2011.*

13.14.3.3 United States

Phyllis Chesler argues that the U.S., as well as in Canada, do not have proper measures in place to fight against honor killings, and do not recognize these murders as a specific form of violence, distinct from other domestic murders, due to fear of being labeled "culturally insensitive". According to her, this often prevents government officials in the United States and the media from identifying and accurately reporting these incidents as "honor killings" when they occur. Failing to accurately describe the problem makes it more difficult to develop public policies to address it, she argues.[195]

She also writes that, although there are not many cases of honor killings within the United States, the overwhelming majority of honor killings are perpetrated by Muslims against Muslims (90% of honor killings known to have taken place in Europe and the United States from 1998 to 2008). In these documented cases the victims were murdered because they were believed to have acted in a way against the religion of the family.[196] In every case, perpetrators view their victims as violating rules of religious conduct and act without remorse.[197] Several honor killings have occurred in the U.S. during recent years. In 1989, in St. Louis, Missouri, 16-year-old Palestina "Tina" Isa was murdered by her Palestinian father with the aid of his wife. Her parents were dissatisfied with her "westernized" lifestyle.[198] In 2008, in Georgia, 25-year-old Sandeela Kanwal was killed by her Pakistani father for refusing an arranged marriage. Amina and Sarah Said, two teenage sisters from Texas were killed, allegedly by their Egyptian father, Yaser Abdel Said, who is still at large. Yaser is currently on the FBI Ten Most Wanted Fugitives, and has been on the list since December 10, 2014. Aasiya Zubair was, together with her husband Muzzammil Hassan, the founder and owner of Bridges TV, the first American Muslim English-language television network. She was killed by her husband in 2009. Phyllis Chesler argued this was an honor killing. In 2009, in Arizona, Noor Almaleki, aged 20, was killed by her father, an Iraqi immigrant, because she had refused an arranged marriage and was living with her boyfriend.

The extent of honor-based violence in the U.S. is not known, as no official data is collected. There is controversy about the reasons why such violence occurs, and about the extent to which culture, religion, and views on women cause these incidents.[199]

---

[195] Phyllis Chesler, Are Honor Killings Simply Domestic Violence?, *Middle East Quarterly*, Spring 2009, pp. 61–69; Meforum.org. Retrieved on 1 October 2011.

[196] Honor Killings: Amnesty USA

[197] *Honor killing" under growing scrutiny in the U.S. – Crimesider. CBS News.*

[198] *Terror and Death at Home Are Caught in F.B.I. Tape". The New York Times. 28 October 1991.*

[199] *CBS News http://www.cbsnews.com/news/honor-killing-under-growing-scrutiny-in-the-us/#*

13.14.3.4 Latin America

Crimes of passion within Latin America have also been compared to honor killings. Similar to honor killings, crimes of passion often feature the murder of a woman by a husband, family member, or boyfriend and the crime is often condoned or sanctioned. In Peru, for example, 70 percent of the murders of women in one year were committed by a husband, boyfriend or lover, and most often jealousy or suspicions of infidelity are cited as the reasons for the murders.[200] The law of Uruguay continues to tolerate crimes of passion due to adultery. However, "while crimes of passion may be seen as somewhat premeditated to a certain extent, honor killings are usually deliberate, well planned and premeditated acts when a person kills a female relative ostensibly to uphold his honor."

The view that violence can be justified in the name of honor and shame exists traditionally in Latin American societies, and machismo is often described as a code of honor. While some ideas originate in the Spanish colonial culture, others predate it: in the early history of Peru, the laws of the Incas allowed husbands to starve their wives to death if they committed adultery, while Aztec laws during early Mexico stipulated stoning or strangulation as punishment for female adultery.[201]

Until a few decades ago, the marriage of a girl or woman to the man who had raped her was considered a "solution" to the incident in order to restore the 'honor'. Indeed, although laws that exonerate the perpetrator of rape if he marries his victim after the rape are often associated with the Middle East, such laws were very common around the world until the second half of the twentieth century, and as late as 1997, 14 Latin American countries had such laws, although most of these Latin American countries have now abolished them. Such laws were ended in Mexico in 1991, El Salvador in 1996, Colombia in 1997, Peru in 1999, Chile in 1999, Brazil in 2005, Uruguay in 2005, Guatemala in 2006, Costa Rica in 2007, Panama in 2008, Nicaragua in 2008, Argentina in 2012, and Ecuador in 2014.

13.14.3.5 Oceania

13.14.3.6 Australia

Jim Spigelman (who served as Chief Justice of the Supreme Court of New South Wales from 19 May 1998 until 31 May 2011) said that Australia's increasing diversity was creating conflicts about how to deal with the customs and traditions

---

[200] http://www.wluml.org/node/4628 Peru Hundreds of Women Murdered in the Name of 'Honor' and 'Passion'

[201] http://www.justice.gc.ca/eng/rp-pr/cj-jp/fv-vf/hk-ch/p3.html

of immigrant populations. He said: "There are important racial, ethnic and religious minorities in Australia who come from nations with sexist traditions which, in some respects, are even more pervasive than those of the West." He said that honor crimes, forced marriages and other violent acts against women were becoming a problem in Australia.[202]

In 2010, in New South Wales, Indonesian born Hazairin Iskandar and his son killed the lover of Iskandar's wife. Iskandar stabbed the victim with a knife while his son bashed him with a hammer. The court was told that the reason for the murder was the perpetrators' belief that extramarital affairs were against their religion; and that the murder was carried out to protect the honor of the family and was a "pre-planned, premeditated and executed killing". The judge said that: "No society or culture that regards itself as civilized can tolerate to any extent, or make any allowance for, the killing of another person for such an amorphous concept as honor".[203]

Pela Atroshi was a Kurdish 19-year-old girl who was killed by her uncle in Iraqi Kurdistan in 1999. The decision to kill her was taken by a council of her male relatives, led by Pela's grandfather, Abdulmajid Atroshi, who lived in Australia. One of his sons, Shivan Atroshi, who helped with the murder, also lived in Australia. Pela Atroshi was living in Sweden, but was taken by family members to Iraqi Kurdistan to be killed, as ordered by a family council of male relatives living in Sweden and Australia, because they claimed she had tarnished the family honor. Pela Atroshi's murder was officially deemed an honor killing by authorities.

13.15 Comparison to Other Forms of Killings

Honor killings are, along with dowry killings (mostly in South Asia), gang-related killings of women as revenge (killings of female members of rival gang members' families—primarily, but not only, in Latin America) and witchcraft accusation killings (Africa, Oceania) some of the most recognized forms of gender based killings.[204] Human rights advocates have compared "honor killing" to "crimes of passion" in Latin America (which are sometimes treated extremely leniently) and also to the killing of women for lack of dowry in India. Some commentators have stressed that the focus on honor killings should not lead to ignoring other forms of gender-based killings of women, in particular those from Latin America ('crimes of passion' and gang related killings); the murder rate of women in this region being extremely high, with El Salvador being reported as the country with the highest murder rate of women in the world. In 2002, Widney Brown, advocacy director for Human Rights Watch, stated that "crimes of passion have a similar dynamic in that

[202]*Honour killings coming to our courts: top judge". WA Today. Retrieved 20 April 2015.*

[203]*Murder verdict over honour killing of wife's lover". ABC News. Retrieved 20 April 2015.*

[204]*Carolyn Fluehr-Lobban. "Cultural Relativism and Universal Rights"*

the women are killed by male family members and the crimes are perceived as excusable or understandable".

13.16 Views on Women

Honor killings are often a result of strongly patriarchal views on women, and the position of women in society. In these traditional male-dominated societies women are dependent first on their father and then on their husband, whom they are expected to obey.[205] Women are viewed as property and not as individuals with their own agency. As such, they must submit to male authority figures in the family—failure to do so can result in extreme violence as punishment. Violence is seen as a way of ensuring compliance and preventing rebellion.[206] According to Shahid Khan, a professor at the Aga Khan University in Pakistan: "Women are considered the property of the males in their family irrespective of their class, ethnic, or religious group. The owner of the property has the right to decide its fate. The concept of ownership has turned women into a commodity which can be exchanged, bought and sold".[207] In such cultures, women are not allowed to take control over their bodies and sexuality: these are the property of the males of the family, the father (and other male relatives) who must ensure virginity until marriage; and then the husband to whom his wife's sexuality is subordinated—a woman must not undermine the ownership rights of her guardian by engaging in premarital sex or adultery.[208]

13.17 Support and Sanction

Actions of Pakistani police officers and judges (particularly at the lower level of the judiciary) have, in the past, seemed to support the act of honor killings in the name of family honor. Police enforcement, in situations of admitted murder, do not always take action against the perpetrator.[209,210] Also, judges in Pakistan (particularly at the lower level of the judiciary), rather than ruling cases with gender equality in mind,

---

[205] *"Violence Against Women and "Honor" Crimes". Human Rights Watch*

[206] Krishan Bir Singh (1 January 1970). "Honour Killing – A Study of the Causes and Remedies in its SocioLegal Aspect". academia.edu. Retrieved 23 December 2013.

[207] "International Domestic Violence Issues". Sanctuary for Families. 2008-10-15. Retrieved 2015-02-15.

[208] http://www.humanrights.ch/upload/pdf/070419_Kvinnoforum_HRV.pdf

[209] *Murat Gezer. "Honor killing perpetrators welcomed by society, study reveals". Today's Zaman*

[210] *Honour Related Violence" (PDF). Humanrights.ch. Kvinnoforum. 2005.*

also seem to reinforce inequality and in some cases sanction the murder of women considered dishonorable.[211]

Often, a suspected honor killing never even reaches court, but in cases where they do, the alleged killer is often not charged or is given a reduced sentence of 3 to 4 years in jail. In a case study of 150 honor killings, the proceeding judges rejected only eight of claims that the women were killed for honor. The rest were sentenced lightly. In many cases in Pakistan, one of the reasons honor killing cases never make it to the courts, is because, according to some lawyers and women's right activists, Pakistani law enforcement do not get involved. Under the encouragement of the killer, police often declare the killing as a domestic case that warrants no involvement. In other cases, the women and victims are too afraid to speak up or press charges. Police officials, however, claim that these cases are never brought to them, or are not major enough to be pursued on a large scale. The general indifference to the issue of honor killing within Pakistan is due to a deep-rooted gender bias in law, the police force, and the judiciary. In its report, "Pakistan: Honor Killings of Girls and Women", published in September 1999, Amnesty International criticized governmental indifference and called for state responsibility in protecting human rights of female victims. To elaborate,

Amnesty strongly requested the Government of Pakistan to take (1) legal, (2) preventive, and (3) protective measures. First of all, legal measures refer to a modification of the government's criminal laws to guarantee equal legal protection of females. On top of that, Amnesty insisted the government to assure legal access for the victims of crime in the name of honor. When it comes to preventive measures, Amnesty underlined the critical need to promote public awareness through the means of media, education, and public announcements. Finally, protective measures include ensuring a safe environment for activists, lawyers, and women's group to facilitate eradication of honor killings. Also, Amnesty argued for the expansion of victim support services such as shelters.

Kremlin-appointed Chechen President Ramzan Kadyrov said that honor killings were perpetrated on those who deserved to die. He said that those who are killed have "loose morals" and are rightfully shot by relatives in honor killings. He did not vilify women alone but added that "If a woman runs around and if a man runs around with her, both of them are killed." In 2007, a famous Norwegian Supreme Court advocate stated that he wanted the punishment for the killing from 17 years in prison to 15 years in the case of honor killings practiced in Norway. He stated that the Norwegian public did not understand other cultures who practiced honor killings, or understand their thinking, and that Norwegian culture "is self-righteous". In 2008, Israr Ullah Zehri, a Pakistani politician in Balochistan, defended the honor killings of five women belonging to the Umrani tribe by a relative of a local Umrani politician. Zehri defended the killings in Parliament and asked his fellow legislators not to make a fuss about the incident. He said, "These are centuries-old traditions, and I will

---

[211] *Femicide: A Gobal Issue that demands Action" (PDF). Genevadeclaration.org. Academic Council on the United Nations System. p. 60.*

continue to defend them. Only those who indulge in immoral acts should be afraid." Nilofar Bakhtiar, Minister for Tourism and Advisor to Pakistan Prime Minister on Women's Affairs, who had struggled against the honor killing in Pakistan, resigned in April 2007 after the clerics accused her of bringing shame to Pakistan by para-jumping with a male and hugging him after landing.

Chapter 14
Early and Forced Marriage

14.1 Abstract

Child marriage is a formal marriage or informal union entered into by an individual before reaching the age of 18. The legally prescribed marriageable age in some jurisdictions is below 18 years, especially in the case of girls; and even when the age is set at 18 years, many jurisdictions permit earlier marriage with parental consent or in special circumstances, such as teenage pregnancy. In certain countries, even when the legal marriage age is 18, cultural traditions take priority over legislative law.[1] Child marriage affects both boys and girls, though the overwhelming majority of those affected are girls, most of who are in poor socioeconomic situations.

Despite this general trend towards increasing the minimum age for marriage in Arab countries, the practice of early marriage is still widespread in many areas. Many countries in the region have a low legal minimum age for marriage, and early marriage sometimes prevents girls from continuing their education. It also undermines the potential of women to participate in the development process, and leads to a consequent increase in spending on health services and treatment. This increase in health spending is attributed to the diseases and injuries experienced by girls as a result of early marriage and pregnancy. Teenage motherhood presents serious health risks, exacerbated in many cases by the unpreparedness of young girls for the role of motherhood.

[1]*Nour, NM (2009). "Child Marriage: a silent health and human rights issue". Reviews in obstetrics and gynecology.*

B. Gerbaka et al., *Child Sexual Abuse, Exploitation and Trafficking in the Arab Region*, Child Maltreatment 13, https://doi.org/10.1007/978-3-030-66507-4_14

14.2 Introduction

Child marriage is related to child betrothal, and it includes civil cohabitation and court approved early marriages after teenage pregnancy. In many cases, only one marriage-partner is a child, usually the female. Causes of child marriages include poverty, bride price, dowry, cultural traditions, laws that allow child marriages, religious and social pressures, regional customs, fear of remaining unmarried, illiteracy, and perceived inability of women to work for money.

Child marriage is one of the main forms of child sexual abuse; UNICEF has stated that child marriage "represents perhaps the most prevalent form of sexual abuse and exploitation of girls"[2]

According to the global partnership "Girls Not Brides," around 14 million girls under 18 (sometimes as young as 8) are married each year. Girls who are forced into child marriages face increased risk of encountering domestic violence, experiencing complications and /or fatality during pregnancy and childbirth, and contracting sexually transmitted infections, including HIV. Additionally, they are denied access to education and in the vast majority of cases live in lifelong poverty.[3]

Although there is a general trend towards raising the minimum age for marriage in Arab countries, early marriage is still widespread in some areas. Many countries of this region reduced the legal age for marriage; in particular, OIC edited recommendations in December 2009 to raise the age of legal marriage to 18 years. Early marriage prevents girls from continuing their education, and reduces women's capacities to participate in the development process, in addition to increased spending on health services and treatment as a result of diseases that expose her as a result of early marriage; furthermore, early pregnancy can lead to severe risks to the health of teenage mothers, in addition to unwillingness of girls at this early age to carry the burden of early motherhood.

14.3 History

Child marriages were common throughout history for a variety of reasons, including poverty, insecurity, as well as for political and financial reasons. Today, child marriage is still fairly widespread in developing countries, such as parts of Africa, South Asia, Southeast Asia, West Asia, Latin America, and Oceania. The incidence of child marriage has been falling in most parts of the world. The countries with the highest observed rates of child marriages below the age of 18 are Niger, Chad, Mali, Bangladesh, Guinea and the Central African Republic, with a rate above 60%.Niger,

---

[2]http://www.unicef.org/chinese/protection/files/Child_Marriage.pdf

[3]Otoo-Oyortey, N. and Pobi, S. (2003) Early Marriage and Poverty: Exploring Links for Policy and Programme Development. London.

Chad, Bangladesh, Mali and Ethiopia were the countries with child marriage rates greater than 20% below the age of 15, according to 2003–2009 surveys.

Historically, child marriage was common around the world. The practice began to be questioned in the twentieth century, with the age of individuals' first marriage increasing in many countries and most countries increasing the minimum marriage age.

In ancient and medieval societies, it was common for girls to be betrothed at or even before puberty. As Friedman claims, "arranging and contracting the marriage of a young girl were the undisputed prerogatives of her father in ancient Israel." Most girls were married before the age of 15, often at the start of their puberty. In the Middle Ages the age at marriage seems to have been around puberty throughout the Jewish world.

Ruth Lamdan writes: "The numerous references to child marriage in the sixteenth-century Responsa literature and other sources, shows that child marriage was so common, it was virtually the norm. In this context, it is important to remember that in halakha, the term 'minor' refers to a girl under twelve years and a day. A girl aged twelve and a half was already considered an adult in all respects."

In Greece, early marriage and motherhood for girls was encouraged. Even boys were expected to marry in their teens. With an average life expectancy between 40 and 45 years, early marriages and teenage motherhood was typical. In Ancient Rome, girls married above the age of 12 and boys above 14. In the Middle Ages, under English civil laws that were derived from Roman laws, marriages before the age of 16 were common. In Imperial China, child marriage was the norm.

14.4 Gender Overview

14.4.1 Boys

Boys are sometimes married as children, although according to UNICEF, "girls are disproportionately the most affected". Research on the effects of child marriage on underage boys is small. As of September 2014, 156 million living men were married as underage boys.[4]

14.4.2 Girls

Child marriage has lasting consequences on girls, from their health, education and social development perspectives. These consequences last well beyond adolescence.

[4] *Strochlic, Nina (18 September 2014). "The Sad Hidden Plight of Child Grooms". Retrieved 9 July 2016.*

One of the most common causes of death for girls aged 15 to 19 in developing countries was pregnancy and child birth. In Niger, which is estimated as having the highest rate of child marriage in the world, about 3 in 4 girls marry before their 18th birthday.[5]

14.5 The Case of Sexual Violence

Marriages involving young teenage girls can be interpreted as cases of sexual violence; they are often forced or arranged. The fact that many countries from the MENA region have sanctions in their legal systems that allow children below the age of 18 to marry is rather worrying and troublesome. It is widely accepted, and moreover sometimes expected of girls to marry before they are 18 years old.

14.6 Causes of Child Marriage

According to UNFPA, factors that promote and reinforce child marriage include poverty and economic survival strategies; gender inequality; sealing land or property deals or settling disputes; control over sexuality and protecting family honor; tradition and culture; and insecurity, particularly during war, famine or epidemics. Other factors include family ties in which marriage is a means of consolidating powerful relations between families.[6]

Providing a girl with a dowry at her marriage is an ancient practice which continues in some parts of the world. This requires parents to bestow property on the marriage of a daughter, which is often an economic challenge for many families. The difficulty to save and preserve wealth for dowry was common, particularly in times of economic hardship, or persecution, or unpredictable seizure of property and savings for discriminatory taxes such as Jizya. These difficulties pressed families to betroth their girl, irrespective of her age, as soon as they had the resources to pay the dowry. Thus, Goitein notes that European Jews would marry their girls early, once they had collected the expected amount of dowry.[7]

A bride price is the amount paid by the groom to the parents of a bride for them to consent to him marrying their daughter. In some countries, the younger the bride, the higher the price she may fetch. This practice creates an economic incentive where girls are sought and married early by her family to the highest bidder. Child

---

[5] *Brides, Girls Not. "Niger – Child Marriage Around The World. Girls Not Brides". Retrieved 9 July 2016.*

[6] *"Marrying Too Young: End Child Marriage" (PDF). UNFPA.*

[7] S.D. Goitein (1978), A Mediterranean Society: The Jewish Communities of the Arab World, Vol. 3, University of California Press.

marriages of girls is a way out of desperate economic conditions, or simply a source of income to the parents. Bride price is another cause of child marriage and child trafficking.

14.6.1 Persecution, Forced Migration, and Slavery

Social upheavals such as wars, major military campaigns, forced religious conversion, taking natives as prisoners of war and converting them into slaves, arrest and forced migrations of people often made a suitable groom a rare commodity. Bride's families would seek out any available bachelors and marry them to their daughters, before events beyond their control moved the boy away. Persecution and displacement of Roma and Jewish people in Europe, colonial campaigns to get slaves from various ethnic groups in West Africa across the Atlantic for plantations, Islamic campaigns to get Hindu slaves from India across Afghanistan's Hindu Kush as property and for work, were some of the historical events that increased the practice of child marriage before the nineteenth century.

A New York Times report and other scholars claim the origin of child marriages in India to be Muslim invasions that began more than 1000 years ago. The invaders raped unmarried Hindu girls or carried them off as booty, prompting Hindu communities to marry off their daughters early to protect them. Similarly, among Sephardi Jewish communities, child marriages became frequent from tenth to thirteenth century as Muslim invasion and rule spread in Spain. This practice intensified after the Jewish community was expelled from Spain, and resettled in the Ottoman Empire. Child marriages among the Eastern Sephardic Jews continued through the nineteenth century in Islamic majority regions.[8]

14.6.2 Fear, Poverty, Social Pressures and Sense of Protection

English stage actress Ellen Terry was married at age 16 to George Frederic Watts who was 46 years old, a marriage her parents thought would be advantageous; later she said she was uncomfortable being a child bride. Terry died at the age of 81, in 1928.

A sense of social insecurity has been a cause of child marriages across the world. For example, in Nepal, parents fear likely social stigma if grown-up adult girls (past 18 years) stay at home. Other fear of crime such as rape, which not only would be traumatic but may lead to less acceptance of the girl if she becomes victim of a crime.

[8]Julia Rebollo Lieberman (2011), Sephardi Family Life in the Early Modern Diaspora, pages 8–10; Brandeis University Press; ISBN 978-1-58465-957-0

For example, girls may not be seen as eligible for marriage if they are not virgins. In other cultures, the fear is that an unmarried girl may engage in illicit relationships, or elope causing a permanent social blemish to her siblings, or that the impoverished family may be unable to find bachelors for grown up girls in their economic social group. Such fears and social pressures have been proposed as causes that lead to child marriages.

Extreme poverty may make daughters an economic burden on the family, which may be relieved by their early marriage,[9] to the benefit of the family as well as the girl herself. Poor parents may have few alternatives they can afford for the girls in the family; they often view marriage as a means to ensure their daughter's financial security and to reduce the economic burden of a growing adult on the family. Child marriage can also be seen as means of ensuring a girl's economic security, particularly if she lacks family members to provide for her. In reviews of Jewish community history, scholars claim poverty, shortage of grooms; uncertain social and economic conditions were a cause for frequent child marriages. Drawings by young Syrian refugee girls in a community center in southern Lebanon promote the prevention of child marriage.

An additional factor causing child marriage is the parental belief that early marriage offers protection. Parents feel that marriage provides their daughter with a sense of protection from sexual promiscuity and safe from sexually transmitted infections. However, in reality, young girls tend to marry older men, placing them at an increased risk of contracting a sexually transmitted infection. Married girls are more likely than unmarried girls to become infected with HIV or the human papilloma virus ('HPV').

Protection through marriage may play a specific role in conflict settings. Families may have their young daughters marry members of an armed group or military in hopes that she will be better protected. Girls may also be taken by armed groups and forced into marriages.

14.6.3 The Social Scenario

Child marriage remains a widely ignored violation of the health and development rights of girls and young women."[10] Many reasons are given by parents and guardians to justify child marriage. Economic reasons often underpin these decisions which are directly linked to poverty and the lack of economic opportunities for girls in rural areas. Girls are either seen as an economic burden or valued as capital for their exchange value in terms of goods, money or livestock. A combination of cultural, traditional and religious arguments are examples utilized to justify child

---

[9] *"Targeting Girls in the Name of Tradition: Child Marriage". U.S. Department of State.*

[10] Ending child marriage, A guide for global policy action, International Planned Parenthood Federation and the Forum on Marriage and the Rights of Women and Girls, 2006, page 6

marriage.[11] The fear and stigma attached to premarital sex and bearing children outside marriage, and the associated family "honor," are often seen as valid reasons for the actions that families take. Finally, many parents tend to curtail the education of their girls and marry them off, due to fear of the high level of sexual violence and abuse encountered in route to, and even at, school.[12]

14.6.4 *The Association with Child Labor*

Child labor and child marriage are still prevalent in MENA.[13] Ten percent of children, ages 5–14, are involved in child labor.[14] Child marriage still occurs in the region with 18 percent of women married under the age of 18. Finally, women and children can still be affected by female genital mutilation. This is very much a country to country issue with 93 percent of women in Djibouti, 91 percent of women in Egypt and 89 percent of women in Sudan having been "circumcised" or cut.

Disputes regarding family issues, which usually cover women and children, are often settled, if at all, in religious courts which mostly favor males.[15] This makes it especially difficult for family legal disputes such as domestic abuse and child custody to be decided in a fair and equitable manner.[16]

14.7 Role of Religion

14.7.1 *Religious Acculturation of Traditions and Norms*

Most religions, over history, influenced the marriageable age. For example, Christian ecclesiastical law forbade marriage of a girl before the age of puberty. Hindu vedic scriptures mandated the age of a girl's marriage to be adulthood which they defined

[11]Davies, Catriona. "Mideast Women Beat Men in Education, Lose out at Work." Inside the Middle East. Cable News Network, 6 June 2012. Web. <http://www.cnn.com/2012/06/01/world/meast/middle-east-women-education>

[12]EARLY MARRIAGES IN MIDDLE EAST AND NORTH AFRICA .Initiative on Violence against Women, Carr Center for Human Rights Policy Harvard Kennedy School of Government; Hayat Bearat, J.D. Candidate, New England Law | Boston.

[13]World Bank. 2013. Opening Doors: Gender Equality and Development in the Middle East and North Africa. Washington DC: World Bank. doi:https://doi.org/10.1596/978-0-8213-9763-3

[14]"Child Protection from Violence, Exploitation and Abuse - MENA Region." UNICEF.org. United Nations Children's Fund, n.d. Web. <h Ibid ttp://www.unicef.org/protection/MENA.pdf>

[15]In Mideast: Career, Family and Activism." WSJ.com. The Wall Street Journal, 17 Nov. 2011. Web.

[16]Ending child marriage, Page 7, http://www.musawah.org/sites/default/files/662_filename_endchildmarriage.pdf

as three years after the onset of puberty. Jewish scholars and rabbis strongly discouraged marriages before the onset of puberty, but at the same time, in exceptional cases, girls ages 3 through 12 (the legal age of consent according to halakha) might be given in marriage by her father.[17]

Some apocryphal accounts state that at the time of her betrothal to Joseph, Mary, the mother of Jesus, was 12–14 years old, but such accounts are unreliable.[18]

Historically within the Catholic Church, prior to the 1917 Code of Canon Law, the minimum age for a dissoluble betrothal (sponsalia de futuro) was 7 years in the contractees. The minimum age for a valid marriage was puberty, or nominally 14 for males and 12 for females. The 1917 Code of Canon Law raised the minimum age for a valid marriage at 16 for males and 14 for females. The 1983 Code of Canon Law maintained the minimum age for a valid marriage at 16 for males and 14 for females. Some Islamic marriage practices have permitted marriage of girls below the age of 10, because Shariat law is based in part on the life and practices of Muhammad, the Prophet, as described in part in Sahih Bukhari and Sahih Muslim. The Prophet married Aisha, his third wife, when she was about age six, and consummated the marriage when she was about age nine. Some mainstream Islamic scholars have suggested that it is not the chronological age that matters; marriageable age under Muslim religious law is the age when the guardians of the girl feel she has reached sexual maturity. Such determination of sexual maturity is a matter of subjective judgment, and there is a strong belief among most Muslims and scholars, based on Sharia, that marrying a girl less than 13 years old is an acceptable practice for Muslims.[19]

14.7.2 Forcing Children Through Religious Concepts

Issues pertaining to women and children are sensitive for many countries, especially throughout the Islamic world and the Arab League. Islam plays a huge role in determining the rights and status of women and children. The varying interpretations and implementations of Quranic principles make it difficult to reach a clear consensus. In Yemen, an 8 year old girl died on her wedding night after suffering internal injuries. She married a 40 year old man in the tribal regions of Yemen, near the border with Saudi Arabia.[20] The issue also remains sensitive because of the social stigmas associated with reporting abuse. In Bahrain, a mother did not report the Special Committee on Arab Human Rights abuse of her 5 year old son by some of

---

[17]*"MAJORITY – JewishEncyclopedia.com". Retrieved 9 July 2016.*

[18]*"Catholic Encyclopedia: St. Joseph".* Newadvent.org. *Retrieved September 30, 2013.*

[19]A. A. Ali, Child Marriage in Islamic Law, The Institute of Islamic Studies, McGill University (Canada), August 2000; see pages 16–18.

[20]Refworld, UN Committee on the Elimination of Discrimination against Women: Sixth Periodic Report of State Parties, Yemen, March 2007, Page 73.

his neighborhood peers because of the shame that might be brought upon her family or her child.[21]

ECM associated with enforcement. Forced marriage is the marriage conducted without full consent of both parties and sometimes with a threat. From human rights point of view, early marriage is considered a violation of human rights conventions. In Arab societies- especially developing countries- early marriage, is considered a means of securing young girls' future and protecting them. Wars and social problems may leads also to early marriage as in Palestine, where the intifada has led to earlier marriage.

Many countries in the world have declared 18 as the minimum legal age of marriage. However, more than millions of young girls are expected to marry in the next decade according to the international statistics.[22]

Early marriage has decreased in many world countries in the last decades. However, it is still common in rural areas and among poor people. Poor parents believe that early marriage will protect their daughters and save their future. Young girls are forced into marriage by their families while they are still children because they think that marriage benefits them and secure their financial and social future.

Early marriage violates children rights because it decreases their human development, leaving them socially isolated with little education, skills and opportunities for employment and self-realization. These conditions ultimately make married girls vulnerable to poverty. Early marriage is a health and human rights violation because it takes place within the context of poverty and gender inequality with social, cultural and economic dimensions.

14.7.3 Religion and International Civil Laws

Although the general marriageable age is 18 in the majority of countries, most jurisdictions allow for exceptions for underage youth with parental and/or judicial consent. Such laws are neither limited to developing countries, nor to state religion. In some countries a religious marriage by itself has legal validity, while in others it does not, as civil marriage is obligatory. For Catholics incorporated into the Latin Church, the 1983 Code of Canon Law sets the minimum age for a valid marriage at 16 for males and 14 for females. In 2015, Spain raised its minimum marriageable age to 16 from the previous 14. In Mexico, marriage under 18 is allowed with parental consent, from age 14 for girls and age 16 for boys. In Ukraine, in 2012, the Family Code was amended to equalize the marriageable age for girls and boys to 18, with courts being allowed to grant permission to marry from age 16-years if it is established that the marriage is in the best interest of the youth. Many states in the

[21]Hamada, Suad. "Child Abuse on the Rise in Bahrain." IPS. Inter Press Service, 25 Sept. 2012. Web.

[22]*Ending child marriage*, Page 7.

USA permit child marriages, with court's permission. Since 2015, the minimum marriageable age throughout Canada is 16. In Canada the age of majority is set by province/territory at 18 or 19, so minors under this age have additional restrictions (i.e. parental and court consent). Under the Criminal Code, Art. 293.2 Marriage under age of 16 years reads: Everyone who celebrates, aids or participates in a marriage rite or ceremony knowing that one of the persons being married is under the age of 16 years is guilty of an indictable offence and liable to imprisonment for a term not exceeding five years. The Civil Marriage Act also states: 2.2 No person who is under the age of 16 years may contract marriage. In the UK, marriage is allowed for 16–17 years old with parental consent in England and Wales as well as in Northern Ireland, and even without parental consent in Scotland. However, a marriage of a person under 16 is void under the Matrimonial Causes Act 1973. The United Nations Population Fund stated the following:

"In 2010, 158 countries reported that 18 years was the minimum legal age for marriage for women without parental consent or approval by a pertinent authority. However, in 146 countries, state or customary law allows girls younger than 18 to marry with the consent of parents or other authorities; in 52 countries, girls under age 15 can marry with parental consent. In contrast, 18 is the legal age for marriage without consent among males in 180 countries. Additionally, in 105 countries, boys can marry with the consent of a parent or a pertinent authority, and in 23 countries, boys under age 15 can marry with parental consent."

Lower legally allowed marriage age does not necessarily cause high rates of child marriages. However, there is a correlation between restrictions placed by laws and the average age of first marriage. In the United States, per 1960 Census data, 3.5% of girls married before the age of 16, while an additional 11.9% married between 16 and 18. States with lower marriage age limits saw higher percentages of child marriages. This correlation between higher age of marriage in civil law and observed frequency of child marriages breaks down in countries with Islam as the state religion. In Islamic nations, many countries do not allow child marriage of girls under their civil code of laws. But, the state recognized Sharia religious laws and courts in all these nations have the power to override the civil code, and often do. UNICEF reports that the top five nations in the world with highest observed child marriage rates—Niger (75%), Chad (72%), Mali (71%), Bangladesh (64%), Guinea (63%)—are Islamic majority countries.

14.7.4 Politics and Financial Relationship

Child marriage in 1697 of Marie Adélaïde of Savoy, age 12 to Louis, heir apparent of France age 15. The marriage created a political alliance.

Child marriages may depend upon socio-economic status. The aristocracy in some cultures, as in the European feudal era tended to use child marriage as a method to secure political ties. Families were able to cement political and/or financial ties by having their children marry. The betrothal is considered a binding contract upon the families and the children. The breaking of a betrothal can have serious consequences both for the families and for the betrothed individuals themselves.

14.8 ECM in the Arab Region

14.8.1 General Overview

Early marriage is common in some of the countries of the region. This practice is considered to increase children's vulnerability to CSEC because it legitimizes early sexual activity. Between 1995 and 2000, a United Nations Population Fund report on young married women between the ages of 15 and 19 showed that, of this age group:

- in Tunisia, 3 per cent of girls are married although the legal age for marriage is 20;
- in Syria 25 per cent are married;
- in Morocco, 13 per cent are married—the legal marriageable age of 15 is in the process of being raised to 18;
- in Jordan 9 per cent of girls aged 15–19 are married (legal age of marriage is 17);
- in Egypt, 14 per cent of 15–19 year-olds are married and the legal age is 16[23];
- in Algeria 10 per cent of under-19 year-olds are married while the legal age is 18.

Early marriage, of course, often also leads to early pregnancy with attendant risks to reproductive health and increased chances of death for both mother and child.

There are other factors that increase the risk of children to sexual abuse and exploitation, or to other hazards of early sexual activity. One is the poor level of sex education in most countries of the region, and low knowledge/understanding of reproductive health and STDs. In Egypt, for example, a national survey of 16–19 year-olds showed that 25 per cent of boys and more than 30 per cent of girls had no knowledge about HIV/AIDS. In Tunisia, 45 per cent of 17–20 year-olds said that they thought HIV/AIDS could be contracted in a swimming pool. Most of the children interviewed for these studies said they wanted more information on puberty, STDs, pregnancy and childbirth. This was also true of children in Gaza and the West Bank.

A 2013 report claims 53% of all married women in Afghanistan were married before age 18, and 21% of all were married before age 15. Afghanistan's official minimum age of marriage for girls is 15 with her father's permission. In all 34 provinces of Afghanistan, the customary practice of *ba'ad* is another reason for child marriages; this custom involves village elders, *jirga*, settling disputes between families or unpaid debts or ruling punishment for a crime by forcing the so-called guilty family to give their 5- to 12-year-old girls as a wife. Sometimes a girl is forced

[23]Livewire Team. "Egypt: Sexual Assaults on Women Protestors Continuing amid the Political Turmoil." Livewire - Amnestys Global Human Rights Blog. Amnesty International, 3 July 2013.

into child marriage for a crime her uncle or distant relative is alleged to have committed.[24]

Over half of Yemeni girls are married before 18, some by the age eight. Yemen government's Sharia Legislative Committee has blocked attempts to raise marriage age to either 15 or 18, on grounds that any law setting minimum age for girls is un-Islamic. Yemeni Muslim activists argue that some girls are ready for marriage at age 9.[25] According to HRW, in 1999 the minimum marriage age 15 for women was abolished; the onset of puberty, interpreted by conservatives to be at age nine, was set as a requirement for consummation of marriage. In practice "Yemeni law allows girls of any age to wed, but it forbids sex with them until the indefinite time they're 'suitable for sexual intercourse "As with Africa, the marriage incidence data for Yemen in HRW report is from surveys between 1990 and 2000. Current data is difficult to obtain, given regional violence.

In April 2008 Nujood Ali, a 10-year-old girl, successfully obtained a divorce after being raped under these conditions. Her case prompted calls to raise the legal age for marriage to 18. Later in 2008, the Supreme Council for Motherhood and Childhood proposed to define the minimum age for marriage at 18 years. The law was passed in April 2009, with the age voted for as 17. But the law was dropped the following day following maneuvers by opposing parliamentarians. Negotiations to pass the legislation continue. Meanwhile, Yemenis inspired by Nujood's efforts continue to push for change, with Nujood involved in at least one rally. In September 2013, an 8-year-old girl died of internal bleeding and uterine rupture on her wedding night after marrying a 40-year-old man.

The widespread prevalence of child marriage in the Kingdom of Saudi Arabia has been documented by human rights groups. Saudi clerics have justified the marriage of girls as young as 9, with sanction from the judiciary.[26] There are no laws in place defining a minimum age of consent in Saudi Arabia, though drafts for possible laws have been created since 2011.

Research by the United Nations Population Fund indicates that 28.2% of marriages in Turkey—almost one in three—involve girls under 18.

Child marriage was also found to be prevalent among Syrian and Palestinian Syrian refugees in Lebanon, in addition to other forms of sexual and gender-based violence. Marriage was seen as a potential way to protect family honor and protect a girl from rape given how common rape was during the conflict.[27] Incidents of child marriages increased in Syria and among Syrian refugees over the course of the conflict. The proportion of Syrian refugee girls living in Jordan who were married

[24] *"United Nations News Centre". UN News Service Section. 20 May 2013.*

[25] *IRIN Middle East – YEMEN: Deep divisions over child brides – Yemen - Gender Issues – Human Rights". IRINnews.*

[26] *Saudi Human Rights Commission Tackles Child Marriages". Asharq Al Awsat. 13 January 2009. Retrieved 19 October 2015.*

[27] *Charles, Lorraine (2013). "Syrian and Palestinian Syrian Refugees in Lebanon: The Plight of Women and Children". Journal of International Women's Studies.*

increased from 13% in 2011 to 32% in 2014. Journalists Magnus Wennman and Carina Bergfeldt documented the practice, and some of its results.

14.8.2 The Concept of Marriage in Arab Families

Understanding how Arab marriage patterns are changing is now particularly important because Arab countries are seeing unprecedented numbers of young adults entering their 20s, when the great majority of people worldwide marry and start families.

14.8.2.1 Overlook on Marriage in Arab Societies

Arab societies are undergoing major changes as new patterns of marriage and family formation emerge across the region. For long decades, early marriage was the common pattern in the Arab world. However, it is no longer the only pattern. The average age of marriage is rising and more Arab women are staying single for long time and sometimes they don't get married at all.

These new marriage trends in the Arab World are part of a world global phenomenon. The changes of marriage trends in the Arab world reflect the social and economic changes taking place in the region. Arab economies moved away from agrarian based systems which supported both early marriage and extended family numbers [Hoda and Magued 2005].

The majority of the Arab populations live in cities working in industrial or service sectors. Today, Arab women are more educated and more likely to work outside their homes for personal and financial independence. These changes create a new image of woman and change her past traditional role as a mother and household.

Marriage is one of the key important factors that determine the social and economic present and future in the Arab countries. Both problems of early marriage and increase of average age of marriage of marriage are explained. Finally, a recommended solutions and actions are proposed in order to naturalize the two problems for decreasing the negative impacts and creation of better Arab societies.

14.8.2.2 Reasons of Early Marriage in Arab Society

There different reasons of early marriage in Arab countries, some of these reasons are referred to cultural reasons; others are referred to economic reasons. Some of these reasons are: High poverty rates, birth rates and death rates, greater incidence of conflict and civil wars, lower levels of overall development, including schooling, employment, health care and believes that early marriage is a means of securing young girls' future and protecting them. Traditional values surrounding girls' virginity and family honor play a major role in Arab families' decisions to marry off their daughters at young ages.

14.8.2.3 Importance of Marriage in Arab Society

Family is the main concern in Arab societies. Family is considered the main social security system for young and elder people in Arab countries. In Arab culture, parents are responsible for children well into those children's adult lives, and children reciprocate by taking responsibility for the care of their aging parents—responsibilities that Arabs generally take on with great pride. Marriage for Arabs is thus both an individual and a family matter.

In Arab societies, marriage is considered the turning point that defines prestige, recognition, and societal approval on both partners, particularly the bride. Marriage in Arab societies is considered the social and economic contract between two families. Marriage is also considered the right form of socially, culturally, and legally acceptable sexual relationship.

14.9 Responding to Early Marriage in Arab Region: More Than One Society

Early marriage is any form of marriage that takes place at age of 18 years. Early marriages are often associated with enforcement. Forced marriage is the marriage conducted without full consent of both parties and sometimes with a threat. From human rights point of view, early marriage is considered a violation of human rights conventions. In Arab societies-especially developing countries-early marriage, is considered a means of securing young girls' future and protecting them. Wars and social problems may leads also to early marriage as in Palestine, where the intifada has led to earlier marriage.

Many countries in the world have declared 18 as the minimum legal age of marriage. However, more than millions of young girls are expected to marry in the next decade according to the international statistics.

Early marriage has decreased in many world countries in the last decades. However, it is still common in rural areas and among poor people. Poor parents believe that early marriage will protect their daughters and save their future. Young girls are forced into marriage by their families while they are still children because they think that marriage benefits them and secure their financial and social future.

Early marriage violates children rights because it decreases their human development, leaving them socially isolated with little education, skills and opportunities for employment and self-realization. These conditions ultimately make married girls vulnerable to poverty. Early marriage is a health and human rights violation because it takes place within the context of poverty and gender inequality with social, cultural and economic dimensions. The percentage of married women and previously married women between the ages 10 and 19 was much higher than among men: 2.6 per cent women compared to 0.2 per cent among men. Between the age group 15 to 19 years old the percentage of married woman is 5.3 per cent compared to 0.4 per cent for men. These numbers prove the existence of early marriages in Lebanon and also indicate that girls marry earlier than boys. This reflects the customs, traditions and belief that marriage shelters girls, protecting them from drifting into extramarital sexual relations. It also reemphasizes the conviction in the traditional role entrusted to woman: namely, the limited biological-role of childbearing. The different studies on early marriages demonstrate that this is an issue found in a number of Arab countries and there are consequences on the woman that include increased levels of illiteracy among them, increased mortality rates of mothers, increased fertility rates, and other problems that hinder the advancement and development of a society.[28] The psychological and health effects of early marriages on girls, justify describing it as a form of sexual abuse against girls and teenagers.

From Yemen where there is currently no minimum age for marriage, to Libya where the minimum age is 20, early marriage is a varying problem in the Middle East and North Africa (MENA).

The MENA region is defined by UNICEF and includes the following 20 states[29]: Algeria, Bahrain, Djibouti, Egypt, Iran, Iraq, Jordan, Kuwait, Lebanon, Libya, Morocco, Oman, Qatar, Saudi Arabia, Palestine, Sudan, Syrian Arab Republic, Tunisia, United Arab Emirates and Yemen. According to the 2014 UNICEF State of the World's Children Report, 3 percent of girls were married before they turned 15-years-old and 18 percent of girls were married before they reached 18-years-old in MENA.[30] This data does not take into account six of the MENA states. All data obviously changes with poverty trends, armed conflicts and social instability.

The Convention on the Elimination of All Forms of Discrimination Against Women (CEDAW), Article 16, paragraph 2, establishes that early marriages are legally void.[31] The article also urges states to take necessary action, including legislation, to specify a minimum age for marriage.[32]

---

[28]Al Shaibany, Saleh. "Shame of Victims over Sex Attacks Is Letting Child Abuse Thrive, Say Doctors." TheNational.ae. The National, 27 June 2011. Web. <http://www.thenational.ae/news/world/middle-east/shame-of-victims-over-sex-attacks-is-letting-child-abuse-thrive-say-doctors>

[29]Information by Country, UNICEF, http://www.unicef.org/infobycountry/northafrica.html

[30]The State of the World's Children 2014 in Numbers: Every Child Counts, Revealing disparities, advancing children's rights, pages 78–83 http://www.unicef.org/sowc2014/numbers/documents/english/SOWC2014_In%20Numbers_28%20Jan.pdf 11 Id. See Bahrain, Kuwait, Oman, Qatar, Saudi Arabia and United Arab Emirates (all six states do not have minimum age limit for marriage).

[31]CEDAW, Article 16, para. 2, http://www.un.org/womenwatch/daw/cedaw/text/econvention.htm#article16 13 Id.

[32]Roudi-Fahimi, Farzaneh. "Child Marriage in the Middle East and North Africa." PRB. Population Reference Bureau, Apr. 2010. Web. <http://www.prb.org/Publications/Articles/2010/menachildmarriage.aspx>

Issues pertaining to women and children are sensitive for many countries, especially throughout the Islamic world and the Arab League. Islam plays a huge role in determining the rights and status of women and children. The varying interpretations and implementations of Quranic principles make it difficult to reach a clear consensus. In Yemen, an 8-year-old girl died on her wedding night after suffering internal injuries. She married a 40-year-old man in the tribal regions of Yemen, near the border with Saudi Arabia.[33] The issue also remains sensitive because of the social stigmas associated with reporting abuse. In Bahrain, a mother did not report the abuse of her 5-year-old son by some of his neighborhood peers because of the shame that might be brought upon her family or her child.[34]

Education, naturally, has been a key factor in reversing these trends by increasing the status of both children and women. Almost two-thirds of universities in MENA countries are comprised of more women than men.[35] Despite this push for women's education, they are significantly underrepresented in the workforce. Much of this has to do with the lack of protections and harassment in the workplace.[36] Only 25 percent of the workforce in the Arab world is female, despite their increased participation in education.[37]

Nearly one in every five Egyptians is between ages 20 and 29, and the United Nations projects that the population in this age group will grow by 20 percent between 2005 and 2025, from 13.5 million to 16.3 million.

Some other Arab countries will experience even faster growth in this age group. By 2025, the number of Iraqis between ages 20 and 29 is expected to grow by 60 percent, and the number of 20-to-29-year-old Yemenis will jump by more than 80 percent.2 Policies related to young adults, women, and families in Arab countries need to take into account the changing marriage patterns and their social and economic implications. This policy brief highlights current trends in marriage patterns of women in the Arab world, emerging policy issues, and links between marriage patterns and other social and demographic trends. Women throughout the Arab region once typically married in their teens or early 20s.

In recent decades, however, early marriage has declined sharply in parts of the region—most notably in Kuwait, Libya,[38] and the United Arab Emirates. In the early

---

[33]Jamjoom, Mohammed, and Hakim Almasmari. "Yemen Minister on Child Marriage: Enough Is Enough." CNN. Cable News Network, 16 Sept. 2013. Web. <http://www.cnn.com/2013/09/15/world/meast/yemen-child- bride/index.html?hpt=hp_t3>.

[34]Hamada, Suad. "Child Abuse on the Rise in Bahrain." IPS. Inter Press Service, 25 Sept. 2012. Web. <http://www.ipsnews.net/2012/09/child-abuse-on-the-rise-in-bahrain/>

[35]Davies, Catriona. "Mideast Women Beat Men in Education, Lose out at Work." Inside the Middle East. Cable News Network, 6 June 2012. Web. <http://www.cnn.com/2012/06/01/world/meast/middle-east-women-education>

[36]Ibid.

[37]World Bank. 2013. Opening Doors: Gender Equality and Development in the Middle East and North Africa.Washington DC: World Bank. doi:https://doi.org/10.1596/978-0-8213-9763-3

[38]analysis of Article 15 of Personal Status Laws, http://www.refworld.org/docid/467138a62.html, and Committee on the Elimination of Discrimination against Women, Second, Third, Fourth and

1970s, around 40 percent of women ages 15 to 19 were married in Kuwait and Libya, but these figures had dropped by the mid-1990s to 5 percent and 1 percent, respectively. The pace of decline has been even faster in the United Arab Emirates, where the percentage of women ages 15 to 19 who were married dropped from 57 percent in 1975 to 8 percent by 1995.

For the region as a whole, women are marrying later (some in their late 20s or early 30s), and some women are not marrying at all. In Tunisia, Algeria, and Lebanon, only 1 percent to 4 percent of women ages 15 to 19 are married, and the percentage of women ages 35 to 39 who have never married in these countries now ranges from 15 percent to 21 percent. The percentage of women ages 35 to 39 who have never married is a good indicator for measuring changes in the universality of marriage, because the likelihood of a single woman marrying after age 40 is quite low. However, the timing of marriage varies within the region. Although less common than before, early marriages are still prevalent in Oman, Yemen, and (to some extent) Egypt, as well as among Palestinians living in Gaza. Around 17 percent of Omani and Yemeni women ages 15 to 19 are married, as are about 60 percent of those ages 20 to 24 in these countries. Among Egyptian women, 10 percent of 15-to-19-year-olds and 52 percent of 20-to-24-year-olds are married. Universal marriage also prevails in Egypt, Oman, and Yemen, where fewer than 5 percent of women ages 35 to 39 have never married.

Palestinians appear to have a unique marriage pattern: early but not universal. According to the 2004 Palestinian Demographic and Health Survey, while 14 percent of 15-to-19-year-old and nearly 60 percent of 20-to-24-year-old Palestinian women are married, 12 percent of Palestinian women ages 35 to 39 had never been married.

However, Gaza and the West Bank have two different marriage patterns. While marriage for women in Gaza is generally early and universal, the opposite is the case for Arab women of the West Bank (including East Jerusalem). One reason for the Palestinian situation could be that only men and not women of the West Bank can marry Jordanians and bring them to the West Bank, which means a higher percentage of female residents of the West Bank will never marry.[39]Overall, more than one-half of married Palestinian women ages 15 to 54 had married by age 19 (see Fig. 2, page 4).3

Finally, the marriage-age gap (the worldwide phenomenon of women commonly marrying older men) is particularly pronounced in Arab societies. One-quarter of recent marriages in Egypt and Lebanon had women at least 10 years younger than their husbands.4.

Although early marriage is on the decline in the Arab world, the number of Arab teenagers who are married is still significant.

Fifth periodic reports of Libya, CEDAW/C/LBY/5, 2008, http://www2.ohchr.org/english/bodies/cedaw/docs/AdvanceVersions/CEDAW.C.LBY.5.pdf

[39]"Making Children's Rights Work: Country Profile on Jordan", International Bureau for Children's Rights, 2007.

In Yemen, for example, the percent of women ages 15 to 19 who are married declined from 27 percent in 1997 to 17 percent in 2003—but this latter figure still represented an estimated 200,000 women.

An estimated 385,000 Egyptians 15 to 19 years old also have already married.

Available data suggests that early marriage is also common practice throughout the region, even in countries that have set the legal age for marriage at above 18.[40] In Morocco, for example, early marriage also remains an issue especially in rural areas, with UNICEF reporting in 2004 that 16 per cent of all marriages were child marriages.[41]

While the Family Code established the minimum age of marriage for women and men at 18 years, judges are still allowed to authorize marriages before that age, including to girls as young as 13, without any mandatory legal conditions having been fulfilled.[42]

In most countries, the legal age of marriage for girls tends to be lower than for boys.[43] In Kuwait, the minimum legal age for marriage remains 15 for girls and 17 for boys, despite the recommendation of the Committee on the Rights of the Child to increase legal age for girls. Within some rural tribal groups, marriage of girls younger than also continue to persist.[44] In Bahrain, there is no defined minimum age for marriage, while in Qatar and Saudi Arabia the minimum age marriage is unclear under the law.[45]

Early marriage stifles the development of girls and often resulting in early pregnancy, constrained decision-making and reduced life choices. In the occupied Palestinian territories, for example, it is estimated that one in every 10 girls or women between the ages of 15 and 19 gives birth every year, while in Syria nearly 3 per cent of women polled had become pregnant before the age of 15, and 30 per cent between 15 and 19.[46]

In the Middle East and North Africa region, several legal systems are implemented.[47] Some countries' legal system is based solely on Islamic Shari'a law (Yemen), while most countries maintain a hybrid legal system combining a

---

[40]See attached table for information on legal age for marriage per country.

[41]"At a Glance: Morocco", UNICEF, http://www.unicef.org/infobycountry/morocco.html

[42]Amnesty International Report 2007 – The State of the World' Human Rights', Amnesty International.

[43]Concluding observations of the Committee on the Elimination of Discrimination against Women: Morocco", Committee on the Elimination of Discrimination against Women, CEDAW/C/MAR/CO/4, 1 February 2008.

[44]"Kuwait – 2004 Country Report on Human Rights Practices", US State Department, 2005.

[45]"Concluding Observations of the Committee on the Rights of the Child: Bahrain", Committee on the Rights of the Child, Consideration of Reports submitted by state parties under article 44 of the Convention, CRC/C/15/Add 175, 7 February 2002.

[46]UNICEF, Op. Cit

[47]UN Committee on the Elimination of Discrimination Against Women (CEDAW), CEDAW General Recommendation No. 21: Equality in Marriage and Family Relations, 1994, available at: http://www.refworld.org/docid/48abd52c0.html [accessed 2 April 2014]

version of French, British or Egyptian legal codes with Shari'a (Iraq, Morocco and Libya).[48] The personal status law, or family code, regulates marriage and is governed in most countries by Shari'a (Yemen, Libya and Iraq).[49]

In examining the legal frameworks for Iraq, Yemen, Morocco and Libya, the local personal status and family laws will be analyzed where available. For states where there is currently an absence of codified family laws or a lack of translation of Arabic personal status laws or recent constitution (Yemen and Libya), references to United Nations, non-governmental organizations (NGOs), local media outlets and academic institutions will be made.[50]

Although there is a general trend towards raising the minimum age for marriage in Arab countries, early marriage is still widespread in some areas. Many countries of this region reduced the legal age for marriage; in particular, OIC edited recommendations in December 2009 to raise the age of legal marriage to 18 years. In countries such as Egypt, Jordan, and Lebanon as well as among the Palestinians, less than one-half of recent marriages fit the traditional pattern in which the husband is more educated than his wife. In these countries, between 0 percent and 36 percent of recent marriages have an educational gap in favor of women.

Early marriage prevents girls from continuing their education, and reduces women's capacities to participate in the development process, in addition to increased spending on health services and treatment as a result of diseases that expose her as a result of early marriage; furthermore, early pregnancy can lead to severe risks to the health of teenage mothers, in addition to unwillingness of girls at this early age to carry the burden of early motherhood.

14.10 Age Allowed to Marry in the Arab Region

Some countries have made remarkable progress in combating early marriage. Across the region, there are discrepancies in the minimum age for marriage, which ranges between 16, 17 and 18 years old in Jordan, Tunisia, Algeria, Oman, Egypt, Morocco and Mauritania, where the age of marriage is fixed at 18 years for both sexes. Qatar, on the other hand, has set the age of marriage at 18 years for males and 16 years for females, while Sudan cited the existence of a law preventing the marriage of minors without specifying age limits. Syria is currently working towards increasing the minimum age for marriage for girls from 17 to 18 years. Bahrain has issued a ministerial decree which describes the inadmissibility of any marriage contract for individuals under the age of 15 for females, and 18 years for males.

[48]15 Regional Overview for the Middle East and North Africa, MENA Gender Equality Profile, Status of Girls and Women in the Middle East and North Africa, UNICEF, 2011.

[49]UNICEF, 2007, Op. Cit

[50]Id.

Egypt has criminalized marriages contracted before the age of eighteen, describing it as child trafficking. The person responsible for concluding a marriage contract including a minor can be prosecuted as a felon. A toll free line has been established to receive reports on incidences of child marriage.

In Yemen, drafted amendments have been submitted to the House of Representatives, requesting legal provisions be enacted to determine the age of marriage. In line with this motion, a programme for support and advocacy for the drafted legal provisions was launched as discussions were held at the Council of Representatives; some resistance has been shown by some members on the adoption of such provisions. A recent ministerial circular directive from the Ministry of Justice has been also sent to religious leaders in order to help prevent illegal marriages by individuals under the age of 17.

In Saudi Arabia, a system to prevent marriages of minors and to identify the suitable age for girls to be eligible to marry is being examined.

According to the Cairo Declaration, a woman is equal to a man in human dignity.[51] However, in MENA, minimum marriage age differs widely and often is lower for girls or women than boys or men. Many of these MENA states permit marriage at an even younger age so long as a judge permits it. The minimum age standards for girls or women vary from no minimum age to 20-years-old.[52]

14.11 The Cases of Poor Response BUT Hope for Implementation

14.11.1 Iraq

Currently, Iraq has one of the most progressive policies for marriage in the MENA region—setting the legal marriage age at 18-years-old.[53]

Iraqi law now sets the legal age for marriage at 18-years-old without parental approval.[54] Girls, as young as 15-years-old, can be married with a guardian's approval.[55] If a 15-year-old person asks to be married, the judge can authorize the marriage if the eligibility and physical ability of the person in question has been proven and after obtaining the approval of the person's legal guardian.[56] The judge

[51]Cairo Declaration on Human Rights in Islam, Article 6(a), August 1990. http://www1.umn.edu/humanrts/instree/cairodeclaration.html

[52]Emory Law School, http://www.law.emory.edu/ifl/region/mideast.html

[53]Law No. 188 of the year 1959, Personal Status Law and amendments, Section 3, Article 7, http://apps.americanbar.org/rol/publications/iraq_personal_status_law_1959_english_translation.pdf

[54]Id.

[55]The Daily Star: Lebanon News, March 15, 2014, http://www.dailystar.com.lb/News/Middle-East/2014/Mar- 15/250339-iraq-bill-slammed-for-legalizing-child-marriage.ashx#ixzz2xjjzbYIr

[56]Law No. 188 of the year 1959, Personal Status Law and amendments, Section 3, Article 8.

can authorize the marriage of a 15-year-old person if it is deemed an "urgent necessity."[57]

However, Iraq is in the process of changing a law enacted in 1959 to lower the minimum marriage age.[58] A contentious draft law being considered, known as the Jaafari Personal Status Law, could open the door to girls as young as nine-years-old getting married.[59] While there is no minimum age for marriage included in the bill, the section on divorce includes rules for divorces of girls who have reached the age of 9 years.[60]

Hanaa Eduar, a prominent Iraqi human rights activist, stated that child marriage is a crime against humanity.[61] "It would deprive a girl of her right to live a normal childhood."[62] In addition, the United Nation's representative to Iraq, Nickolay Mladenov has also condemned the legislation and stated that the pending bill "risks constitutionally protected rights for women and international commitment."[63]

Supporters of the draft say it merely regulates customs already in place.[64] In addition, officials stated that there has been a rise in the marriage of girls under the age of 18-years-old since the overthrow of Saddam Hussein in 2003.[65]

Parliament must still ratify the bill before it can become the law.[66] However, elections are scheduled for April 30, 2014, and so it is unlikely that this will take priority until after elections are completed.[67]

---

http://apps.americanbar.org/rol/publications/iraq_personal_status_law_1959_english_translation.pdf

[57]Id.

[58]Id.

[59]"Ja'fari Law Takes the Iraqi Government's Violation of Women's Rights to a New Level," Iraqi Civil Society Solidarity Initiative, April 2014, http://www.iraqicivilsociety.org/archives/3022

[60]"Iraq: Don't legalize Marriage for 9-Year-Olds,"Iraqi Al-Amal Association, http://www.iraqi-alamal.com/ArticleShow.aspx?ID=236

[61]Id.

[62]Id.

[63]Id.

[64]Id.

[65]Id.

[66]"Ja'fari Law Takes the Iraqi Government's Violation of Women's Rights to a New Level," Iraqi Civil Society Solidarity Initiative, April 2014, http://www.iraqicivilsociety.org/archives/3022

[67]"Iraq: Don't legalize Marriage for 9-Year-Olds,"Iraqi Al-Amal Association, http://www.iraqi-alamal.com/ArticleShow.aspx?ID=236

14.11.2 Yemen

The UN estimates that one in three Yemeni girls are married before reaching age 18.[68] In Yemen there is currently no minimum age for marriage set.[69] In 1999, Yemen's parliament abolished article 15 of Yemen's Personal Status Law, which set 15 as the minimum age for marriage.[70] This has led to the practice of marrying girls at a young age.[71] "The greatest problem facing Yemeni women today is child marriages," says Wafa Ahmad Ali of the Yemeni Women's Union (YWU), one of several local NGOs trying to change the prospects of young girls by ensuring they remain unmarried and in school until they are at least 18.[72]

According to the UN and Yemeni government data from 2006, 52 percent of girls were married, often to—much—older men, before age 18, and 14 percent before age 15.[73] Yemen has the fourth highest percentage of women, between ages 20 and 24-years-old, who were married by age 18.[74] Early marriages often result in increased drop-out rates, dying in childbirth, and a higher risk of physical and sexual abuse when comparing to women who marry at 18 or later.[75] Another concern of having no minimum age set is that marriage at such a young age leads to girls as young as 8 years-old dying on their wedding night due to bleeding to death.[76]

Wafa, was married at 11-years-old to a 40-year-old who raped and tortured her.[77] Fortunately, a lawyer hired by Equality Now and the Yemeni Women Union managed to arrange for her divorce.[78] Fawziya, another 11-year-old, died during

[68]UNICEF, Table 9: Child Protection, http://www.unicef.org/sowc2013/files/Table_9_Stat_Tables_SWCR2013_ENGLISH.pdf

[69]Refworld, UN Committee on the Elimination of Discrimination against Women: Sixth Periodic Report of State Parties, Yemen, March 2007, Page 73, analysis of Article 15 of Personal Status Laws, http://www.refworld.org/docid/467138a62.html

[70]"How Come You Allow Little Girls to Get Married?" Human Rights Watch, 2011, http://www.hrw.org/sites/default/files/reports/yemen1211ForUpload_0.pdf

[71]Id.

[72]Women in the World Today, Changing Hearts and Minds: Averting Child Marriage in Yemen, Chap. 12, Dalia-Al- Eryani and Laurel Lundstrom, IIP Digital http://iipdigital.usembassy.gov/st/english/publication/2012/02/20120228131454ael0.8837789.html#axzz2zDXucU Ho

[73]Yemen, Monitoring the situation of children and women, Multiple Indicator Cluster Survey 2006, page 56–57, http://www.childinfo.org/files/MICS3_Yemen_FinalReport_2006_Eng.pdf

[74]"Marrying Too Young, End Child Marriage," United Nations Population Fund, page 23. https://www.unfpa.org/webdav/site/global/shared/documents/publications/2012/MarryingTooYoung.pdf

[75]Yemen, Monitoring the situation of children and women, Multiple Indicator Cluster Survey 2006, page 56–57.
http://www.childinfo.org/files/MICS3_Yemen_FinalReport_2006_Eng.pdf

[76]"How Come You Allow Little Girls to Get Married?" Human Rights Watch, 2011.
http://www.hrw.org/sites/default/files/reports/yemen1211ForUpload_0.pdf

[77]Yemen: End child marriages by enacting and enforcing a minimum age of marriage law, Equality Now, September 2013, http://www.equalitynow.org/take_action/adolescent_girls_action344

[78]Id.

childbirth.[79] Salwa, a 12-year-old girl, killed herself by throwing herself off a roof.[80] And the recent, widely-reported case, which was not officially corroborated, of an eight-year-old girl said to have died of internal injuries after her wedding night, prompted renewed calls for action.[81]

Until now, Yemen has been one of the few countries in the region without any minimum age for marriage.[82] In 2008, a majority of the Parliament voted to set 17 as the minimum marriage age, but a strong minority comprised of conservatives was able to shelve the bill indefinitely.[83] However, there is opportunity for change, as Yemen has taken the initiative to construct a new constitution.[84] This new constitution could provide the change needed to combat violence against girls in Yemen by passing a minimum age of marriage

14.12 The Cases of Strong Response BUT Threats on Implementation

14.12.1 Morocco

Morocco has recently changed their marriage laws to raise the minimum age to 18-years- old.[85] Prior to this change, the minimum marriage age was 18 years for males and 15 for females.[86] In addition, the compatibility of age in marriage is defined as the wife's right.[87] The government also organized a large-scale media campaign—involving Islamic law experts, intellectuals and political representatives—to raise awareness of the new law and encourage changes in behavior.[88]

A Family Affairs Judge may authorize the marriage of a girl or boy below the age of 18 in a "well-substantiated decision explaining the interest and reasons justifying the marriage, after having heard the parents of the minor who has not yet reached the

[79]Id.

[80]Id.

[81]Id.

[82]"How Come You Allow Little Girls to Get Married?" Human Rights Watch, 2011, http://www.hrw.org/sites/default/files/reports/yemen1211ForUpload_0.pdf

[83]Id.

[84]Id.

[85]Human Rights Education Associates, Moroccan Family Code (Moudawana) of February 5, 2004, Title Two, Chap. 1, Article 19, http://www.hrea.org/moudawana.html#11

[86]51Emory Law School, http://www.law.emory.edu/ifl/legal/morocco.htm

[87]Id.

[88]Middle East Media Research. "King of Morocco Calls for Fundamental Reform in Family Law." November 7, 2003, http://www.icrw.org/files/images/Child-Marriage-Fact-Sheet-Laws.pdf

age of capacity or his/her legal tutor, with the assistance of medical expertise or after having conducted a social enquiry."[89]

Even though Article 19 of the family code adopted in 2004 prohibits marriage for anyone below 18-years-old, child marriage is still a reality in Morocco.[90] It continues to expand, and creates irreparable negative social consequences. According to AFP TV, official figures show that the number of child marriages in Morocco rose to more than 35,000 in 2010 up from 30,000 two years before. In March 2012, Morocco was shocked by the suicide of Amina Filali, a 16-year-old girl, who was forced to marry the man who had raped her. He remained a free man in accordance with Article 475 of the country's penal code that allows a rapist to escape prison by marrying his victim.[91] This death called for a change in the law to be made. Fortunately, in January 2014, Moroccan lawmakers enacted legal reforms to strengthen punishments for child marriages.[92] Articles were removed from the Personal Status Law that allowed a judge to endorse early marriage under the legal age. Although, the marriage age minimum is 18-years-old in Morocco, judges continue to approve marriages of younger individuals.[93] Although the parliament has taken measures in responding to some of the demands of women's rights activists regarding early marriages and sexual violence, more needs to be done to ensure that the law in place is being implemented. A bill has been proposed by the Moroccan government threatening prison sentences of up to 25 years for perpetrators of violence against women, yet it is still in the drafting stage. This bill could provide the opportunity needed by criminalizing early and forced marriages.

14.12.2 Libya

Child marriages are rare in Libya.[94] In looking at the percentage of Libyan women, ages 20 to 24, who married before their 18th birthday, only 2 percent of them were

---

[89]Human Rights Education Associates, Moroccan Family Code (Moudawana) of February 5, 2004, Title Two, Chap. 1, Article 20, http://www.hrea.org/moudawana.html#11

[90]"Morocco considers law on child marriage," Morocco World News, March 10, 2013 http://www.moroccoworldnews.com/2013/03/81696/morocco-considers-law-on-child-marriage/

[91]"Morocco considers law on child marriage," Morocco World News, March 10, 2013 http://www.moroccoworldnews.com/2013/03/81696/morocco-considers-law-on-child-marriage/, Morocco: Girl's Death Highlights Flawed Laws, March 23, 2012, http://www.hrw.org/news/2012/03/23/morocco-girl-s-death- highlights-flawed-laws

[92]Morocco: Enact legal reforms to strengthen punishments for sexual violence & prevent child marriage, Equality Now, January 28, 2014, http://www.equalitynow.org/category/country/morocco

[93]"Morocco repeals 'rape marriage law'," Al Jazeera English, January 23, 2014, http://www.aljazeera.com/news/africa/2014/01/morocco-repeals-rape-marriage-law-2014123254643455.html

[94]Ending Child Marriage in the Arab Region, Population Reference Bureau, June 2013. http://www.prb.org/Publications/Reports/2013/child-marriage-mena.aspx

married. This percentage places Libya as the state with the lowest percentage of child marriages in the MENA region.

Libya has recently changed their marriage laws to raise the minimum age to 20-years- old.[95] The minimum marriage age is the same for both men and women. Judicial discretion for marriages below that age is granted on the grounds of benefit or necessity and with Wali agreement (someone who possesses or has been granted the authority to perform a marriage contract). In addition, a guardian may not force a girl, boy, woman or man into a marriage or prevent him or her from marrying. If a guardian withholds consent, a minor may take the matter to the court to obtain permission.

Libya is an example of a state that has changed its legal framework by maintaining that 20 be the minimum age for marriage, but also has been able to implement the legal enforcement of its law by showing that a small percentage of its population was married before international legalized marriage age. There has been a remarkable progress by some States to prevent early marriage; there is, however, a discrepancy in the minimum age for marriage between the ages of 16 and 18 years. In Jordan, Algeria, Oman, Qatar, Egypt, and Morocco the minimum age of marriage is determined at 18 years for both sexes, except Qatar that set the age of 18 years for males and 16 years for females. Algeria set a minimum age of marriage at 19 years, while Sudan referred to a law to prevent the marriage of a minor without specifying the age of the minor, and Syria is currently working to prepare a law to prevent the marriage before the age of 18 years. In march 2011, The HRC released three studies covering child marriages in the Kingdom of Saudi Arabia. Those studies will address the religious, health and social issues associated with child marriages and will also recommend a minimum age for marriage in Saudi Arabia as well as criminalizing the act.

In the United Arab Emirates, the average age at marriage for women with secondary or higher education is 27, compared with age 18 for those with no education. In Oman, those with high school diplomas marry on average at age 25, while those who never went to school are married by age 19 on average. In other countries in the region, however, the differential in age at marriage by education is smaller. In Egypt, the average age at marriage for women who are at least high school graduates is 24—only three years higher than that for women with no education and two years higher than that for women with some elementary or high school education.[96]

Despite this legislative attention, the age of marriage is still young and is not linked to other important variables such as education. The age determined as an age

[95]Committee on the Elimination of Discrimination against Women, Second, Third, Fourth and Fifth periodic reports of Libya, CEDAW/C/LBY/5, 2008, http://www2.ohchr.org/english/bodies/cedaw/docs/AdvanceVersions/CEDAW.C.LBY.5.pdf

[96]The "No Lost Generation" campaign ("NLG") was initially launched in September 2013 at the United Nations General Assembly by UNICEF, UNHCR, Save the Children, World Vision and other partners. The "NLG" campaign has grown considerably since its inception, with many additional partners in various sectors joining the initiative.

of marriage is when young people are about to go to university; even then, it is clear that marriage may be a reason to stop learning or not to continue it.

14.12.3 Lebanon

In Lebanon, almost18 per cent of surveyed female youth aged 15 to 18 years were married[97]11 and, in Jordan, the proportion of registered marriages involving Syrian children rose from 18 to 25 per cent between 2012 and 2013. Of these, 48 per cent involved marriages between Syrian girls and husbands who were 10 or more years older than them. In Turkey, some 4.5 per cent of refugee children are married.[98] Further complications may arise when the marriage cannot be legally registered because the parties to the marriage are below the minimum age permitted by law. This can further erode the legal and social security of the girls concerned by jeopardizing their rights to alimony, inheritance, and—in certain circumstances—child custody. Furthermore, the lack of a valid marriage certificate is an impediment to register a new birth.

14.13 Threats and Opportunities

Unrest in the Arab World has been at the forefront of many discussions since 2011 and the beginning of the "Arab Spring". Women and children participated in many of these demonstrations and protests. For instance, Egyptian women played a vital role in the initial removal of Mubarak and continued to play a role in the recent protests over Muhammad Morsi.[99] However, testimonies from many female protestors detail abuse and harassment by their male counterparts. Some women reported their veils being ripped off, their breasts groped and weapons used to threat and intimidate them.[100]

Children in MENA can also fall victim to sexual and physical abuse—sometimes even from family members. The shame felt by the victim and their family following

[97]4.1 per cent of women aged 15–49 years were married before the age of 15 years, while 21.2 per cent of women aged 20–49 years were married before the age of 18 years.

22 Of 778 Palestinian girls in South Lebanon, the NGO Nabaa found that 46.75 per cent of 17 year olds and around 32 per cent of 16 year olds were already married.

[98]RRP6 MYR, July 2014.

[99]Livewire Team. "Egypt: Sexual Assaults on Women Protestors Continuing amid the Political Turmoil." Livewire – Amnestys Global Human Rights Blog. Amnesty International, 3 July 2013. Web. <http://livewire.amnesty.org/2013/07/03/sexual-assaults-on-women-protestors-continuing-amid-the-political- turmoil/>.

[100]Ibid.

these attacks often prevents them from reporting the incident to the police.[101] Child marriage is also another issue for many female children in the region. The minimum legal age for marriage varies between country and some of these ages are well above 18 years of age.[102] Despite these laws, women in many countries marry before their 18th birthday or before it is legal. There has been a remarkable progress by some States to prevent early marriage; there is, however, a discrepancy in the minimum age for marriage between the ages of 16 and 18 years. In Jordan, Algeria, Oman, Qatar, Egypt, and Morocco the minimum age of marriage is determined at 18 years for both sexes, except Qatar that set the age of 18 years for males and 16 years for females. Algeria set a minimum age of marriage at 19 years, while Sudan referred to a law to prevent the marriage of a minor without specifying the age of the minor, and Syria is currently working to prepare a law to prevent the marriage before the age of 18 years.

Despite this legislative attention, the age of marriage is still young and is not linked to other important variables such as education. The age determined as an age of marriage is when young people are about to go to university; even then, it is clear that marriage may be a reason to stop learning or not to continue it. Early marriage is an issue facing various refugee populations in MENA but which has been most pronounced during the Syrian refugee crisis. The conflict and the resulting displacement, increased poverty, fears of sexual violence and harassment, and uncertainty about the future have increased the prevalence of early marriage among girls in particular. Abusive home environments may create additional pressures for adolescent girls to enter into early marriages, which may be seen as a means to escape violence within the home. Notably, a 2014 UNICEF study found that all female survey respondents who had married below the age of 18 years did not want their own daughters to marry at an early age. Despite legislative emphasis on early marriage issues, the age of marriage remains low, and key issues such as education have not been fully considered. Due to the correlation between the legal age of marriage and the age at which girls complete their secondary schooling, early marriage could present a hindrance to the completion of secondary education and progression to university.

Preventing and Responding to Early Marriage. UNHCR focuses on preventing early marriage and mitigating the risks faced by children who are already married. Prevention is undertaken through a wide range of actions including: assisting socio-economically vulnerable families; supporting women, girls, boys and men to advocate for change to social norms that condone early marriage and to raise awareness of the risks of early marriage; promoting girls participation in education; and strengthening legal and policy frameworks to discourage early marriage. For instance, in

---

[101] Al Shaibany, Saleh. "Shame of Victims over Sex Attacks Is Letting Child Abuse Thrive, Say Doctors." TheNational.ae. The National, 27 June 2011. Web. <http://www.thenational.ae/news/world/middle- east/shame-of-victims-over-sex-attacks-is-letting-child-abuse-thrive-say-doctors>.

[102] Roudi-Fahimi, Farzaneh. "Child Marriage in the Middle East and North Africa." PRB. Population Reference Bureau, Apr. 2010. Web. <http://www.prb.org/Publications/Articles/2010/menachildmarriage.aspx>

Algeria, UNHCR uses school attendance records to identify girls and boys who are at risk of early marriage or who are already married and, subsequently, provides multi-sectoral assistance to them. Multi-sectoral assistance includes legal aid, psychosocial support, protection monitoring, and specialized child protection services.

14.14 The International Data on Child Marriage by Region

A UNFPA report stated that, "For the period 2000–2011, just over one third (an estimated 34 per cent) of women aged 20 to 24 years in developing regions were married or in union before their eighteenth birthday. In 2010 this was equivalent to almost 67 million women. About 12 per cent of them were married or in union before age 15." The prevalence of child marriage varies substantially among countries.

14.14.1 Africa

According to UNICEF, Africa has the highest incidence rates of child marriage, with over 70% of girls marrying under the age of 18, in three nations. Niger has one of the highest rates of early marriage in sub-Saharan Africa. Among Nigerian women between the ages of twenty and twenty-four, 76% reported marrying before the age of 18 and 28% reported marrying before the age of fifteen. This UNICEF report is based on data that is derived from a small sample survey between 1995 and 2004, and the current rate is unknown given lack of infrastructure and in some cases, regional violence.

African countries have enacted marriageable age laws to limit marriage to a minimum age of 16 to 18, depending on jurisdiction. In Ethiopia, Chad and Niger, the legal marriage age is 15, but local customs and religious courts have the power to allow marriages below 12 years of age. Child marriages of girls in West Africa and Northeast Africa are widespread. Additionally, poverty, religion, tradition, and conflict make the rate of child marriage in Sub-Saharan Africa very high in some regions.

In many tribal systems a man pays a bride price to the girl's family in order to marry her (comparable to the customs of dowry and dower). In many parts of Africa, this payment, in cash, cattle, or other valuables, decreases as a girl gets older. Even before a girl reaches puberty, it is common for a married girl to leave her parents to be with her husband. Many marriages are related to poverty, with parents needing the bride price of a daughter to feed, clothe, educate, and house the rest of the family. In Mali, the female:male ratio of marriage before age 18 is 72:1; in Kenya, 21:1.

The various reports indicate that in many Sub-Saharan countries, there is a high incidence of marriage among girls younger than 15. Many governments have tended to overlook the particular problems resulting from child marriage, including obstetric fistulae, premature births, stillbirth, sexually transmitted diseases (including cervical cancer), and malaria.

In parts of Ethiopia and Nigeria many girls are married before the age of 15, some as young as 7. In parts of Mali 39% of girls are married before the age of 15. In Niger and Chad, over 70% of girls are married before the age of 18.

As of 2006, 15–20% of school dropouts in Nigeria were the result of child marriage. In 2013, Nigeria attempted to change Sect. 29, subsection 4 of its laws and thereby prohibit child marriages. This was opposed by Islamic states of Nigeria, who called any attempts to prohibit child marriages as un-Islamic. Christianity and Islam are practiced by roughly 50%–50% of its population respectively, and the country continues with personal laws from its British colonial era laws, where child marriages are forbidden for its Christians and allowed for its Muslims. Child marriage is a divisive topic in Nigeria and widely practiced. In northern states, predominantly Muslim, over 50% of the girls marry before the age of 15.

In 2016, during a feast ending the Muslim holy month of Ramadan, the Gambian President Yahya Jammeh announced that child and forced marriages were banned.[103]

In 2015, Malawi passed a law banning child marriage, which raises the minimum age for marriage to 18. This major accomplishment came following years of effort by the Girls Empowerment Network campaign, which ultimately led to tribal and traditional leaders banning the cultural practice of child marriage.

In Morocco, child marriage is a common practice. Over 41,000 marriages every year involve child brides. Before 2003, child marriages did not require a court or state's approval. In 2003, Morocco passed the family law (Moudawana) that raised minimum age of marriage for girls from 14 to 18, with the exception that underage girls may marry with the permission of the government recognized official/court and girl's guardian. Over the 10 years preceding 2008, requests for child marriages have been predominantly approved by Morocco's Ministry for Social Development, and have increased (~29% of all marriages).[104] Some child marriages in Morocco are a result of Article 475 of the Moroccan penal code, a law that allows rapists to avoid punishment if they marry their underage victims. Article 475 was amended in January 2014 after much campaigning, and rapists can legally no longer avoid sentencing by marrying their victim.[105]

In South Africa the law provides for respecting the marriage practices of traditional marriages, whereby a person might be married as young as 12 for females and 14 for males. Early marriage is cited as "a barrier to continuing education for girls (and boys)". This includes absuma (arranged marriages set up between cousins at birth in local Islamic ethnic group), bride kidnapping and elopement decided on by

---

[103] *Gambia's leader says ban on child marriage 'as from today'"*. Bigstory.ap.org. *Retrieved 2016-07-11.*

[104] *Morocco: Child marriages continue despite law to curb practice – Adnkronos Culture And Media"*. adnkronos.com

[105] *Morocco amends controversial rape marriage law". BBC News. 23 January 2014.*

the children. In 2016, the Tanzanian High Court—in a case filed by the Msichana Initiative, a lobbying group that advocates for girls' right to education—ruled in favor of protecting girls from the harms of early marriage. It is now illegal for anyone younger than 18 to marry in Tanzania. A 2015 Human Rights Watch report stated that in Zimbabwe, one-third of women aged between 20 and 49 years old had married before reaching the age of 18. In January 2016, two women who had been married as children brought a court case requesting a change in the legal age of marriage to the Constitutional Court, with the result that the court declared that 18 is to be the minimum age for a legal marriage for both men and women (previously the legal age had been 16 for women and 18 for men). The law took effect immediately, and was hailed by a number of human rights, women's rights, medical and legal groups as a landmark ruling for the country.[106]

14.14.2 *Asia and Oceania*

More than half of all child marriages occur in the South Asian countries of India, Pakistan, Bangladesh, and Nepal. There was a decrease in the rates of child marriage across South Asia from 1991 to 2007, but the decrease was observed among young adolescent girls and not girls in their late teens. Some scholars believe this age-specific reduction was linked to girls increasingly attending school until about age 15 and then getting married.[107]

14.14.2.1 India

According to UNICEF's "State of the World's Children-2009" report, 47% of India's women aged 20–24 were married before the legal age of 18, with 56% marrying before age 18 in rural areas.[108] The report also showed that 40% of the world's child marriages occur in India. As with Africa, this UNICEF report is based on data that is derived from a small sample survey in 1999. The latest available UNICEF report for India uses 2004–2005 household survey data, on a small sample, and other scholars report lower incidence rates for India.

According to Raj et al., the 2005 small sample household survey data suggests 22% of girls ever married aged 16–18, 20% of girls in India were married between 13–16, and 2·6% were married before age 13. According to 2011 nationwide census of India, the average age of marriage for women in India is 21. The child marriage

[106]*Landmark ruling hailed | The Herald".* www.herald.co.zw. *Retrieved 2016-01-23*

[107]*Raj, Anita (2012). "Changes in Prevalence of Girl Child Marriage in South Asia". JAMA. 307. doi:*https://doi.org/10.1001/jama.2012.3497

[108]http://www.unicef.org/sowc09/docs/SOWC09_Table_9.pdf

rates in India, according to a 2009 representative survey, dropped to 7%.[109] In its 2001 demographic report, the Census of India stated zero married girls below age 10, 1.4 million married girls out of 59.2 million girls in the age 10–14, and 11.3 million married girls out of 46.3 million girls in the age 15–19 (which includes 18–19 age group). For 2011, the Census of India reports child marriage rates dropping further to 3.7% of females aged less than 18 being married.[110]

The Child Marriage Restraint Act, 1929 was passed during the tenure of British rule on Colonial India. It forbade the marriage of a male younger than 21 or a female younger than 18 for Hindus, Buddhists, Christians and most people of India. However, this law did not and currently does not apply to India's 165 million Muslim population, and only applies to India's Hindu, Christian, Jain, Sikh and other religious minorities. This link of law and religion was formalized by the British colonial rule with the Muslim personal laws codified in the Indian Muslim Personal Law (Shariat) Application Act of 1937. The age at which India's Muslim girls can legally marry, according to this Muslim Personal Law, is 9, and can be lower if her guardian (*wali*) decides she is sexually mature. Over the last 25 years, All India Muslim Personal Law Board and other Muslim civil organizations have actively opposed India-wide laws and enforcement action against child marriages; they have argued that Indian Muslim families have a religious right to marry a girl aged 15 or even 12. Several states of India claim specially high child marriage rates in their Muslim and tribal communities. India, with a population of over 1.2 billion, has the world's highest total number of child marriages. It is a significant social issue. As of 2016, the situation has been *legally* rectified by The Prohibition of Child Marriage Act, 2006. According to "National Plan of Action for Children 2005", published by Indian government's Department of Women and Child Development, set a goal to eliminate child marriage completely by 2010. In 2006, "The Prohibition of Child Marriage Act, 2006"was passed to prohibit solemnization of child marriages. This law states that men must be at least 21 years of age and women must but be at least 18 years of age to marry. Some Muslim organizations planned to challenge the new law in the Supreme Court of India. In latter years, various High courts in India—including the Gujarat High Court, the Karnataka High Court and the Madras High Court—have ruled that the act prevails over any personal law (including Muslim personal law).

14.14.2.2 Pakistan

According to two 2013 reports, over 50% of all marriages in Pakistan involve girls less than 18 years old. Another UNICEF report claims 70 per cent of girls in Pakistan

---

[109] K. Sinha Nearly 50% fall in brides married below 18 The Times of India (February 10, 2012).

[110] *Percentage of Female by age at effective marriage and by residence India and bigger States, 2011, chapter 2: Population Composition, Table Statement 12, India totals for < 18, 2011 Census of India, Government of India (2013), page 26" (PDF).*

are married before the age of 16.[111] As with India and Africa, the UNICEF data for Pakistan is from a small sample survey in the 1990s. The exact number of child marriages in Pakistan below the age of 13 is unknown, but rising according to the United Nations. Andrew Bushell claims rate of marriage of 8- to 13-year-old girls exceeding 50% in northwest regions of Pakistan.[112] Another custom in Pakistan, called swara or vani, involves village elders solving family disputes or settling unpaid debts by marrying off girls. The average marriage age of swara girls is between 5 and 9. Similarly, the custom of watta satta has been cited as a cause of child marriages in Pakistan. According to Population Council, 35% of all females in Pakistan become mothers before they reach the age of 18, and 67% have experienced pregnancy—69% of these have given birth—before they reach the age of 19. Less than 4% of married girls below the age of 19 had some say in choosing her spouse; over 80% were married to a near or distant relative. Child marriage and early motherhood is common in Pakistan.

14.14.2.3 Bangladesh

Child marriage rates in Bangladesh are amongst the highest in the world. Every 2 out of 3 marriages involve child marriages. According to statistics from 2005, 49% of women then between 25 and 29 were married by the age of 15 in Bangladesh. According to the "State of the World's Children-2009" report, 63% of all women aged 20–24 were married before they were 18. According to a 2008 study, for each additional year a girl in rural Bangladesh is not married she will attend school an additional 0.22 years on average.[113] The later girls were married, the more likely they were to utilize preventative health care. Married girls in the region were found to have less influence on family planning, higher rates of maternal mortality, and lower status in their husband's family than girls who married later. Mia's Law was enacted in 2006 to protect child brides from abuse following the torture and murder of Mia Armador, an 11-year-old who was killed by her abusive 48-year-old husband. This law requires all marriages under 13 to require special government permission. The Ministry of Women and Children Affairs is making progress in increasing women's education and employment opportunities. This, combined with specific education about child marriage and cooperation with religious leaders, is hoped to decrease child marriage.

[111] *"Pakistan's child brides: suffering for others' crimes".* thestar.com. *26 August 2013.*

[112] *Child Marriage in Afghanistan and Pakistan". America Magazine.*

[113] *Field, Erica; Ambrus, Attila (2008). "Early Marriage, Age of Menarche, and Female Schooling Attainment in Bangladesh" (PDF). Journal of Political Economy. 116: 881–930. doi:*https://doi.org/10.1086/593333

14.14.2.4 Nepal

UNICEF reported that 28.8% of marriages in Nepal were child marriages as of 2011.[114] A UNICEF discussion paper determined that 79.6 percent of Muslim girls in Nepal, 69.7 percent of girls living in hilly regions irrespective of religion, and 55.7 percent of girls living in other rural areas, are all married before the age of 15. Girls who were born into the highest wealth quintile marry about two years later than those from the other quintiles.

14.14.3 Oceania

A couple after celebrating their child marriage in Indonesia, about 1939.

Hill tribes girls are often married young. For the Karen people it is possible that two couples can arrange their children's marriage before the children are born.[115]

About 22% of Indonesian girls experience child marriage every year, and 12% get married before age 15, according to 2012 United Nations Population Fund report. There are many reports of Muslim clerics taking multiple underage wives, some less than 12 years old. Indonesian prosecutors have attempted to stop this practice by demanding prison terms for such clerics, however local courts have issued soft sentences. In Indonesia the 1974 Law on Marriage stipulates that a woman must be at least 16 years old and a man must be at least 19 years old to marry. With the popular rise of social networking sites like Facebook underage marriage appears to be increasing in areas like Gunung Kidul, Yogyakarta. Couples have reported becoming acquainted through Facebook and continuing their relationships until girls became pregnant. Among the Atjeh of Sumatra girls formerly married before puberty. The husbands, though usually older, were still unfit for sexual union. Among the islanders of Fiji, also, marriage took place before puberty.[116]

The Marquesas Islands have been noted for their sexual culture. Many sexual activities seen as taboo in Western cultures are viewed appropriate by the native culture. One of these differences is that children are introduced and educated to sex at a very young age. Contact with Western societies has changed many of these customs, so research into their pre-Western social history has to be done by reading antique writings. Children slept in the same room as their parents and were able to witness their parents while they had sex. Intercourse simulation became real penetration as soon as boys were physically able. Adults found simulation of sex by children to be funny. As children approached 11 attitudes shifted toward girls. When

---

[114]*Rabi, Amjad (2014). "Cost of Inaction: Child and Adolescent Marriage in Nepal" (PDF). UNICEF Nepal Working Paper Series.*

[115]Marshall, H. I., (1922) The Karen of Burma. Bangkok: White Lotus (Reprinted, 1997).

[116]*Metchnikoff, Elie (1903). The Nature of Man: Studies in Optimistic Philosophy. New York: Putnam. p. 90.*

a child reaches adulthood, they are educated on sexual techniques by a much older adult. Yuri Lisyansky in his memoirs reports that: The next day, as soon as it was light, we were surrounded by a still greater multitude of these people. There were now a hundred females at least; and they practiced all the arts of lewd expression and gesture, to gain admission on board. It was with difficulty I could get my crew to obey the orders I had given on this subject. Amongst these females were some not more than ten years of age. But youth, it seems, is here no test of innocence; these infants, as I may call them, rivalled their mothers in the wantonness of their motions and the arts of allurement. Adam Johann von Krusenstern in his book about the same expedition as Yuri's, reports that a father brought a 10-to 12-year-old girl on his ship, and she had sex with the crew. According to the book of Charles Pierre Claret de Fleurieu and Étienne Marchand, 8-year-old girls had sex and other unnatural acts in public.

14.14.4 Latin America

Child marriage is common in Latin America and the Caribbean island nations. About 29% of girls are married before age 18. The child marriage incidence rates varies between the countries, with Dominican Republic, Honduras, Brazil, Guatemala, Nicaragua, Haiti and Ecuador reporting some of the highest rates in the Americas. Bolivia and Guyana have shown the sharpest decline in child marriage rates as of 2012. Brazil is ranked fourth in the world in terms of absolute numbers of girls married or co-habitating by age fifteen.[117] Poverty and lack of laws mandating minimum age for marriage have been cited as reasons of child marriage in Latin America. In an effort to combat the widespread belief among poor, rural, and indigenous communities that child marriage is a route out of poverty, some NGOs are working with communities in Latin America to shift norms and create safe spaces for adolescent girls.

14.14.5 North America

14.14.5.1 Canada

Since 2015, the minimum marriageable age throughout Canada is 16. In Canada the age of majority is set by province/territory at 18 or 19, so minors under this age have additional restrictions (i.e. parental and court consent). Under the Criminal Code, Art. 293.2 Marriage under age of 16 years reads: *Everyone who celebrates, aids or*

[117] *Women Around the World » Child Marriage in Latin America". Council on Foreign Relations – Women Around the World. Retrieved 2015-12-10.*

participates in a marriage rite or ceremony knowing that one of the persons being married is under the age of 16 years is guilty of an indictable offence and liable to imprisonment for a term not exceeding five years. The Civil Marriage Act also states: *2.2 No person who is under the age of 16 years may contract marriage.*[118]

14.14.5.2 United States

Child marriage, as defined by UNICEF, is observed in the United States. The UNICEF definition of child marriage includes couples who are formally married, or who live together as a sexually active couple in an informal union, with at least one member—usually the girl—being less than 18 years old. The latter practice is more common in the United States, and it is officially called cohabitation. According to a 2010 report by National Center for Health Statistics, an agency of the United States government, 2.1% of all girls in the 15–17 age groups were in a child marriage. In the age group of 15–19, 7.6% of all girls in the United States were formally married or in an informal union. The child marriage rates were higher for certain ethnic groups and states. In Hispanic groups, for example, 6.6% of all girls in the 15–17 age group were formally married or in an informal union, and 13% of the 15–19 age group were. Over 350,000 babies are born to teenage mothers every year in the United States, and over 50,000 of these are second babies to teen mothers.[119]

Laws regarding child marriage vary in the different states of the United States. Generally, children 16 and over may marry with parental consent, with the age of 18 being the minimum in all but two states to marry without parental consent. Those under 16 generally require a court order in addition to parental consent. Until 2008 the Fundamentalist Church of Jesus Christ of Latter Day Saints practiced child marriage through the concept of "spiritual marriage" as soon as girls were ready to bear children, as part of its polygamy practice, but laws have raised the age of legal marriage in response to criticism of the practice. In 2008 the Church changed its policy in the United States to no longer marry individuals younger than the local legal age. In 2007 church leader Warren Jeffs was convicted of being an accomplice to statutory rape of a minor due to arranging a marriage between a 14-year-old girl and a 19-year-old man. In March 2008 officials of the state of Texas believed that children at the Yearning For Zion Ranch were being married to adults and were being abused. The state of Texas removed all 468 children from the ranch and placed them into temporary state custody. After the Austin's third Court of Appeals and the Supreme Court of Texas ruled that Texas acted improperly in removing them from the YFZ Ranch, the children were returned to their parents or relatives. Musician Jerry Lee Lewis's third wife, Myra Gale Brown, was Lewis's first cousin once removed and was only 13 years old at the time.

[118]http://laws-lois.justice.gc.ca/eng/acts/c-31.5/page-1.html

[119]Breaking the Cycle of Teen Pregnancy CDC, US Government (April 2013)

14.14.6 Europe

14.14.6.1 General Overview

Each European country has its own laws; in both the European Union and the Council of Europe the marriageable age falls within the jurisdiction of individual member states. The Istanbul convention, the first legally binding instrument in Europe in the field of violence against women and domestic violence,[120] only requires countries which ratify it to prohibit forced marriage (Article 37) and to ensure that forced marriages can be easily voided without further victimization (Article 32), but does not make any reference to a minimum age of marriage.

14.14.6.2 Scandinavia

In April 2016, Reuters reported "Child brides sometimes tolerated in Nordic asylum centers despite bans." For example, at least 70 girls under 18 were living as married couples in Sweden; in Norway, "some" under 16 lived "with their partners". In Denmark, it was determined there were "dozens of cases of girls living with older men," prompting Minister Inger Stojberg to state she would "stop housing child brides in asylum centers."[121]

14.14.6.3 Netherlands

The Dutch government's National Rapporteur on Trafficking in Human Beings and Sexual Violence against Children wrote that "between September 2015 and January 2016 around 60 child brides entered the Netherlands." At least one was 14 years-old. The Washington Post reported that asylum centers in the Netherlands were "housing 20 child brides between ages 13 and 15" in 2015.[122]

14.14.6.4 Belgium

The Washington Post reported in April 2016 that "17 child brides" arrived in Belgium in 2015 and a further 7 so far in 2016. The same report added that "Between 2010 and 2013, the police registered at least 56 complaints about a forced marriage."

---

[120] https://www.oas.org/es/mesecvi/docs/CSW-SideEvent2014-Flyer-EN.pdf

[121] *Doyle, Alister (21 April 2016). "Child brides sometimes tolerated in Nordic asylum centers despite bans". Reuters (Oslo). Retrieved 22 April 2016.*

[122] *Ishaan, Ishaan (1 April 2016). "Refugee child bride went on a hunger strike after Belgium separated her from husband". The Washington Post. Retrieved 22 April 2016.*

14.14.6.5 United Kingdom

The marriageable age in Scotland is 16, and no parental consent is required.

In the UK girls as young as 12 have been smuggled in to be brides of men in the Muslim community, according to a 2004 report in The Guardian. Girls trying to escape this child marriage can face death because this breaks the honor code of her husband and both families. As with the United States, underage cohabitation is observed in the United Kingdom. According to a 2005 study, 4.1% of all girls in the 15–19 age group in the UK were cohabiting (living in an informal union), while 8.9% of all girls in that age group admitted to have been in a cohabitation relation (child marriage per UNICEF definition), before the age of 18. Over 4% of all underage girls in the UK were teenage mothers.

In July 2014, the United Kingdom hosted its first global Girl Summit; the goal of the Summit was to increase efforts to end child, early, and forced marriage and female genital mutilation within a generation.

14.15 Consequences of Child Marriage

Child marriage has lasting consequences on girls, which last well beyond adolescence. Women married in their teens or earlier, struggle with the health effects of getting pregnant at a young age and often with little spacing between children. Early marriages followed by teen pregnancy also significantly increase birth complications and social isolation. In poor countries, early pregnancy limits or can even eliminate their education options. This affects their economic independence. Girls in child marriages are more likely to suffer from domestic violence, child sexual abuse, and marital rape.

14.15.1 Social Effects

Although the trend of early marriage is decreasing in the Arab world, the number of young girls in Arab countries teenagers who are married is still high. Early marriage is generally associated with early childbearing and high fertility, both of which pose health risks for women and their children. Young mothers are at greater risk than older mothers of dying from causes related to pregnancy and childbirth. And the younger a bride is, the more significant the age gap with her husband tends to be—which exacerbates her disadvantage in negotiating with her husband on matters such as her own health care needs.

Young wives are required to do a many hard domestic duties, including new roles and responsibilities as wives and mothers. The young bride's status in the family is dependent on her demonstrating her fertility within the first year of marriage when she is not physiologically and emotionally prepared. Young wives are forced to be responsible for the care and welfare of their families and future generations while they are still children themselves.

They have no decision making powers, restricted mobility and limited economic resources. Early marriage is a direct cause of woman poverty and wide age gaps between younger married girls and their spouses create unequal power relations between the young bride and her older and more experienced husband, resulting in husbands having total control over sexual relations and decision-making.

Young wives are often unable to make wise plans for their families and may be forced to select between one of two hard choices: either to tolerate husbands' violence or to make crimes (killing them). AIDS epidemic increases in young women due to the combination socioeconomic, cultural and political factors that put young women at greater risk of HIV infection due to the lack of sexual knowledge and limited access to information and resources. Younger women may face unsuccessful marriages and divorce could happen as a result of lack of maturity, incomplete independence, limited time to get prepared for marriage and having kids, dealing with education/career building and family formation at the same time.

14.15.2 Health

Child marriage threatens the health and life of girls.[123] Complications from pregnancy and childbirth are the main cause of death among adolescent girls below age 19 in developing countries. Pregnant girls aged 15 to 19 are twice as likely to die in childbirth as women in their 20s, and girls under the age of 15 are five to seven times more likely to die during childbirth. These consequences are due largely to girls' physical immaturity where the pelvis and birth canal are not fully developed. Teen pregnancy, particularly below age 15, increases risk of developing obstetric fistula, since their smaller pelvises make them prone to obstructed labor. Girls who give birth before the age of 15 have an 88% risk of developing fistula. Fistula leaves its victims with urine or fecal incontinence that causes lifelong complications with infection and pain. Unless surgically repaired, obstetric fistulas can cause years of permanent disability, shame to mothers, and can result in being shunned by the community. Married girls also have an increased risk of sexually transmitted diseases, cervical cancer, and malaria than non-married peers or girls who marry in their 20s.

Child marriage not only threatens the mother's health, it also threatens the lives of offspring. Mothers under the age of 18 years have 35 to 55% increased risk of delivering pre-term or having a low birth weight baby than a mother who is 19 years old. In addition, infant mortality rates are 60% higher when the mother is under

[123] *Yemeni child bride, 8, dies of internal injuries on first night of forced marriage to groom, 40 – Daily Mail Online". Mail Online.*

18 years old. Infants born to child mothers tend to have weaker immune systems and face a heightened risk of malnutrition.

Prevalence of child marriage may also be associated with higher rates of population growth, more cases of children left orphaned, and the accelerated spread of disease.

14.15.3 Illiteracy and Poverty

Child marriage often ends a girl's education, particularly in impoverished countries where child marriages are common.[124] In addition, uneducated girls are more at risk for child marriage. Girls that have only a primary education are twice as likely to marry before age 18 than those with a secondary or higher education, and girls with no education are three times more likely to marry before age 18 than those with a secondary education. Early marriage impedes a young girl's ability to continue with her education as most drop out of school following marriage to focus their attention on domestic duties and having or raising children. Girls may be taken out of school years before they are married due to family or community beliefs that allocating resources for girls' education is unnecessary given that her primary roles will be that of wife and mother. Without education, girls and adult women have fewer opportunities to earn an income and financially provide for themselves and their children. This makes girls more vulnerable to persistent poverty if their spouses die, abandon, or divorce them.[125] Given that girls in child marriages are often significantly younger than their husbands, they become widowed earlier in life and may face associated economic and social challenges for a greater portion of their life than women who marry later.

14.15.4 Domestic Violence

Married teenage girls with low levels of education suffer greater risk of social isolation and domestic violence than more educated women who marry as adults. Following marriage, girls frequently relocate to their husband's home and take on the domestic role of being a wife, which often involves relocating to another village or area. This transition may result in a young girl dropping out of school, moving away from her family and friends, and a loss of the social support that she once

[124]International Center for Research in Women (2005), Too young to wed: education & action toward ending child marriage. Washington DC

[125]*Davidson, Helen (26 November 2013). "Papua New Guinea takes first steps to combat 'epidemic' of abuse". Guardian News and Media Limited. Retrieved 9 March 2014.*

had.[126] A husband's family may also have higher expectations for the girl's submissiveness to her husband and his family because of her youth. This sense of isolation from a support system can have severe mental health implications including depression.

Large age gaps between the child and her spouse makes her more vulnerable to domestic violence and marital rape. Girls who marry as children face severe and life-threatening marital violence at higher rates. Husbands in child marriages are often more than ten years older than their wives. This can increase the power and control a husband has over his wife and contribute to prevalence of spousal violence. Early marriage places young girls in a vulnerable situation of being completely dependent on her husband. Domestic and sexual violence from their husbands has lifelong, devastating mental health consequences for young girls because they are at a formative stage of psychological development. These mental health consequences of spousal violence can include depression and suicidal thoughts. Child brides, particularly in situations such as vani, also face social isolation, emotional abuse and discrimination in the homes of their husbands and in-laws.

14.15.5 Women's Rights

The United Nations, through a series of conventions has declared child marriage a violation of human rights. The Convention on the Elimination of all Forms of Discrimination of Women ('CEDAW'), the Committee on the Rights of the Child ('CRC'), and the Universal Declaration of Human Rights form the international standard against child marriage. Child marriages impact violates a range of women's interconnected rights such as equality on grounds of sex and age, to receive the highest attainable standard of health, to be free from slavery, access to education, freedom of movement, freedom from violence, reproductive rights, and the right to consensual marriage. The consequences of these violations impact not only the woman, but her children and broader society.

14.15.6 Development

High rates of child marriage negatively impact countries' economic development because of early marriages' impact on girls' education and labor market participation. Some researchers and activists note that high rates of child marriage prevent significant progress toward each of the eight Millennium Development Goals and global efforts to reduce poverty due to its effects on educational attainment, economic and political participation, and health.

---

[126]May-Chahal and Herczog 2003.

A UNICEF Nepal issued report noted that child marriage impacts Nepal's development due to loss of productivity, poverty, and health effects. Using Nepal Multi-Indicator Survey data, its researchers estimate that all girls delaying marriage until age 20 and after would increase cash flow among Nepali women in an amount equal to 3.87% of the country's GDP. Their estimates considered decreased education and employment among girls in child marriages in addition to low rates of education and high rates of poverty among children from child marriages.

14.16 Prevalence Data

Percentage of women aged 20–24 who were married or in union before the age of 18 is listed in the table below. The data from International Center for Research on Women (ICRW) and UNICEF, if traced all the way to the ultimate sources, is from surveys that are 10 to 20 years old. The UN data is between 10 and 15 years old.

Country	% girls married before 18 ICRW-UNICEF data[a,b] (Year of data)	% girls married before 18 (UN data)[c]
Niger	76 (2012)	62
Chad	68 (2010)	49
Central African Republic	68 (2010)	42
Bangladesh	65 (2011)	48
Mali	55 (2010)	50
Guinea	52 (2012)	46
Malawi	50 (2010)	37
Mozambique	48 (2011)	47
Madagascar	41 (2012)	34
Sierra Leone	44 (2010)	47
Burkina Faso	52 (2010)	35
India	47 (1999–2005)	30
Somalia	45 (1998–2006)	38
Nicaragua	41 (2000–2006)	32
Zambia	42 (2002–2007)	24
Eritrea	41 (2010)	38
Uganda	40 (2011)	32
Ethiopia	41 (2011)	30
Nepal	41 (2011)	40
Dominican Republic	41 (2009–2010)	29
Afghanistan	40 (2012)	29

[a]Jasmine Abdulcadira, et al., "Care of women with female genital mutilation/cutting", Swiss Medical Weekly, 6(14), January 2011. doi:10.4414/smw.2011.13137 PMID 21213149
[b]Rigmor C. Berg, Vigdis Underland, "Immediate health consequences of female genital mutilation/cutting (FGM/C)", Kunnskapssenteret (Norwegian Knowledge Centre for the Health Services), systematic review no. 8, 2014, pp. 4–5 (full text). ISBN 978-82-8121-856-7
[c]Dan Reisel, Sarah M. Creighton, "Long term health consequences of Female Genital Mutilation (FGM)", Maturitas, 80(1), January 2015 (pp. 48–51), p. 49. PMID 25466303 doi:10.1016/j.maturitas.2014.10.009

14.17 International Initiatives to Prevent Child Marriage

In December 2011 a resolution adopted by the United Nations General Assembly (A/RES/66/170) designated October 11 as the *International Day of the Girl Child.* On October 11, 2012 the first *International Day of the Girl Child* was held, the theme of which was ending child marriage.

In 2013 the first United Nations Human Rights Council resolution against child, early, and forced marriages was adopted; it recognizes child marriage as a human rights violation and pledges to eliminate the practice as part of the U.N.'s post-2015 global development agenda.

In 2014 the UN's Commission on the Status of Women issued a document in which they agreed, among other things, to eliminate child marriage.

The World Health Organization recommends increased educational attainment among girls, increased enforcement structures for existing minimum marriage age laws, and informing parents in practicing communities of the risks associated as primary methods to prevent child marriages.

Programs to prevent child marriage have taken several different approaches. Various initiatives have aimed to empower young girls, educate parents on the associated risks, change community perceptions, support girls' education, and provide economic opportunities for girls and their families through means other than marriage. A survey of a variety of prevention programs found that initiatives were most effect when they combined efforts to address financial constraints, education, and limited employment of women. Girls in families participating in an unconditional cash transfer program in Malawi aimed at incentivizing girls' education got married and had children later than their peers who had not participated in the program. The program's effects on rates of child marriage were greater for unconditional cast transfer programs than those with conditions. Evaluators believe this demonstrated that the economic needs of the family heavily influenced the appeal of child marriage in this community. Therefore, reducing financial pressures on the family decreased the economic motivations to marry daughters off at a young age. The Haryana state government in India operated a program in which poor families were given a financial incentive if they kept their daughters in school and unmarried until age 18. Girls, in families who were eligible for the program, were less likely to be married before age 18 than their peers. A similar program was operated in 2004 by the Population Council and the regional government in Ethiopia's rural Amhara region. Families received cash if their daughters remained in school and unmarried during the two years of the program. They also instituted mentorship programs, livelihood training, community conversations about girls' education and child marriage, and gave school supplies for girls. After the two-year program, girls in families eligible for the program were three times more likely to be in school and one tenth as likely to be married compared to their peers. Other programs have addressed child marriage less directly through a variety of programming related to girls' empowerment, education, sexual and reproductive health, financial literacy, life skills, communication skills, and community mobilization.

14.18 Tipping Point Analysis

Researchers at the International Center for Research on Women found that, in some communities, the rates of child marriage increase significantly when girls are a particular age. This "tipping point", or age at which rates of marriage increase dramatically, may occur years before the median age of marriage. Therefore, the researchers argue prevention programs should focus their programming on girls who are pre-tipping point age rather than only girls who are married before they reach the median age for marriage.

14.19 Implications

"Child marriage cuts across countries, cultures, religions and ethnicities."[127] Eighteen percent of girls under 18 are married in the Middle East and North Africa. This is a violation of all the rights of the child. It forces girls to assume responsibilities for which they are typically not physically and psychologically prepared for. States must increase the minimum age to marry to 18 years of age for both girls and boys. In addition, child marriages should be criminalized and should not be justified on traditional, religious, cultural or economic grounds. Lastly, there needs to be public awareness highlighting the nature and harm caused by forced and early marriages and community programs to help detect, provide advice, rehabilitation and shelter where necessary.

[127]International Day of the Girl Child, October 2012, Joint Statement* by a group of UN human rights experts to mark the first International Day of the Girl Child, Thursday, 11 October 2012, https://www.un.org/en/events/girlchild/2012/hrexperts.shtml

Chapter 15
Sexual Violence

15.1 Abstract

Sexual violence against children is a form of child abuse. It includes harassment and rape, as well as the use of children in prostitution or pornography.

Sexual violence is a serious infringement upon a child's rights, and one which can result in significant physical and psychological trauma to the victim. A 2002 WHO study approximated that 223 million children have been victims to sexual violence involving physical contact. Yet, due to the sensitivity of the issue and the tendency of the crime to stay hidden, the true figure is likely to be much higher.

15.2 Children

Girls are more frequent targets for sexual abuse than boys. The WHO study found that 150 million girls were abused compared to 73 million boys. Other sources also conclude that girls face a greater risk of sexual violence, including prostitution.[1]

Children are exposed to sexual abuse that might occur in the family or school and in various institutions. Sexual violence is reported in 8 countries: Jordan, United Arab Emirates, Sudan, Oman, Qatar, Lebanon, Egypt, Morocco, and Yemen, where the existence of laws that prevent violence and sexual exploitation are not specifically available. In Yemen, there is a draft of an amendment to the Children's Act, which is in the process of development.

[1]Pinheiro, P. (2006). Rights of the Child: Report of the Independent Expert for the United Nations Study on Violence Against Children. Office of the United Nations High Commissioner for Human Rights.

B. Gerbaka et al., *Child Sexual Abuse, Exploitation and Trafficking in the Arab Region*, Child Maltreatment 13, https://doi.org/10.1007/978-3-030-66507-4_15

15.3 Perpetrators

There is no stereotypical profile of sexually violent persons. Perpetrators may be coming from various backgrounds, and they may be someone known by the victim like a friend, a family member, an intimate partner, an acquaintance, or they may be a complete stranger. The primary motivators behind sexually violent acts are believed to be power and control, and not, as it is widely perceived, a sexual desire. Sexual violence is rather a violent, aggressive and hostile act aiming to degrade, dominate, humiliate, terrorize and control the victim. Some of the reasons for committing sexual violence are that it reassures the offender about his sexual adequacy, it discharges frustration, compensates for feelings of helplessness, and achieves sexual gratification.

Data on sexually violent men are somewhat limited and heavily biased towards apprehended rapists, except in the United States, where research has also been conducted on male college students. Despite the limited amount of information on sexually violent men, it appears that sexual violence is found in almost all countries (though with differences in prevalence), in all socioeconomic classes and in all age groups from childhood onwards. Data on sexually violent men also show that most direct their acts at women whom they already know. Among the factors increasing the risk of a man committing rape are those related to attitudes and beliefs, as well as behavior arising from situations and social conditions that provide opportunities and support for abuse.

15.4 Consequences

Sexual violence is a serious public health problem and it has both short and/or long-term negative physical and psychological effects on health and well-being. There is evidence that male and female victims of sexual violence may experience similar mental health, behavioral and social consequences. Watts et al. (2013) reported that 72.4% of the victims had at least one gynecological complaint. 52.2% suffered from chronic lower abdominal pain, 27.4% from abnormal vaginal bleeding, 26.6% from infertility, 25.3% from genital sores, and 22.5% from swellings in the abdomen. 18.7% of the participants also suffered from severe psychological and surgical morbidity including alcoholism. 69.4% showed significant psychological distress, 15.8% attempted suicide, 75.6% had at least one surgical complaint. 4.8% of the participants had a positive HIV status.

In child sexual abuse (CSA) cases, the child may suffer mental health disorders that can extend into adult life especially if sexual abuse involved actual intercourse. Studies on abused boys have shown that around one in five continue in later life to molest children themselves. CSA may lead to negative behavioral patterns in later life, learning difficulties as well as regression of/or slower development.

The table below gives some examples of possible physical and psychological consequences of sexual violence:

<table>
<tr><th colspan="4">Examples of fatal outcomes related to sexual violence</th></tr>
<tr><td colspan="4">• Suicide
• Homicide
• AIDS-related</td></tr>
<tr><th colspan="4">Examples of non-fatal outcomes related to sexual violence</th></tr>
<tr><th colspan="2">Physical consequences</th><th colspan="2">Psychological consequences</th></tr>
<tr><td>• Unwanted pregnancy
• Infertility
• Sexual dysfunction
• Chronic pelvic pain
• Sexually transmitted infections (stis), including hiv/aids
• Obesity or anorexia</td><td>• Urinary tract infections
• Gastrointestinal disorders
• Gynecological and pregnancy complications
• Migraines and other frequent headaches
• Fatigue
• Nausea</td><td>• Rape trauma syndrome
• Post-traumatic stress disorder
• Social phobias
• Shock
• Increased substance use or abuse;
• Denial</td><td>• Fear
• Confusion
• Anxiety
• Guilt
• Depression</td></tr>
</table>

In addition to the above-mentioned outcomes, in some cases victims of sexual violence may also be stigmatized and ostracized by their families and others. Societal perceptions that the victim provoked sexual violence lead to a lack of disclosure of sexual assault which is associated with even more severe psychological consequences, particularly in children. Thus, more interventions are needed in order to order to change societal attitudes towards sexual violence as well as efforts designed to educate those to whom the survivors may disclose the assault.

One of the reasons for non-reporting is that children lack independent access to resources. They normally require the cooperation of one of their parents who may refuse to believe their child, or may, in fact, be the perpetrator.

Data on sexual violence typically come from police, clinical settings, nongovernmental organizations and survey research. The relationship between these sources and the global magnitude of the problem of sexual violence may be viewed as corresponding to an iceberg floating in water (see diagram). The small visible tip represents cases reported to police. A larger section may be elucidated through survey research and the work of nongovernmental organizations.

15.5 Culture and Acculturation

Sexual violence occurs in all cultures with varying definitions of what constitutes it. It is possible that in cultures where man and his manly role are prized better, additional perceived or real power may encourage them to think of their "rights." If a woman resists sexual intercourse, it may be perceived as a direct threat by men to their masculinity, triggering a crisis of male identity and contributing to sexual control and violence as it is seen as a way of resolving this crisis. It has been reported that victims who attempt resistance or escape from the situation are more likely to be brutalized by the offender,[2] thereby giving an inflated sense of power to the abuser as was seen in the New Delhi gang rape case of *Nirbhaya* in December 2012. It is likely that in patriarchal cultures, any resistance from the woman victim is perceived by the offender as an insult to his "manhood" further provoking him to resort to more violent means to control the victim.

There is a theory that explains sexual violence as socioculturally constructed which disproves the biological framework that suggests sexual violence is a result of a man's sexual urges. This theory looks to prove that sexual violence is a natural behavior that originates from the "biological propensity to reproduce have a net positive effect on the person's (resorting to sexual violence) reproductive success.[3] The sociocultural theory takes into account gender power equations, moral values, male dominance, and attitudes toward violence."

15.6 Social Background of Sexual Violence

15.6.1 History

15.6.1.1 General

Sexual violence can be traced back to the Greeks and Romans where women were seen as property without any rights over their bodies or sexual integrity. Rape of women during peace times was therefore considered as property crime only affecting their owners: the husbands, sons or brothers.[4] During armed conflict sexual violence, particularly rape, was perceived as a normal byproduct of war, as "a socially acceptable behavior well within the rules of warfare".

In Ancient Greece, women were sometimes the reason for the attack of a city, conquering women as new wives or concubines, legitimate booty, as slaves or as trophies. The fact that sexual violence to women was commonplace during both war and peace times led to the negligence of any indications of what the methods, aims and magnitude of such violence was; it was face- and nameless.

---

[2]Usta, J., Mahfoud, Z., Chahine, G. and Anani, G. CHILD SEXUAL ABUSE: The situation in Lebanon. KAFA (enough) Violence & Exploitation. Save the Children: Sweden, 2008. 15

[3]"Child Protection from Violence, Exploitation and Abuse - MENA Region." UNICEF.org. United Nations Children's Fund, n.d. Web. <http://www.unicef.org/protection/MENA.pdf>.

[4]Melissa A. Polusny; Victoria M. Follette (1995). "Long-term correlates of child sexual abuse: Theory and review of the empirical literature". Applied and Preventive Psychology. Elsevier Ltd. 4 (3): 143–166.

15.6.1.2 Middle Ages

The Middle Ages strongly reflected the patriarchal sexual violence view. During times of peace, female spouses had no right to refuse sex with their husbands. Even though laws punishing rapes existed, sexual violence was usually considered as justified or inconsequential. Usually, depending on the elite's views, which perceived sexual violence as a minor issue, sexual violence was not prosecuted. This view was also transferred to the colonies.

In Alta California, for example, the Catholic clergy relied heavily on corporal punishment such as flogging, placing in the stocks or shackling of Amerinindian women within their programs of Christianization. Within this context of trying to restore a certain social order, women were often the victims of sexual violence if politically active and posing a threat to the existing order. With regard to times of war, jurists, writers and scholars argued that as soon as war is just, no boundaries would be set towards methods used in order to achieve victory. However, with Alberico Gentili (1552–1608) discussions started that suffering of women should be reduced and rape prohibited during peace and war times. However, this view was not accepted for a long time, as women and children not participating in the fighting were still considered as being the enemy and the patriarchal view on women prevailed during peace and war times.

15.7 Codification of Laws of War on Gender-Related Crimes

Gradually, over the centuries laws and customs of war changed in direction of a wider understanding of sexual violence and the need to protect the victims. During the American civil war, the US started to codify the customary rules regulating land-based wars. With the Lieber Code of 1863, President Lincoln tried to regulate the conduct of Union soldiers and prohibited explicitly rape.[5] The first-ever Geneva Convention one year after and the Fourth Hague Conventions 1907 followed this line by advocating the protection of family rights and honor, implying specifically also the prohibition of rape. But the only enforcement mechanisms were the military commanders themselves, having the right to execute the soldiers immediately.

After World War I, a War Crimes Commission was established in order to bring war criminals before justice. Forced prostitution and rape was seen as grave violation of the customs and laws of war. Under the International Military Tribunal at Nuremberg (IMT) and the International Military Tribunal for the Far East at Tokyo (IMTFE), the spectrum of sexual violence as war crime was widened even though rape was not explicitly mentioned. The transcripts of the trials contain

[5]Neumann, D.A., Houskamp, B.M., Pollock, V. and Briere, J. The long-term sequelae of childhood sexual abuse in women: A meta-analytic review. Child Maltreatment 1996; 1: 6–16.

evidence of rape, sexual slavery, sexual torture, forced prostitution, forced sterilization, forced abortion, pornography, sexual mutilation, forced nudity and sexual sadism. But only after the Tokyo Tribunal, when Japanese commanders were prosecuted the first time based on the chain of command for not having prevented rape and sexual slavery of comfort women during the Second World War, was sexual violence gradually considered as a grave war crime in itself. This view was the first time expressed after Nuremberg and Tokyo in the second series of trials for the prosecution of "lesser" war criminals where the Control Council Law No. 10 explicitly listed rape constituting a crime against humanity.

15.8 Sexual Violence Trends in the Arab Region

15.8.1 Country Reports

The sexual abuse of children may occur within the family, in school, and in various other settings and institutions.

In reference to this issue, 13 countries (Jordan, UAE, Tunisia, Sudan, Syria, Oman, Palestine, Qatar, Lebanon, Libya, Egypt, Morocco, and Yemen) have described existing laws that aim to end violence and sexual torture; other countries did not provide information on this subject.

Bahrain has formed a national committee to combat human trafficking and a commission to assess the state of victims of human trafficking.

Tunisia, in addition to the laws that prevent and punish sexual abuse, has enacted a Child Protection Code (Chap. 20) which focuses on sexual exploitation as a threat to children requiring the intervention of a child protection officer. A bill also provides special protection for child victims of physical violence and sexual abuse at all stages of inquiry and prosecution, with provisions for legal rights, and free treatment and psycho-social rehabilitation.

Sudan's Children's Rights Law, or "Child Act" (2010 Chap. Ix) includes provisions banning the use of children in prostitution and pornography; these criminal acts are punishable by death sentences or imprisonment accompanied by a fine for twenty years for rape or harassment, or for harming or engaging a child in sex acts.

In Syria, Decree No. 3/2010 on human trafficking provides special protection for female and child victims of trafficking. Such trafficking includes the sexual exploitation of a child in any form or manner (including photographing of the child's genitalia or creation of pornographic images to meet unsolicited demand directly or indirectly).

In Palestine, the Palestinian Child Law prohibits all forms of sexual abuse of children as well as the engagement of children in pornography and prostitution.

Within the framework of separate legislation to criminalize human trafficking, an ad hoc committee was established by the Egyptian Council of Ministers in 2007 to formulate an open-ended statement addressing the issue of sexual exploitation of children. The Committee is linked to the National Coordinating Committee and is meant to combat and prevent human trafficking and to prepare an integrated draft law to criminalize human trafficking. Such a law will focus on the various aspects of trafficking and the implications of the fragmented provisions that exist currently within several laws. This effort comes in line with a global trend towards dealing effectively with the issue of Trafficking.

In Yemen, a draft amendment to the Children's Rights Act is in the pipeline for ratification by the House of Representatives; the Act incorporates provisions for punitive action against various forms of sexual exploitation of children.

All member states that ratified the Optional Protocol to the Convention on the Rights of the Child on child trafficking child prostitution and child pornography have committed themselves to the development of measures and preliminary procedures for the protection of children from sexual violence. These measures are to be included as part of laws on children and in provisions in criminal law and operational procedures in order to develop an effective mechanism to reduce sexual violence against children.

15.8.2 The Burden

Education, naturally, has been a key factor in reversing these trends by increasing the status of both children and women. Almost two-thirds of universities in MENA countries are comprised of more women than men. Despite this push for women's education, they are significantly underrepresented in the workforce. Much of this has to do with the lack of protections and harassment in the workplace. Only 25% of the workforce in the Arab world is female, despite their increased participation in education.

Unrest in the Arab World has been at the forefront of many discussions since 2011 and the beginning of the "Arab Spring". Women and children participated in many of these demonstrations and protests. For instance, Egyptian women played a vital role in the initial removal of Mubarak and continued to play a role in the recent protests over Muhammad Morsi. However, testimonies from many female protestors detail abuse and harassment by their male counterparts. Some women reported their veils being ripped off, their breasts groped and weapons used to threat and intimidate them.

Children in MENA can also fall victim to sexual and physical abuse—sometimes even from family members. The shame felt by the victim and their family following these attacks often prevents them from reporting the incident to the police.12 Child marriage is also another issue for many female children in the region. The minimum legal age for marriage varies between country and some of these ages are well above 18 years of age. Despite these laws, women in many countries marry before their 18th birthday or before it is legal.

One in three women will encounter sexual violence in her lifetime, and every year millions of children are sexually abused. Sexual abuse results in a range of damaging physical and emotional effects, including: depression, suicide, post-traumatic stress disorder, reproductive health issues, and potential exposure to sexually transmitted infections and HIV. Sexual and domestic violence simultaneously results from and reproduces low levels of education, exposure to and normalization of violence, drug and alcohol abuse, and a culture that subordinates women and girls.

15.8.3 The Response

In connection with sexual violence, it is worth noting that all member states who have ratified the Optional Protocol to the Convention on the Rights of the Child on the sale of children, child prostitution and pornography, have committed to the development of measures and initiate actions to protect children from some form of sexual violence, in laws penalties and operational procedures embodied in laws of childhood and relevant legislation. This process ranks first in terms of importance to reduce sexual violence on children.

In terms of legal framework, member states who have ratified the Optional Protocol to the Convention on the Rights of the Child on the sale of children, child prostitution and pornography, have committed to the development of measures and initiate actions to protect children from sexual violence, in laws penalties and operational procedures embodied in laws of childhood and relevant legislation. This process ranks first in importance to reduce sexual violence on children, together with the promotion of the universal ratification of the Optional Protocols to the CRC, systematic data collection and a global survey to assess progress, addressing violence in the context of education and administration of justice, accessible and child-sensitive counselling, complaint and reporting mechanisms, positive developments and persisting challenges.

Strategic initiatives include the adoption of the Global Plan of Action to Combat Trafficking in Persons and the endorsement of the Roadmap for Achieving the Elimination of the Worst Forms of Child Labor, including sexual abuse and exploitation. In the area of the institutionalization of regional governance structures and the development of regional strategies to prevent and address violence against children, critical progress is made, including political commitments and monitoring mechanisms.

The United Nations Children's Fund also supports the three priority areas identified by the Special Representative: the development of a national comprehensive strategy in each State, the introduction of a legal ban on all forms of violence against children in all settings and the promotion of a national data collection system and research agenda on violence against children, while including child-sensitive counselling, complaint and reporting mechanisms. The European are also strongly committed to transform policy objectives into action, through "A European Union Agenda for the Rights of the Child", as well as the "Commission's Strategy" for the effective implementation of the Charter of Fundamental Rights of the European Union, the "European Union Guidelines on the Rights of the Child" and the "European Forum for the Rights of the Child".

Furthermore, the Organization of the Islamic Conference condemns all forms of violence against children, including physical, mental, psychological as well as sexual violence and recognizes that VAC is surrounded by stigma and secrecy. In view of a need for effective and child-sensitive counseling mechanisms to prevent or respond to violence, the OIC supports culture-sensitive child-counseling adapted to age, maturity, gender and circumstances, with child-centered mechanisms. Counseling and reporting services at the community level could encourage children and family members to speak out against the VAC, while addressing education as well as administration of justice.

Slave trade, including trade of sex slaves, fluctuated in certain regions in the Middle East up until the twentieth century (see also Arab slave trade). These slaves came largely from Sub-Saharan Africa (mainly Zanj), the Caucasus (mainly Circassians),[6] Central Asia (mainly Tartars), and Central and Eastern Europe (mainly Saqaliba).[7] The Barbary pirates also captured 1.25 million slaves from Western Europe between the sixteenth and nineteenth centuries.[8,9]

In contrast to the Atlantic slave trade where the male-female ratio was 2:1 or 3:1, the Arab slave trade usually had a higher female:male ratio instead, suggesting a general preference for female slaves. Concubinage and reproduction served as incentives for importing female slaves (often Caucasian), though many were also imported mainly for performing household tasks.[10]

More recently, in Pakistan, young girls have been sold by their families to brothels as sex slaves in big cities.

Often this happens due to poverty or debt, whereby the family has no other way to raise the money than to sell the young girl.[11] Cases have also been recorded where wives and sisters have been sold to brothels to raise money for gambling, drinking or consuming drugs. Many sex slaves are also bought by 'agents' in Afghanistan who trick young girls into coming to Pakistan for well-paying jobs. Once in Pakistan they are taken to brothels (called Kharabat) and forced into sexual slavery for many years.

Sexual slavery also exists in the Arab states of the Persian Gulf, where women and children are trafficked from the post-Soviet states, Eastern Europe, Far East,

---

[6]Pedophilia". Psychology Today. Sussex Publishers, LLC. 7 September 2006.

[7]Ward, Tony; Hudson, Stephen M.; Marshall, William L. (1995). "Cognitive Distortions and Affective Deficits in Sex Offenders: A Cognitive Deconstructionist Interpretation1". Sexual Abuse: A Journal of Research and Treatment.

[8]Groth, A. Nicholas; Birnbaum, H. Jean (1978). "Adult sexual orientation and attraction to underage persons". *Archives of Sexual Behavior*. 7 (3): 175–81. doi:https://doi.org/10.1007/BF01542377. PMID 666571.

[9]This is based on ideas that somehow incest is different from other forms of CSA and this is largely not true. Some incest fathers/stepfathers are abusing children outside of their home. Some rape adult women.

[10]Child Abuse Negl. 2010 Aug;34(8):570–5. doi: 10.1016/j.chiabu.2010.01.011. Epub 2010 Jun 2.

[11]kdeniz, Yaman (2008). Internet child pornography and the law: national and international responses. Ashgate Publishing, Ltd.. p. 11. ISBN 0754622975.

Africa, South Asia and other parts of the Middle East.[12,13,14] Many of the Iraqi women fleeing the Iraq War turned to prostitution, while others were trafficked abroad, to countries like Syria, Jordan, Qatar, the United Arab Emirates and Turkey. Prostitution in Syria alone accounts for an estimated 50,000 Iraqi refugee girls and women, many of them widows.[15] Cheap Iraqi prostitutes have helped to make Syria a popular destination for sex tourists. The clients come from wealthier countries in the Middle East. Higher prices are offered for virgins.

In connection with sexual violence, it is worth noting that all member states who have ratified the Optional Protocol to the Convention on the Rights of the Child on the sale of children, child prostitution and pornography, have committed to the development of measures and initiate actions to protect children from some form of sexual violence, in laws penalties and operational procedures embodied in laws of childhood and relevant legislation. This process ranks first in terms of importance to reduce sexual violence on children.

15.8.4 Succinct Case Management

In the emergency room, emergency contraceptive medications are offered to women raped by men because about 5% of such rapes result in pregnancy.[16] Preventative medication against sexually transmitted infections are given to victims of all types of sexual assault (especially for the most common diseases like chlamydia, gonorrhea, trichomoniasis and bacterial vaginosis) and a blood serum is collected to test for STIs (such as HIV, hepatitis B and syphilis). Survivors with abrasions are immunized for tetanus if 5 years have elapsed since the last immunization. Short-term treatment with a benzodiazepine may help with acute anxiety and antidepressants may be helpful for symptoms of PTSD, depression and panic attacks.

---

[12]Anda, R., Felitti, V., Bremner, J., Walker, J., Whitfield, C., Perry, B., Dube, S. and Giles,W. The enduring effects of abuse and related adverse experiences in childhood. European Achieves of Psychiatry and Neuroscience 2006; *256* /3:174-186.

[13]Melissa A. Polusny; Victoria M. Follette (1995). "Long-term correlates of child sexual abuse: Theory and review of the empirical literature". Applied and Preventive Psychology. Elsevier Ltd. 4 (3): 143–166.

[14]Understanding child sexual abuse: education, prevention, and recovery. American Psychological Association Retrieved 30 October 2012.

[15]Anderson, James; Mangels, Nancie; Langsam, Adam (2004). "Child Sexual Abuse: A Public Health Issue". The Justice Professional. 17: 107.

[16]Varcarolis, Elizabeth (2013). Essentials of psychiatric mental health nursing. St. Louis: Elsevier. pp. 439–442.

15.8.5 Principles of Prevention

The number of initiatives addressing sexual violence is limited and few have been evaluated. The approaches vary with most interventions being developed and implemented in industrialized countries. How relevant they may be in other settings is not well known. Early interventions and the provision of psychological support may prevent or minimize many of the harmful and lasting psychological impacts of sexual assault.

There is also a public health approach to prevention. Because sexual violence is widespread and directly or indirectly affects a community as whole, a community-oriented approach encourages not just victims and advocates to spread awareness and prevent sexual violence, but allocates responsibility to wider community to do so as well The CDC's report on Sexual Violence Prevention: Beginning the Dialogue suggests following its four step model.

1. Define the Problem: Collect data about the victims, perpetrators, where it's occurring, and how often it's happening.
2. Identify Risk and Protective Factors: Research the risk factors that may put people at risk for victimization of perpetration.
3. Develop and Test Prevention Strategies: Work with community leaders, practitioners to test different sexual violence prevention strategies.
4. Ensure Widespread Adoption: Implement and spread awareness about the successful prevention strategies.

The interventions that have been developed can be categorized as follows.

Initiatives to prevent sexual violence

Individual approaches	Health care responses	Community based efforts	Legal and policy responses
Psychological care and support	Medico-legal services	Prevention campaigns	Legal reform
Programmes for perpetrators	Training for health care professionals	Community activism by men	International treaties
Developmental approaches	Prophylaxis for HIV infection	School-based programmes	
	Centres providing comprehensive care to victims of sexual assault		

15.8.6 Why Statistics Are Poor?

Sexual violence is a widely underreported phenomenon, therefore available statistics are unlikely to inform about the true scale of the problem. The available data are scanty and fragmented. Police data, for instance, are often incomplete and limited. Data from medico-legal clinics, on the other hand, may be biased towards the more violent incidents of sexual abuse. In addition, the proportion of people who seek medical services for immediate problems related to sexual violence is also relatively small.

Reasons for non-reporting include shame and embarrassment, fear of not being believed, fear of the perpetrator of the crime, fear of the legal process, or disbelief that the police would be able to do anything to help them. Men are even more reluctant to report sexual violence due to extreme embarrassment and concerns about opinions of other people, their masculinity and the fact that they were unable to prevent the assault. Thus information about the extent of sexual violence against males is especially limited. Child sexual abuse is also largely underreported. Most of the data comes from asking adults about their past experiences.

Chapter 16
Violence in Armed Conflicts and Natural Disasters: A Link to CSAET

16.1 Abstract

Many Arab states are suffering from the devastating effects of political conflicts, occupation and wars within the region, and particularly in the last 3 years of disturbances. The region also faces challenges of decades-long political conflicts, including the on-going Arab-Israeli conflict, which have resulted in multiple occupations and wars and left the Arab region in a state of instability.[1]

The lack of accurate statistical information on the number of child fatalities, amount of displacement, and number of injured or refugee children as a result of these conflicts does not limit the clear truth reflected by the media, child rights organizations and humanitarian aid, which is that children in Arab countries are targeted, being arrested, suffering and dying. They are also being exploited through participation in demonstrations and actions that have political dimensions, and are used as tools to fuel conflicts and divisions rather than being raised in a non-violent and accepting culture.

16.2 Gender-Based Violence

Areas affected by conflict and natural disasters also see high rates of GBV. Violent rape and torture is often used as a weapon in warzones, such as in the Democratic Republic of Congo and South Sudan, and can result in severe injuries and trauma. Natural disasters also put women at high risk for sexual assault; a March 2010 UNFPA survey in Port-au-Prince, Haiti found that 3% of the city's population had

[1]The Report of the Special Representative of the Secretary-General on violence against children, Marta Santos Pais, (A/HRC/16/54) The Report of the Special Rapporteur on the sale of children, child prostitution and child pornography, Najat M'jid Maalla, (A/HRC/16/57).

B. Gerbaka et al., *Child Sexual Abuse, Exploitation and Trafficking in the Arab Region*, Child Maltreatment 13, https://doi.org/10.1007/978-3-030-66507-4_16

been sexually assaulted in the three months that had passed since the January 12th, 2010 earthquake had struck. Individuals in war and disaster zones may have difficulty accessing potentially life-saving medical, legal, and mental health services after surviving GBV.

16.3 Sexual Harassment in the MENAG Region

At the time when almost all the Arab countries are suffering from this same crime, it is still difficult to break the silence of women and it was not an easy task for many of them, particularly in the absence of studies that could help identify the strategy to be undertaken.

As a result of this communication and experience with sharing a number of studies, an opportunity emerged that indicated the extensiveness of the problem in other countries. In Algeria 27% of female university students confirmed that they were subject to molestations and sexual misbehaviors by their professors. 44.6% of them complained about verbal utterances, whereas 13.8% said they were subject to physical harassment. In Qatar 21.1% of young girls revealed their vulnerability to the same thing. Almost 30% of working-women were subjected to sexual harassment in their work places. In Saudi Arabia 22.7% of children face the same matter, as well official reports and statistics showed that in 2002, 9580 ethical incidents included 997 crimes of harassment. In Yemen, 90% of women complained of harassment, whether in public or work places.

A closer coordination with women's associations is needed, in various countries such as KSA, Bahrain, Syria, Palestine, Tunisia, Morocco, Sudan and others, in order to share experiences and uphold the draft laws. An example is a draft law put forward to the Shoura Council in Saudi Arabia that criminalizes sexual harassment.

16.4 Impact on Children

The many different armed conflicts, as well as social conflicts in Lebanon, Gaza, West Bank, Iraq, Somalia and Sudan have had significant impacts on children. Many crimes have added to the forms of violence which are suffered by the rest of the children in the Arab region and the world.[2] Since the structural violence exercised directly influence and lead to an escalation of violence within Palestinian society resulting in even more poverty and frustration and a need to ventilate that frustration

[2]Child Sexual Abuse in Lebanon during War and Peace. Usta, J., and J. Farver. 2010. "Child Sexual Abuse in Lebanon during War and Peace." *Child: Care, Health and Development* 36 (3): 361–68. doi:https://doi.org/10.1111/j.1365-2214.2010.01082.x

against whoever is available among the family members. Accordingly women and children become the immediate target.

16.5 Who Is Defined as Child?

The definition of a child is a concern: for example, it is applied according to the convention on Israeli children, while Palestinian children are subject to military laws. Such definitional issues are also a concern in Sudan and Darfur.

The Convention on the Rights of the Child (CRC), in its concluding observations for the year 2011 on Bahrain, expressed its concerns about inadequate protection for children during the period of political turmoil experienced by the country, and demanded that the state develop a legal and institutional system for the protection of children.

The CRC also urged the Egypt to strengthen the protection of children during its phase of political transition. The Special Representative of the United Nations Secretary-General for VAC demanded that Syria secure the protection of children from violence and keep its commitment to the CRC and the 2010 Marrakesh Declaration of the Fourth High Level Conference on the Rights of the Child. UNICEF has also demanded that all parties respect their obligations towards the CRC, as well as International Humanitarian Law, by taking necessary steps to protect children from the direct and indirect effects of violence.

16.6 The Violations in Country Reports

Children in the Arab region remain prone to serious rights violations as a result of the significant existing gaps related to their protection. Their participation in armed conflict is an additional risk factor, as highlighted by the annual report of the Secretary-General on Children and Armed Conflict issued in 2013.

Libya: In Libya, children suffered harm, and were widely involved in armed conflict. Attacks took place against schools and damage was incurred by health facilities.

Syria: Children in Syria continue to be killed, wounded and maimed as a result of heavy artillery, air raids and war remnants such as explosives. This was a result of the on-going conflict between government and opposition forces. A number of children were tortured and sexually abused, while others aged 15–17 were recruited for fighting or support. Hospitals and schools were also targeted within the conflict.

Palestine: In the period the report covers, 50 Palestinian children were killed and 665 wounded in the occupied Palestinian territories. In the West Bank, four Palestinian children were killed and 552 wounded, while 46 were affected in Gaza. The arrest and detention of Palestinian children by Israeli forces continued in 2012, on the basis that they had committed security violations for which they were to be tried in martial courts for juveniles. Palestine highlighted its existing national and local mechanisms, which were recorded by the Palestinian Child Act for the year 2011 and are concerned with cases of emergency. A national committee was formed to follow up on children who are the victims of violence under the occupation, and they are all connected to the child protection system for referrals and on-going follow up.

Jordan referred to the memorandum of understanding it signed with the UN Refugee Agency (UNHCR) in 1998. The National Council for Family Affairs in cooperation with UNICEF and UNHCR also sought to improve procedures for protecting children in times of crisis and emergency, and pursued their ratification by all of the international and national institutions working with Syrian and Iraqi refugees.

Iraq: In 2012, regional working teams reported 355 major violations against children; these included 178 cases of killing and maiming of children. Children aged 14–17 were also recruited to battle. Women and girls from Iraq's Yazidi minority have been raped, sold into sexual slavery and abused by the Islamic State (IS) group in a systematic ethnic cleansing drive, according to an Amnesty International report released Tuesday.

In a report titled, "Escape From Hell," Amnesty International detailed the ordeals of 42 women and girls who managed to escape from their captors, who included fighters with the IS group (also known as ISIS or ISIL) as well as IS supporters such as local businessmen in northern Iraq.

Months after IS fighters swept through swathes of northern Iraq in a lightening summer offensive, details of the crimes against humanity being perpetrated in the areas they control are gradually emerging. But the full extent of the atrocities is still not known. In 2014, IS militants abducted thousands, of Yazidi men, women and children, according to the Amnesty report. Many men were killed or forced to convert under the threat of the death. For the women and children, a nightmare of almost unimaginable proportions had begun. Separated from their families, sold into sexual enslavement, forced to convert, raped and sometimes tortured, the victims—including girls as young as 12—have endured abuses that constitute war crimes and crimes against humanity, according to Amnesty International.

Lebanon: The UN documented 24 violations against children, most of which were comprised of killing children and maiming them. The UN also received reports of the participation of children in the armed confrontations that took place between opposing political factions in Lebanon. In Lebanon there is no ready plan or any clear and definite official framework for dealing with emergency cases. There are, however, government initiatives that are still being examined but have not yet been officially ratified. Through available national mechanisms, work is done on evolving the model that is applicable to protecting children in cases of emergency. This applies specifically to displaced Syrian and Iraqi children. A number of measures and procedures have been undertaken regarding them.

Bahrain's Ministerial Council issued a resolution establishing a national committee whose role would be to propose detailed plans and programs focusing on crisis management and mitigation 2000. The national committee would also put in place safety guidelines and mechanisms for coordination, and would delineate ministries' tasks. It would also put forward suggestions for modification and development, and raise reports to concerned parties. The Bahraini Child Law also stipulates "the child would be given priority in receiving protection and assistance, in case of disasters whether natural, man-made or resulting from warfare".

In Saudi Arabia, the Ministry of Interior, in cooperation with several actors, is currently implementing a work mechanism that will guarantee the establishment of a national plan for crisis management. This endeavor is being undertaken with the aim of offering the full range of assistance services to different social groups' discrimination. In 2012 the Saudi Ministry of Education also launched a program of safety from fire inside schools, whose aim was to protect and educate students regarding the risks of fire accidents, and how to curtail them.

Oman: The Ministry of Social Development established a plan for rescue operations in cooperation with concerned ministries and quarters, the National Centre for Managing Emergencies and the National Committee for Civil Defense. The plan would thus cover natural, industrial and environmental threats, and aims to rescue those afflicted, provide refuge centers and secure basic needs, guidance and psychological support.

Qatar: The Qatari cabinet issued a decree in 2011 stipulating the formation of a permanent committee for emergencies in the Ministry of the Interior. Headed by the General Director of Public Security, the committee would be composed of concerned ministries and councils. In addition to this, a special decree was issued, ratifying a memorandum of cooperation in the field of prevention, and facing emergencies and catastrophes between Qatar and Belarus in 2011. A committee for international humanitarian law was also formed.

Yemen: The recruitment of children for combat purposes has continued. In 2012, 53 children aged 13–17 were recruited to combat. The report also showed that 50 children were killed and 165 were maimed in 2012. Many casualties among children were the result of land mines, unexploded ammunition and remnants of war explosives. In the same period, 165 cases were recorded of attacks on schools and 11 cases of attacks on hospitals. These necessitate non-deportation or removal and extending their periods of stay. In Yemen, with the support of UNICEF, has prepared an emergency preparedness plan for protecting children in cases of emergency. This covered a number of areas related to children, including undertaking quick surveys of afflicted areas, training and rehabilitation, and capacity building. The plan also included providing recuperation services and psychological and social rehabilitation, as well as health and educational services. Social committees for the protection of children have also been suggested.

Somalia: In 2012, the Qatari Task Force for Monitoring and Reporting documented 4660 cases of violations against children in Somalia. 2051 cases were related to the recruitment and use of children in armed actions and 213 cases of sexual violence against 210 girls and 3 boys were attributed to the National Armed Forces and various armed groups.

Sudan and South Sudan: Widespread violations of children in South Sudan and Darfur also continue. In Sudan, The National Council for Childhood in Sudan is coordinating between national mechanisms and international organizations working in the field of child protection in emergencies (e.g. the Unit for Child Rights in the Armed Forces, the Consultative Council for Human Rights, the National Commission for Voluntary Return and Displacement, local child protection groups, and local police units for the protection of family and children). UN Security Council Resolution 1612 on Children in Armed Conflict also established an assistance committee. These mechanisms are all linked to a national protection service. With regard to displaced children the National Council for Childhood in collaboration with international organizations established a program for the reunification of families and unaccompanied children, to provide them with care and protection, to search for their families and integrate them into society. This was begun after the separation of South Sudan in July 2011, through a memorandum of understanding to bring families together, establish a database for children, and undertake steps for familial screening.

16.7 The MENA Region Specificities

The refugees' related problems concern millions of people in the MENA region and provoke religious and demographic instability; it also creates hot areas of armed violence, uncontrolled by some states. The humanitarian conditions inside the camps and slumps affect important numbers of children, exposed to community violence, customs and discrimination that may even be irrelevant with legislation. Qualitatively, the situation of children is also highly concerning. Some reports—shadow reports—bring information about the condition of children in such housings and social settings, where commercial and sexual exploitation are current, adding violence over violence to poverty, clan violence, discrimination and religious confrontations. The situation of children also addresses the insufficiency of the international community in carrying out Article 1 obligation to "ensure respect" for the Geneva Conventions and the protection of civilians during armed conflicts throughout the Arab region, . . .to pass a resolution denouncing the deteriorating respect for international humanitarian law in the Arab region, including in Iraq, the OPTs, Darfur and Yemen.

The responses of Arab countries have revealed a scarcity of existing mechanisms available on the national level to protect children in cases of emergency. One notable exception to this lack can be found in countries existing in an on-going state of emergency. There is a sizeable global effort to establish policies and strategies that curtail rights violations in emergency contexts, and to design methodologies and tools to develop and build emergency responders. It would be useful for Arab states to interact with specialized international agencies to draw on available international experience. The Women, Family and Childhood Department, with its connections to international community organizations, can contribute to the development of national plans and strategies for child protection in emergency situations. The department adopted the document for "Guiding Principles on Guaranteeing Children's Rights in Cases of Emergency" in cooperation with Save the Children

16.8 Conflict Zones and Natural Disasters Challenges

- The lack of a legal framework to protect children during armed conflicts and emergency situations, or even for asylum-seekers:
  - Resort to various forms of violence against and torture of children during the recent political events experienced by some Arab countries.
  - Strengthen the legal and institutional system for the protection and promotion of children's rights during emergencies, especially in the context of legal proceedings.
  - Ensure that no child is subjected to torture or any other form of cruel, inhumane, or degrading treatment.
  - Establish an effective system for receiving of complaints and collecting data on torture or other forms of abuse of children who are deprived of their freedom. In addition, immediate investigations should be made into all allegations of torture or other forms of abuse, and the perpetrators should be prosecuted.
  - Stop Impunity for people who have violated children's rights and not bringing them to justice.
- Data collection
  - The absence of a centralized system for data collection on the national level, which would cover all areas of the convention.
  - The total absence of data classified according to geographic location, social and economic status, and categories of children who suffer from fragility of situation, in addition to data on exposure to violence, abuse, and exploitation.
  - In most cases, policy-makers' use of unreliable national data in assessing the situation.
- Child helplines:
  - The presence of various child helplines, some run by organizations of civil society and others supported by the state.
  - The majority of calls received by these helplines are from adults and not the children themselves.

16.9 Recommendations

The Arab region is experiencing multiple types of armed conflict and political turmoil, which reflect negatively on the rights of the child. The right to protection and the right to live in a safe environment away from violence, death and exploitation are particularly affected. The presence of such conflicts and turmoil necessitates the organization of appropriate national responses in a coherent formal institutional framework with child protection at its core. The responses of countries in this regard, shown by their answers in the questionnaire, are limited to some initiatives taken by international organizations. Governmental government commitment is nearly non-existent. In countries witnessing armed conflicts there is a need to adopt a monitoring and reporting system for cases of children who are affected or at risk of being affected by the conflict. This requires a clear political decision, supported by the allocation of other resources. In countries where there is turmoil, preventive legislative methods are necessary to limit the suffering of children. Exploitation within activities and events that are not age-appropriate and cause harm to child development, personalities, and behavior in social life must be stopped. The Bahrain initiative to include an article in its Child Act highlighting the inadmissibility of the use of children in demonstrations and political acts is a positive example of such legislation.

Some Arab countries witnessing armed conflicts insisted, with the technical help of UN agencies and international organizations, on creating communal and central protection mechanisms for the protection of children. They also initiated programs of rehabilitation and reintegration for recruits and family screening programs, and introduced specialized units in this regard.

The Arab region is experiencing multiple types of armed conflict and political turmoil, which reflect negatively on the rights of the child. The right to protection and the right to live in a safe environment away from violence, death and exploitation are particularly affected. The presence of such conflicts and turmoil necessitates the organization of appropriate national responses in a coherent formal institutional framework with child protection at its core. Arab countries are limited to some initiatives taken by international organizations. Governmental government commitment is nearly non-existent. In countries witnessing armed conflicts there is a need to adopt a monitoring and reporting system for cases of children who are affected or at risk of being affected by the conflict. This requires a clear political decision, supported by the allocation of other resources. In countries where there is turmoil, preventive legislative methods are necessary to limit the suffering of children. Exploitation within activities and events that are not age-appropriate and cause harm to child development, personalities, and behavior in social life must be stopped. The Bahrain initiative to include an article in its Child Act highlighting the inadmissibility of the use of children in demonstrations and political acts is a positive example of such legislation.

Part V
International Efforts and the UNVAC in the MENA Region

Chapter 17
Principles and Practices in Prevention of Child Sexual Abuse

17.1 Abstract

International professional organizations have contributed to the global effort for the prevention of child abuse and neglect: identification of efficient procedures in respective backgrounds, increasing the knowledge base, reducing the acceptance threshold of CAN, thus enhancing the quality of national visions in terms of child oriented policies. In some areas of the Arab world, initiatives are hindered by armed conflicts, with many violations to the CRC, the EU Guidelines and the Geneva conventions. They are also challenged by unstable socio-political situations in many counties of the MENA region

17.2 Role for ISPCAN and the Arab Professionals' Society for the Prevention of Violence Against Children

The mission of professionals—at academic or informal levels—aims at the prevention of maltreatment as well as the identification and management of abused and neglected children. Established in taskforces, they accomplish such missions within multidisciplinary teams, such as law enforcement personnel, child welfare and mental health specialists in addition to research resources and health professionals. However, and unless controlled by reliable monitoring systems, professional training and societal implication, increase of violence against children can be expected in many countries of the Arab region—in view of the alarming rates of associated risk factors.

Responsibility for prevention of child sexual abuse is shared by parents, schools, communities and government and the broader society. In seeking to prevent sexual violence against children, it is important to recognize that some risk factors—such as poverty and lack of access to education—must be addressed at policy and practice

B. Gerbaka et al., *Child Sexual Abuse, Exploitation and Trafficking in the Arab Region*, Child Maltreatment 13, https://doi.org/10.1007/978-3-030-66507-4_17

levels. Poly-victimization and the co-occurrence of other forms of abuse must also be acknowledged in the formulation of prevention strategies. Response to situations of conflict, post-conflict and natural disasters must consider evidence that the prevalence of sexual violence often increases in contexts of these conditions and respond adequately.

Sexual exploitation of children including 'sex tourism' requires the involvement of all aspects of government, and its prevention is not the sole responsibility of child protection services. Greater attention should be paid to innovative efforts that try to address multiple risk factors, such as armed conflicts and sectal riots. Greater emphasis should be placed on primary prevention—preventing violence from ever taking place—as opposed to secondary or tertiary prevention. There is also a need to strengthen the service provision network (e.g., health care sector needs to be trained to identify and care for cases). Secondary and tertiary prevention should be evidence-based, identifying ways in which victims can continue to be re-victimized and victims can become people who harm others. Evidence-based research is needed regarding the risk and protective factors associated with both perpetration and victimization in order to develop effective preventive strategies. Prevention strategies need to be rigorously evaluated at all levels and takes into account the range of social contexts of vulnerable children. Primary prevention of sexual violence may require adaptation to different manifestations of sexual violence, different profiles of potential perpetrators and different groups of vulnerability for victimization of children and families.

Prevention strategies should include a combination of provision of information (e.g., on children's human rights), building skills (e.g., what to do, who to talk to) and provision of resources (e.g., hotlines).

17.3 Health Services for CSA in the Arab Region

Arab countries provide a range of accessible health care services in the areas of pre-hospitalization and emergency care. A range of programs and pilot projects are offered in this area, including development of procedures and protocols governing coordination amongst participants, the creation of specialized fixed or mobile units to deal with violence, and programs promoting maternal and child health. Other examples include training programs for health workers and doctors to identify the signs and symptoms of violence, trainings and assignment of staffers specialized in the detection of early symptoms of violence and in reporting.

Jordan has developed procedures and protocols with the Ministry of Health to deal with cases of domestic violence. A specialized unit within the ministry handles issues of violence via a forensic medicine clinic within the Family Protection Department, which provide specialized medical services. All medical services are provided free of charge to victims of domestic violence. The Council of Ministers decided in 2004 to provide treatment and services free of charge to victims of domestic violence referred to hospitals and health centers by the Department of Family Protection.

Tunisia has installed a toll-free telephone number dedicated to helping battered women. Child protection officers can also be contacted by phone or e-mail in cases where children become victims of violence.

In Algeria 1212 units exist to screen for health issues in schools, in addition to 48 units to protect children in difficult circumstances and to integrate them in the society. Saudi Arabia (KSA) has formed social protection committees in the country to provide care in cases of violence. Saudi Arabia has also established health units within the Department of Medical Supervision for clinical and psychological care. Relevant services and appropriate care are provided to students. The Department undertakes special programs, workshops and seminars tackling violence and problems relating to childhood and adolescence, and trains educational personnel in relevant skills.

In Syria, the Directorate of School Health at the Ministry of Education designated clinics to each cluster of schools; these facilities serve several functions: providing medication, a program for psychosocial support and child protection, and psychological evaluation, clinical and supportive psychotherapy and pharmacotherapy services. The National Centre for Forensic Medicine within the Ministry of Health provides specialized services and has branches in all Syrian governorates.

In Oman, all schools have designated health services facilities. An ad hoc form has been designed to document and report cases of abuse in health centers, and task forces have been formed to study and follow-up on cases of abuse across the governorates of Oman

Qatar has opened two offices for The Qatar Foundation for Protection of Women and Children and to receive reports of offenses at the Emergency Department of Hamad Medical Corporation and within the Directorate of Security in the capital city

In Egypt, the centers affiliated with the Ministry of Health offer general health care, including preventive and emergency services; critical cases are referred to the secondary level of Ministry of Health hospitals in accordance with the Child Act, Article (7) bis. Mobile units to provide on-site emergency health services for street children at their gathering places have been established

Morocco has developed 18 medical units to receive female and child victims of violence, and has created units for child protection providing support, coping with urgent health issues and keeping current with legal and social services for the children victims of violence or those threatened by violence.

In 2006, Yemen launched a program for prevention of injuries and violence. Obviously those settings have been dismantled by the raging conflict within the country.

17.4 Principles and Practices for a Holistic Approach to Children Affected by CSA

- Training of the professionals responsible for the first contact with the child.
- Integrated and interdisciplinary approach should include the Judiciary.
- Strong leadership for coordination is needed to set guidelines for intervention, including the Judiciary bodies.[1]
- Written and binding protocols signed by the head of the agencies are recommended with some flexibility to adapt to local conditions.
- Written and biding protocols should state that the child has a right to be heard, as in her wishes as opposed to parental wishes where there is conflict.
- Ensure the implementation of the protocols through interdisciplinary training (including the legal system) and supervision (including judges and other professionals).
- When collecting evidence it is important to rely on the child statement without excluding other evidence (investigation should focus on the protection of the children not only on the requirements of the punitive criminal proceedings).
- Children's allegations should be assessed through appropriate forensic interviews, where the number of interviews by different professionals are reduced to the minimum. Children should therefore be interviewed but not interrogated.[2]
- Victims should have a party status in the process with the right of a defender to grant his/her rights within the proceedings (e.g., to deal with the impact of cross examination in those countries that allow it).[3]
- Criminal courts specialized in crimes against child victims and integrated court for family issues (criminal, family and civil) are needed.
- Integration is a process and not only a goal. Observation of the rights of the child and an integrated systemic approach is less traumatizing for the child.
- Different programs need to be developed for young and adult offenders and for first-time and chronic offenders.

---

[1]The law is the primary guideline for the judiciary; there is a need for guidelines in areas of judicial discretion (e.g. placement of children, judge allowing unscientific testimony (e.g. Parent Alienation Syndrome).

[2]There is actually limited data that the number of interviews is harmful to children. Some children benefit from multiple interviews. The issue is interviewing vs. interrogation. This is an investigation model. It needs to be validated in regions and professional settings.

[3]The victim is not going to be a party in a criminal matter against the offender. Even if the child is somehow a party (which would be a fundamental change in criminal law), the issue of cross examination is solved by modifications as having the child interview outside of the presence of the accused, allowing a professional to interview and ask questions submitted by both sides, etc.

17.5 Education and Training Issues: Professionals, Schools, Communities

- All victims of child sexual abuse and sexual exploitation and their families have the right to have access to knowledgeable and skilled service providers regardless of their discipline.
- Since child sexual abuse and sexual exploitation is an ever-evolving field, children deserve competent practitioners who acknowledge the importance of continuing education.
- The dissemination of knowledge may occur through many different strategies, including:
  - Regional, national and international conferences;
  - Development of a resource library;
  - Core discipline specific training to address needs tailored to the developmental stage of a given program, consultation and networking.
- The world-community continues to learn about the definition, prevention, assessment, and the treatment of child sexual abuse.
- As evidenced based understanding of core principles, guidelines, and standards evolve for the medical, legal, and social sciences there is a need to disseminate this information world-wide through education and training initiatives.
- If we are to significantly reduce the prevalence of child sexual abuse and sexual exploitation in its many manifestations, such efforts must be designed by and for the relevant individuals and systems in a state, country, or community.
- Any such training and education efforts shall remain open to the inclusion and adoption of culturally sensitive and culturally relevant alternatives.

17.6 Medical Care Domains

17.6.1 Best Practices in Medical Care of Child Sexual Abuse

- Much has been learned about best practices in the substantiation of allegations of child sexual abuse, building of medical diagnostic and treatment services and addressing the mental health needs of child victims.
- This said the challenge remains adapting this core knowledge in a way that is relevant to a given country, the resources available and priority given to this issue.

17.6.2 Integration of the Health Care Professional

- Health professionals have both an opportunity and responsibility to objectively evaluate children who are alleged to experience child sexual abuse.
- The medical diagnosis of CSA is an important first step that can address the health and welfare of child victims. It is not an isolated and unique intervention. It needs to be articulated with other professional interventions with the medical profession and in other health and socio-legal resources.
- Without a diagnosis the ability to intervene, protect and ultimately provide the medical and mental health services necessary to address the impact of victimization will be compromised.
- Although the medical component is an important piece of the diagnostic process, it is the collective insights of the numerous disciplines that will result in the most complete understanding and evaluation of a child's experience, as well as the required next steps.
- Children suspected of experiencing child sexual abuse are entrusted to health professionals with the responsibility to objectively assess the concerns when they present to formulate a "medical diagnosis" that is balanced and defensible. Even in hazy circumstances and conditions, the lack of a medical diagnosis need not keep child protection or intervention specialists from deciding a child has been abused.
- Systems need to acknowledge that as many as 70 to 90% of child sexual abuse is not confirmed through medical evaluation by itself; CSA may not confirmed by "physical examination alone." Although the physical examination may not be diagnostic, when the medical history and examination are considered together, the medical diagnosis of CSA may increase the probability of evidence or substantiation.

Key Elements

- Medical diagnosis of suspected child sexual abuse and sexual exploitation can be critical to the substantiation process.
- Medical diagnosis must be balanced, objective and defensible.

17.6.3 Need for Health Care Professionals to Provide Diagnosis and Treatment

- For the child suspected of being sexually abused regardless of the conduit to which the concerns present themselves all children should have access to skilled health care professionals who can address the potential adverse health effects of child sexual abuse and sexual exploitation whether there be extra-genital or penetrative injuries, pregnancy in adolescents or the acquiring of a sexually transmitted infection (STI).
- Equally important is the need to address concerns that could be viewed as altered body images/body intactness questions that are commonly associated following sexual victimization.
- The need for child victims to know that their bodies are "normal" in spite of their experience is critical to their long-term psychological well-being. The medical evaluation can be the first step to therapeutic intervention, through the assurance provided by the health care provider about body image, risk of pregnancy, sexually transmitted infections, or other fears.

Key Elements

- Diagnosis and treatment of physical injuries and sexually transmitted infections following child sexual victimization is an essential component of the health care of child sexual abuse and sexual exploitation victims.
- Diagnosis of "normality" or physical intactness is critical to the long-term mental health of child victims.

17.6.4 Health Providers' Approach

- Health professionals can apply their tried and true approach to the diagnosis of any disease in order to substantiate a specific diagnosis. A public health approach algorithm and training package has been also developed by ISPCAN and WHO, in order to help professionals globally, in the process of the diagnosis of child sexual abuse and sexual exploitation; the public health approach was found to be helpful in the diagnostic process, and was consequently translated and developed in the Arab region, allowing a better understanding of the clinical expression of sexual victimization in girls and boys of varying ages.
- As with any form of victimization there is a spectrum of experiences from contact that is minimally physically intrusive to very intrusive and physically traumatic. By understanding that sexual victimization has the potential for both physical and

emotional health consequences the health care provider can tailor their clinical approach to improve their competence in addressing CSA.[4]

- The single most important skill set that health care professionals must have is the ability to obtain a medical history [pediatrician, psychologist, etc.] from suspected child victims in a developmentally appropriate manner that is non-judgmental, facilitating and empathetic. When children are asked about their experiences in a manner that allows them to tell their story there will be an opportunity to obtain the best insight into their experience. Equally important is the thorough documentation of both the questions asked by the historian and the child's verbatim response.
- Some children will experience physical injuries and contract sexually transmitted infections requiring health care providers to diagnose both acute and heal residual to sexual contact and meet the treatment needs and follow-up care. The medical diagnosis is the result of the successful integration of medical history, physical examination findings and laboratory findings.
- The ability to evaluate child victims requires a very specific set of knowledge and skills that are not intuitive to health care professionals and few are capable of meeting without specific professional training.

Key Elements

- The medical history is the single most important element of making the diagnosis of child sexual abuse and sexual exploitation.
- Obtaining and documenting the medical history is a critically important skill set.

[4]Understanding effects is one aspect of treatment. Other aspects are less clear: The point about consequences appearing at any time in development including in adulthood is also a good one. What is not clear is what is treated to prevent these negative consequences. The models for treatment do not directly target many of the consequences. Additionally some of the long term adult consequences of CSA (e.g. medical problems) are not developmentally stage salient when the child is seen. Understanding consequences and good treatment are therefore two different undertakings.

17.6.5 Health Care or a Forensic Role?

- The health provider is well grounded in their ability to provide diagnosis and treatment. A well-crafted and defensible medical opinion can have significant forensic value. Evidence can be found in the child's history, physical examination findings and/or "forensic" testing. It is the collective professional and collaborative input of all disciplines that ultimately will provide the most complete understanding and allow for child protection and law enforcement to address their discipline specific responsibilities. Health care providers best serve child victims when they see themselves as responsible for meeting the health care needs of the child and not as an agent of child protective services or law enforcement.

Key Elements

- When health care professionals address the health needs of child victims they also meet the forensic needs that are important to child protective services/law enforcement ability to substantiate allegations to their respective discipline specific standards.
- Working in a multi-disciplinary manner while knowing the limits of one's respective discipline is critical to substantiation.

17.6.6 Developing Health Care Capacity to Serve Medical Diagnostic Needs

- The child protective services (or child welfare services) response in many communities has traditionally been focused on the issues of protection rather than addressing the health needs of child victims. Societal emphasis on prosecution does not necessarily encompass the needs of victims, unless specific policies, practices, and laws require victim assistance. As a result there is variability in the accessibility to specialized medical expertise.
- With shared experience with the medical community, child protective services and law enforcement professionals begin to understand the critical importance of the health care role. These non-health care professionals must identify health care professionals in their community to provide needed care.
- If medical resources are not immediately apparent then protective services and law enforcement authorities need to strategically plan how to secure and support medical resources. In most communities a physician and/or nurse can be identified who have special demonstrated leadership and special interest in serving the needs of sexually abused children and should be invited to participate in a discussion as to how best to integrate them into the system of care.
- In most communities there are greater demands for medical services than capacity to meet the need. Through dialogue an opportunity can be created to prioritize

which children receive services. A protocol can be established for both the type of cases that will receive care and the timing of any medical response.

Key Elements

- Child protective services/law enforcement must identify health care providers within their community to provide medical services.
- Health care professionals have a reciprocal duty to advocate for and assist in identification of committed health providers and their training
- Where medical services do not exist a strategic plan to develop such must be implemented collaboratively.
- Policies and protocols to access medical services once developed must be implemented.

17.6.7 Sharing Responsibility and Shared Decision Making

- Each and every discipline has a responsibility to perform with the highest level of professionalism knowing the limitations of their discipline and provide objective defensible opinions.
- Each discipline has the right to know the special skills and responsibilities of each partners involved in intervening when child sexual victimization is suspected and to hold each other responsible.
- Therefore professional education both discipline specific and interdisciplinary should be integral to a culture of developing and improving professional expertise to deal with child sexual abuse and sexual exploitation.
- All effective systems of health care recognize that providing care to child victims of abuse has the potential for vicarious traumatization, causing emotional trauma for the caregivers, and that special efforts must be made to take of care of the care providers.

Key Elements

- Each discipline has the responsibility to perform with the highest level of expertise and professionalism.
- Professional development is an ongoing process and should be collectively supported and shared to serve the best interests of children and society.
- Vicarious trauma is a work hazard and should be both recognized and addressed to maintain a healthy work force.

17.6.8 Implications for Health Services

- The health professional can provide a unique and critical input and expertise into understanding a child's experience when allegations of sexual abuse arise.
- The health care provider's opinion can be an important piece of the puzzle of understanding whether abuse has occurred and simultaneously meet the health care needs of the child.
- Any successful system of care must integrate medical services into the fabric of how care is provided.
- It is the child protection systems ability to meet the medical and mental health care needs of child victims that promises the greatest return on investment, a child's life-long optimization of their physical and emotional development.
- This document serves simply to emphasize the importance of addressing the health care needs of children suspected of experiencing sexual victimization. Once the system of child protection and law enforcement acknowledges the important role of health there is then an opportunity to develop systems of care that incorporate this invaluable resource in a meaningful manner.

17.7 Social Services for CSA in the Arab Region

The majority of Arab countries have implemented toll-free telephone line services to receive complaints and provide guidance and counselling services to victims of violence. Private institutions have also been established to receive reports about and follow-up on cases of violence against children.

In Jordan, the "Protection against Abuse" office at the Ministry of Education receives reports on cases of abuse of students at schools through its toll-toll-free hotline and website. Social workers are appointed to follow-up on abuse issues, and agreements have been signed with civil society organizations along with the signing of agreements with civil society organizations to monitor cases of abuse, in addition to the outstanding efforts exerted by NGOs in this area.

The Bahrain Centre for Child Protection offers a one stop shop for legal, health and social services in a child-friendly environment. In Bahrain, toll-free lines are being established to allow children to report cases of abuse or violence. The hotline has been dubbed 'hotline and child support' and will be reachable by children at an easy-to-remember number, 998. A number of specialists in the fields of health, psychological and social guidance and counselling have been assigned the task of receiving calls to the hotline. A home has also been set up to provide shelter, security, health care, and psycho-social support to women and children exposed to violence. This is in addition to the introduction of Batelco House Children's Fund, and the opening of a private clinic to receive children experiencing violence, at Sulaymaniyeh Medical Centre, Ministry of Health.

Algeria has established offices within each municipality for social activities, providing social and economic assistance for families in need. These offices rely on the National Committee on Solidarity and its existing local branches across 48 states, in addition to toll-free hotlines to receive complaints and provide guidance and counselling services.

Syria has established family protection units; such units receive child abuse complaint cases, and investigate and forward them to the competent authorities. Some units have also embarked on setting up a shelter facility to protect—in a center dedicated for child victims—the children who cannot be reintegrated in their communities without receiving physical and psychological rehabilitation; a re-evaluation of the environment in which they live would follow rehabilitation.

In Palestine, a protocol on child protection across networks, including public and private institutions involved in child protection, has been concluded. Child protection services are implemented based on full partnership and interaction among institutions. Children's issues are mediated through a child protection system of interventions, programs and services. The system represents a child protection program, with centers for child protection, and protection teams for children, which receive calls and complaints. Referral of children is made in writing or over the phone; children are then placed following a plan devised to provide protection and care for victims of domestic violence. The system also ensures rehabilitation and reintegration of child victims in their families and communities. The emphasis put on these plans is meant to avoid committing children into justice systems; pre-trial detention is proposed only in extreme cases according to the amendments made to the Palestinian Child Act, which has recently increased the minimum age of criminal accountability from 9 to 12 years.

In Qatar, several institutions have created programs to end violence and provide social support, psychological counselling and behavioral change programs for children and their families, in addition to the availability of protection and refuge and alternative family care when necessary.

In Egypt, the offices of social defense, family and children at the Ministry of Solidarity monitor the role of NGOs in monitoring, control and inspection, and oversee care provision in relation to children's issues. Incidences of exposure to risk and violence are detected by these offices and complaint boxes have been installed in social welfare units, allowing children to lodge complaints of violence by their caregivers. School doctors and psychologists detect and follow-up on cases such, work on character development and assist the children in solving the problems they encounter. Egypt has also established committees at the provincial level, with a mandate to monitor cases of exposure to risk, receive complaints and undertake direct interventions to confront the dangers children face. Recently, in addition to the existing child rescue line, another special line was installed to address family issues.

In Yemen, the Supreme Council for Motherhood and Childhood, in cooperation and coordination with governmental and non-governmental organizations, has established a range of networks and national commissions for children, including the National Network on Violence against Children, and the National Network for the Care of Children in Conflict with Law. In 2008, the two networks were integrated into a single national network, under the name 'National Network for Child Protection'. This Network aims to contribute to the provision of a safe environment to meet the needs of children. This goal can be furthered through strengthening the legal framework for child protection, raising community awareness about child protection, and providing psycho-social and legal support for child victims of violence, abuse, neglect and exploitation. It can also be accomplished through monitoring, reporting and follow-up on cases of violence and abuse, neglect and exploitation. The services are based on coordination of efforts among members of the network and its affiliated entities. Currently, the establishment of child protection networks in ten governorates is underway. The first stage is the completion of network development and regulation of the networks for child protection at the provincial level. Recently, the Yemeni journalists' network to end violence against children was also established.

Those social services have also been broken down by the conflict and the emerging health priorities, including epidemics and spreading violence.

17.8 Child Welfare Domains: Psycho-Social and Family Support

17.8.1 Principles and Practices in the Child Welfare Practices in Child Sexual Abuse

- Child protection professionals usually have the responsibility of ensuring that a child is safe in terms of their protection within a family or institution.
- In some countries these professionals and community workers may undertake a protection role. They gather evidence of risk and safety and seek to enhance the well-being of children who have been sexually abused or are at risk of sexual abuse.
- In some countries these professional will interview using forensic protocols and within the context of policies of the country.
- The child welfare approach is at times undertaken in conjunction with the criminal approach as many times it is not possible to seek protection using a criminal approach.
- The child protection approach seeks to engage the child's support network in promoting immediate and long term safety, access to therapy and access to appropriate educational, medical and relationship development services.
- Case management is often a child protection role. Child protection practitioners should act therapeutically and seek to ensure that the child is not further harmed by the system.
- Ethical practices are essential for ensuring that the children and their family are able to access good enough and evidence based practice.

- In those cases where the offenders are juvenile, child protection professionals should ensure an approach promoting access to therapy and access to appropriate educational, medical and relationship development services as well as immediate and long-term safety.

17.8.2 Mental Health Domains

- Although many definitions of child sexual abuse define the act[s] with accuracy, there is some difficulty in **defining the impact of abusive events** on the child or young person themselves; DSM is one way to do so.
- More harmful effects of sexual abuse can be seen in combination with other forms of maltreatment: CS exploitation, worst forms of child labor, Cinderella syndrome, etc. Management of the effects of child sexual abuse may require management of the effects of other forms of maltreatment (physical violence towards children by a parent/guardian and exposure to family violence).
- Children and young people who have been sexually abused are at risk of developing mental health, behavioral, developmental, emotional, and relationship difficulties. Young people who have been sexually abused may also be at risk of developing harmful behavior towards others, or may continue to be vulnerable to further abuse both within the family and within the community.
- An interdisciplinary assessment framework, including the family interactions, is an important part of ensuring the safety and well-being of children and families, thus promoting resilience. The assessment needs to include a full assessment of the child's needs, the nature and level of harm experienced by the child, the parenting capacity, family and environmental factors both in intrafamilial and extra-familial abuse.
- Children need to be protected from the impact of investigations when their allegations need to be assessed. Safe child-friendly contexts are needed for investigations to take place, based on guidelines to ensure the interdisciplinary process is effective and enhances the safety and well-being of the child. These are important so that mental health of children and families is not compromised.
- It is essential that community arrangements for the investigation of sexual abuse be well established and the interdisciplinary approach well developed. It is helpful if each community has:
  - a structure to represent all professionals, police, education, health, and to establish and train designated professionals who carry out investigations of different forms of maltreatment including sexual abuse;
  - safe child friendly contexts where investigations take place; and
  - Guidelines for how the interdisciplinary process works in practice.
- In many countries interviewing children and young people who may have been abused is carried out by skilled interdisciplinary interviewers. Police, social workers and forensic interviewers need to be trained to use established protocols

and utilize knowledge about the development of children's capacity to recall and share experiences.

- Recording interviews can protect children from having to give repetitive accounts. The basic principle is that all professionals in contact with children who may have been sexually abused should "listen" and to be trained how to help children describe their experiences.
- Mental health professionals have an important role in:
  - therapeutic interventions with children who have been abused;
  - therapeutic interventions with young people who are victims;
  - therapeutic interventions with young people responsible for sexually harmful behavior;
  - therapeutic interventions with adults responsible for sexually abusive actions; and
  - Therapeutic interventions with potentially supportive family members.
- It is essential that any therapeutic intervention uses evidence based modules which have been demonstrated to be effective, and uses evidence based assessments of a wide range of functioning to assess whether intervention has been effective using a consistent feedback process to monitor the course of therapeutic work.
  - Many psychotherapeutic approaches have been used to treat victims of child sexual abuse.
  - The Trauma-Focused Cognitive Behavior Therapy (TF-CBT) for children and young people who have experienced extensive maltreatment and abuse has proven successful and has been widely adopted.
  - There are similarly sets of modules which have a role in working with young people who are responsible for sexually harmful behavior. It takes a general view in encouraging them to develop a 'Good Life,' ensures the availability of good quality parenting, remedial education and individual, group and family interventions.
- Parents and non-offending caregivers who are supporting children and young people who have been sexually abused need to:
  - have psycho-educational models to help them understand processes associated with abusive action;
  - understand and support and manage their children's anxiety, anger, depression and post-traumatic symptomatology;
  - reflect on the impact on themselves and their relationships;
  - understand the ways in which they have been inducted into disbelieving the statements of children and believing abusive parents;
  - challenge the maladaptive, abusive attitudes and responses of young people responsible for sexually harmful behavior or adults who abuse;
  - Understand processes such as grooming, sexualization and the way in which children and young people have been sexually abused may become

responsible for abusive behavior in turn; and Repair attachments damaged by abusive individuals who undermine the relationship between children, young people and potentially caring parent figures.

- Mental health professionals who work with adult sexual offenders base their interventions on:
  - Programs that employ Multi-Component Cognitive Behavior Therapy within a Relapse Prevention framework;
  - Techniques that analyze and challenge distorted thinking to promote behavioral, thinking and emotional change;
  - Group work programs that target deviant sexual arousal, distorted cognitions, social skills deficit, empathy deficits, impulse control, emotional regulation, poor interpersonal relationships, substance abuse, and pro-offending attitudes;
  - Behavioral techniques that address deviant arousal and extinguish the link between sexual arousal and deviant fantasies and analyze the links which lead to offending behavior to establish a relapse prevention plan;
  - The 'Good Lives Plan' helps construct a more balanced, pro-social, personal identity; and
  - A multi-modal self-regulatory approach to all aspects of functioning.

17.9 Legal Services for CSA in the Arab Region

With regard to programs for legal assistance to children and their families, some countries that responded to the questionnaire provided data concerning the provision of legal aid. Such provision is made through a variety of mechanisms and programs, including projects intended to protect and care for children in the criminal justice system, and programs meant to provide legal assistance and counselling for children and their families. One of the programs has provided judicial services to children, as well as police and legal assistance; meanwhile, certain NGOs provide legal services, assistance and advice, including:

- Legal advice.
- Judicial assistance (assigning volunteer lawyers to plead) in cases where clients are unable to retain counsel.
- Communication with security services for follow-up purposes to ensure safety on one hand, and secure legal proceedings on the other.

The available data show that the majority of countries assign, within the framework of legal assistance for children and families, volunteer lawyers to represent them and provide advice free of charge. We also noted some experimental programs directed towards the development of public institutions to provide legal aid and allocate grants to NGOs to undertake ad hoc projects and provide legal assistance to children.

In the context of suitable legal provisions for child victims of violence, Jordan has ensured that abused children have access to the necessary technology to give their testimony without becoming subject to undue psychological pressure. Jordan also plans to provide protection and care services for children in the criminal justice system in order to provide guidance and legal assistance to a number of correctional centers and institutions. This is in addition to the implementation of the.

“Nour” legal aid and counselling program for children accused of breaking the law.

The UAE prepared a bill on protection of children’s rights, detailing the specific functions of the law and the role of social workers who provide legal assistance to children and families at risk of violence. The Dubai Foundation for Women and Children also plays an important role in sheltering and providing health, social and legal assistance to victims of sexual violence.

Tunisia developed a new system that provides an advisor to every child appearing in a court of first instance to provide support and legal advice free of charge.

In Algeria, a council offers support to children at all stages of the judicial process. In Oman, the Ministry of Social Development proposed an act on accountability regarding juveniles, detailing the role of the probation officer, who manages probation, visits the juvenile offender at their place of residence, and provides advice and assistance.

In Lebanon, a child friendly setting, equipped with audio-visual technical media, was created in the Justice Palace in Beirut; the aim is to listen to the child victim of sexual abuse and exploitation, thus avoiding repeated interrogations. The bill to protect children against abuse and neglect introduces mechanisms for protection at the national level, such as the social guide, specialized police and others.

In Egypt, the law stipulates that parties must present a lawyer conversant with trials to defend the accused child; expenses are borne by State. The National Council for Childhood and Motherhood in Egypt provides some internationally funded grants to ensure legal aid to children through civil society organizations.

In Mauritania, a special department to secure judicial protection for children was created at the Ministry of Justice. A legal aid system is also in place and a private room has been designated within the courthouse for juveniles in conflict with the law. The law also provides for judicial protection of the child; for example, interrogation of a child by police must be conducted in the presence of a social worker and a lawyer.

Yemen has begun to activate after-care services through the establishment of offices for after-care and social protection services in the governorates of Taiz and Hodeida; this motion will be scaled up to include the provinces of Sana’a and Aden. A family protection unit at the Police General Directorate has recently been established to serve women and children at the Interior Ministry. The Ministry of Justice is currently examining a proposal on the establishment of family courthouses in a number of provinces.

17.9.1 Legal Domains in Multidisciplinary Settings

- Many groups are relevant to the task of developing an optimal legal approach to Child Sexual Abuse. These groups and individuals include:
- judges,
- lawyers,
- police,
- other law enforcement personnel,
- forensic health and mental health professionals domain, and
- Health professionals giving evidence.

While these individuals are most likely to become involved in the daily work of the legal system, legislators, policy makers, many different interest groups, and the general public will necessarily influence the laws that are enacted and the degree to which the laws are obeyed.[5]

17.9.2 Different Legal Systems and Different Kinds of Law Within Each Type of Legal System

- The world's nation states operate within domestic legal systems and legal cultures that can be quite different from one another.
- Even when a country ratifies a treaty or reaches another form of agreement to be bound by various international standards, compliance with international law is limited by any number of factors including reservations to treaties that are ratified in general but not ratified with respect to specific portions of the international convention or other form of international law.
- With this in mind, the legal section includes examples of both criminal and non-criminal law practices tried in various countries so that practices that appear suitable can be adapted and then adopted for use by any nation state trying to improve its response to child sexual abuse.
- Two major cultures of law found in the world are sometimes characterized as "common law" and "code" with the latter category including Napoleonic law, Islamic law and the Romano-Germanic law. In addition to these populous examples of legal culture, there are many possible forms of "indigenous law".
- Comparing these traditions, except in the broadest terms, is fraught with difficulty because each tradition can have many exceptions to the general tradition. The common law is set apart by its emphasis on the independent role of judges, who can act even in the absence of clear statutory guidance and create a "precedent" that becomes the law for other judges who follow unless the decision is overridden by legislative, other political authority, or through appeal to a higher court.

---

[5]Iman, Izz. 2004. Violence against Children: A Field Study in Institutions of Delinquent Juveniles.

- While binding judges to follow prior judicial decisions* is standard in common law countries, other countries emphasize that the governing Code, Constitution or Statutes of the country is completely sovereign and each case should be interpreted by the judge only in terms of the governing Code. The decision of judges in other cases under the same Code system of law does not necessarily bind a later court. On the other hand, the work of prior scholars or jurists can be influential even if not binding, as illustrated by the example of Islamic law or Sharia.
- No matter what legal culture is examined, it is at least theoretically possible for one legal culture to "borrow" one aspect of "foreign law" and implement that aspect of another system. This can occur even when there is no ratified international treaty requiring a change in domestic law·
- All legal cultures have some form of criminal law and the modern development of various forms of non-criminal law sometimes referred to as "civil" law.
- An important example of a form of law that has developed everywhere in its fullest form mostly in the last two centuries is public health law. Public health law is marked by a special focus on the status of populations, individuals, and specific locations, as either being healthy, unhealthy, or within a spectrum of risk. Rather than "accusing" or even "denouncing" a place, the public health authority permits government, under scientifically and thus legal prescribed circumstances, to "clean up" the person, place or populations to prevent the spread of disease or toxins. Public health law has parallel examples in mental health law, the law of chemical dependence and the law of civil child protection. All four types of law are clearly "ameliorative" rather than "punitive" in primary intention.

17.9.3 Principles and Practices in the Legal Domain

- In investigation and prosecution law plays a key role in preventing and responding to child sexual abuse (CSA). To be effective, law must be coordinated at multiple levels with medicine, mental health, social welfare, education, and other systems, no matter what type of legal system governs.
- Most countries have found that legislation is needed to provide the robust legal framework and foundation required for an effective legal response to child sexual victimization. No matter what system of law is being considered, it is possible to analyze and develop the legal response that is needed to protect children from a harm that historically was poorly addressed.
- Countries that ignore the problem place their children and future at risk, no matter what form of legal system they follow if they do not realistically and effectively address child abuse and neglect.
- The United Nations Convention on the Rights of the Child (CRC), supplemented by the Optional Protocol on the Rights of the Child on the Sale of Children, Child Prostitution, and Child Pornography (Optional Protocol), provide logical starting places for a necessary legal framework. Countries with quite different historical,

ethnic, religious, geographical, and political traditions have chosen to endorse these agreements. In so doing, they have also endorsed the principle that "the best interests of the child shall be a primary consideration" in all actions regarding children (Article 3(1)).

- The CRC emphasizes the importance of comprehensive laws, administrative procedures, and social and educational measures to protect children from all forms of extrafamilial and intrafamilial sexual exploitation and sexual abuse.
- Recognizing the importance of the family, the CRC states that a child may not be removed from her or his parents against the parents' wishes except to protect the child from maltreatment, and pursuant to fair procedures and judicial review (Article 9(1)). The CRC reinforces the importance of services to help child victims of sexual exploitation and abuse recover and lead happy, productive lives (Article 39). Note, however, that these aspirational standards leave to nation-states the problem of balancing family integrity and child safety.
- The Optional Protocol reinforces the CRC emphasis on protecting children from sexual exploitation by requiring states parties to "prohibit the sale of children, child prostitution and child pornography" (Article 1). The Optional Protocol contains valuable measures to protect the rights of child victims of sexual exploitation (Article 8). This protocol addresses a form of child sexual abuse that should not impinge on the family except to the extent it is the family itself that is profiting from the child's use as a commodity.
- In addition to the CRC and the Optional Protocol, an effective response to child sexual abuse and sexual exploitation requires detailed domestic laws on the following subjects: (1) Statutes criminalizing specific forms of child sexual victimization, and (2) Statutes creating and funding a workable, and to the extent possible, comprehensive child protection system to ensure that child sexual victimization is detected, reported, and investigated by properly trained professionals from law enforcement and child protection.

17.9.4 Child Sexual Abuse as a Crime

- It is difficult to imagine that most adults would ever endorse child sexual abuse as a 'good thing'. However, deciding what is sexually abusive and deciding what acts should be punished varies from society to society and within societies: legal consequences may vary from sect to sect; such consequences include marrying the perpetrator and the victim, with or without further victimization, with poor legal rights for the child, including divorce procedures.
- There are individuals and groups that justify sexual contact between adults and children and portray such acts as misunderstood or as a positive good. Such individuals even share methods of propagandizing their activities in an effort to induce other adults to permit sexual abuse of children to continue.
- One method for undermining efforts to prevent child sexual abuse is to define it in a confusing way. Another method for disruption of child protection is to define it

in such a limited way that virtually no sexual contact with a child is considered child sexual abuse.

- Aside from deliberate efforts to undermine regulation of child sexual abuse, legal definitions of child sexual abuse vary to some degree throughout the world. However, some core concepts are universal:
  - Children below a certain age, usually known as "the age of consent" are too immature to consent to sexual activity of any kind, and any sexual contact with an underage child constitutes abuse;
  - Any use of children in the production or distribution of pornography is abuse.
- Commercial sexual exploitation of children is a crime in most countries that have enacted laws on the subject.
- Given that all sexual abuse is not the same, the legal consequences for perpetrators should reflect the severity of the abuse, the use of enticement or force, the misuse of a position of authority over the child by any adult (e.g. school teacher, coach, clerical figure, legal or judicial figure or any other person acting under the mantle of official responsibility for the child). Laws must be tailored intelligently to ensure justice and protection for victims, protection of society, and punishment and rehabilitation for offenders. This is most especially true for the youngest offenders and it is very important to provide not only accountability but treatment for the youngest perpetrators of child sexual abuse.

17.9.5 Legal Aspects of a Child Protection System

- Every state should establish in law a comprehensive child protection system. The exact configuration of a state's child protection system depends on cultural, practical, and legal considerations. A comprehensive and effective system must provide mechanisms to detect sexual abuse and report it to proper authorities so that the incidence of CSA can be monitored but especially to assure accountability for ameliorative intervention on behalf of the victim child.
- Thus mechanisms must be created to protect children in danger, to prevent contact between the offender and the child, to remove the offender from the child's home and provide appropriate out of home care for children who cannot live safely at home. The law should require interdisciplinary cooperation among the various professions concerned with the problems of child abuse and neglect. Finally, a child protection system cannot operate effectively without sufficient funding.

17.9.6 Children as Interviewees and Witnesses

- In most cases of sexual abuse there is no medical or physical evidence of the abuse. The child's description of events is often the most compelling evidence of maltreatment. Because children's statements can be vital to the ability to protect them, care must be taken to interview children properly and to document professional and forensic interviews.
- When legal proceedings are commenced, children may need to testify under some legal regimes, and steps are required to reduce the stress of testifying while, at the same time, protect the rights of the accused.
- In many countries, specifically in non-common law countries, a criminal proceeding can usually be maintained without the child becoming a witness. This fact is viewed by some as a "child's rights" advantage in non-common law countries, for example countries governed by Napoleonic Code traditions.
- There are also legal cultures where children of any age will not be heard, where the voice of children is not valued and where the child might not be permitted to give evidence even if psychologically competent to do so. Thus the legal system of any country committed to protecting children from child sexual abuse and sexual exploitation must be flexible enough to protect the child through some approach, for example through documentation of a failure to protect by the caregiver.
- A voluminous literature exists on the advantages of interviewing children [video] for forensic purposes, and there is an increasing consensus on most aspects of proper interviewing. Forensic interviews should be memorialized, preferably by video recording, or recognized legal scripting. States should support high quality forensic interviewing by highly qualified interviewers.
- When children must testify in court, which is not a requirement under some legal systems, steps are required to prepare them to testify and to support them through the experience. The Optional Protocol of the U.N.C.R.C. contains useful guidelines, reproduced below:
  - States Parties shall adopt appropriate measures to protect the rights and interests of child victims of [child sexual abuse] at all stages of the criminal justice process, in particular by:
  - Recognizing the vulnerability of child victims and adapting procedures to recognize their special needs, including their special needs as witnesses;
  - Informing child victims of their rights, their role and the scope, timing and progress of the proceedings and of the disposition of their cases;
  - Allowing the views, needs and concerns of child victims to be presented and considered in proceedings where their personal interests are affected, in a manner consistent with the procedural rules of national law;
  - Providing appropriate support services to child victims throughout the legal process;

  - Protecting, as appropriate, the privacy and identity of child victims and taking measures in accordance with national law to avoid the inappropriate dissemination of information that could lead to the identification of child victims;
  - Providing, in appropriate cases, for the safety of child victims, as well as that of their families and witnesses on their behalf, from intimidation and retaliation;
  - Avoiding unnecessary delay in the disposition of cases and the execution of orders or decrees granting compensation to child victims.
  - States Parties shall ensure that uncertainty as to the actual age of the victim shall not prevent the initiation of criminal investigations, including investigations aimed at establishing the age of the victim.
  - States Parties shall ensure that, in the treatment by the criminal justice system of children who are victims (...), the best interest of the child shall be a primary consideration.
  - States Parties shall take measures to ensure appropriate training, in particular legal and psychological training, for the persons who work with victims of the offences prohibited under the present Protocol.
  - Nothing in the present article shall be construed to be prejudicial to or inconsistent with the rights of the accused to a fair and impartial trial.

- Because CSA can occur in many different settings, including close family and among more "distant" relatives, in religious settings, sports activities, schools, and when accessing two-way electronic communications, different methods of management for child sexual victimization must be considered.

17.9.7 Child Sexual Victimization Within the Family

- Even in a country with criminal and civil laws to deal with child abuse and neglect, it is important to realize that criminal complaints are not inevitable. While many cases are not filed in court, the availability of the court proceeding for more serious cases appears to be crucial as a statement of community morals, standards, and commitment to the well-being of children.
- Specifically with respect to child sexual abuse cases, another study of over four hundred CSA cases found that certain factors affected the decision to file, among these support of the child by the mother, use or threat of force, severity of the abuse, and the overall availability of evidence. Most, but not all, cases involving child sexual abuse within the family challenge legal authorities with a conundrum.

17.9.8 Child Sexual Victimization Outside the Family

- In all countries familiar to the study group, child sexual victimization that occurs to children outside of the family is addressed with rare exceptions through a criminal justice process.
- Among the people who have been prosecuted in the past several decades in different parts of the world are teachers, religious figures, youth group advisors, parents and other adults known to the victim child's family, as well as judges, police officers, and mental health professionals. Effectively these are individuals, usually but not always men, from every background and walk of life. Adult sex offenders against children, especially if they target both boys and girls, can commit a very large number of crimes against children unless they are incarcerated.
- The advent of the digital age, especially the World Wide Web, has increased the access that sexual offenders have to children, either for the purpose of setting up direct contact with the child or engaging the child on-line for the purposes of sexual exploitation.
- Child sexual abuse and sexual exploitation are known to cross international boundaries. "Sex tourists" are known to travel internationally to prey on children. "Sex trafficking" that involves the commercial use of children for sexual purposes has been documented. Just as a country defends its men, women and children against other threats, each country is challenged with keeping its children safe from sexual exploitation by foreign perpetrators.

17.10 Multi-Disciplinary Teams[6]

Significant variability persists in the response to allegations of child sexual abuse between professional disciplines, national jurisdictions, cultural groups, and religious sects; this phenomenon is globally observed, although with some regional increased prevalence, such as FGM and ECM.[7]

Responses to allegations of child sexual abuse within and between these groups is often unpredictable—and dependent upon the existence of informal systems, local expertise and vagaries of local resource and funding.

The establishment of the first multi-disciplinary "Child Protection Teams" and "Child Protection Units" [CPU] marked the beginning of modern success in identifying and responding to child physical abuse. When child sexual abuse was

[6]Lombardo, L. and Polonko, K. Interdisciplinary Contributions to the Prevention of Child Maltreatment. International Journal of Interdisciplinary Social Sciences 2010; 4: 89–112.

[7]Gerbaka. B: Building a Multisectoral Taskforce in Lebanon for the Prevention of Child Abuse and Neglect; Public Health Approaches to Child Maltreatment: Prevention as a Priority. Town and Country Resort and Conference Center. San Diego, California, U.S. January 23, 2006.

identified as a systemic issue in the 1970's, it became clear that this multidisciplinary model of collaboration between disciplines and agencies was essential to effectively investigate, manage, treat and prevent child sexual abuse; many examples exist in the Arab region, from municipal to hospital based CPUs, since the 2005 UNVAC Arab regional consultation held in Cairo.

Investigations that are coordinated between child protective services, criminal justice agencies, health and forensic services, and treatment services can reduce stress on children, prevent conflicts between the agencies, allow treatment resources to be shared, and allow agencies to support each other, as well as hold each other accountable on behalf of child victims and the public.

Over the last decades, and since Finkelhor recent studies in the 70s, published research in the western hemisphere indicates that recommendations generated by Child Protection Teams:

- increase the likelihood that service for the child or family will be carried out;
- reduce worker 'burnout' and attrition; and
- improve collegial relationships between case workers, physicians, and lawyers;

These capacities building tools have also shown to be effective in different countries of the Arab region: Municipal Units I Morocco, Hospital units in Lebanon, regional units in KSA, state supported NGO based units in Jordan and Lebanon.

Regional Child Protection Consulting Teams provide missing expertise, reduce ambiguity and increase confidence for the local team. In up to 30% of case, appropriate resolution without the consultation would not have occurred.

Essential agencies include health, public health, child protective services, mental health, civil law, and criminal justice.

As with any complex system, systematized evaluation of the activities of specific professions and agencies against defined outcome measures is essential to define and refine best practice models.

The advantage of interdisciplinary work is that it provides a means for sharing knowledge and resources, and endorses working together so that complementary approaches can be integrated for the benefit of children, parents and society.

Managing the boundaries between individuals from different disciplines is a key element to the practices and principles or interdisciplinary collaborative work. The contribution of each individual's professional discipline needs to be recognized; have its appropriate role, and assist with the development of shared skills which will enhance the protection and interventions for children and their families.

17.11 Roles and Responsibilities of the Parties Concerned to Stop Violence Against Children

This section presents a comparative analysis of the recommendations contained in the Arab countries to the questionnaires for the roles and responsibilities of the parties concerned to stop violence against children.

There have been a series of recommendations linked to sites of violence, scenes of violence which has been divided into five, namely: family and home, and educational institutions, care institutions and the judiciary, and the local community and the street, including the workplace.

The recommendations included on the location of violence against children, which had been drawn at each site as follows:

17.11.1 In the Home and Family

Sexual violence and abuse within the family is rarely reported and children themselves are largely silent on this issue. Laws in some of the countries also make reporting by children unlikely. For example, under the **Jordanian** penal code, complaints from a child can only be accepted if they are supported by the parents or guardian. Complaints from third parties—teachers, social workers, child rights workers—are not usually accepted.

Some laws also tolerate violence in the family: for example, Article 220 of the **Iranian** penal code recognizes only a light sentence and fine for a father who kills his child in the course of administering 'educational' punishment.

One in three women will encounter sexual violence in her lifetime, and every year millions of children are sexually abused. Sexual abuse results in a range of damaging physical and emotional effects, including: depression, suicide, post-traumatic stress disorder, reproductive health issues, and potential exposure to sexually transmitted infections and HIV. Sexual and domestic violence simultaneously results from and reproduces low levels of education, exposure to and normalization of violence, drug and alcohol abuse, and a culture that subordinates women and girls.

Given the important role played inside the home in the care and upbringing of children, States must concentrate their efforts to stop violence against children on programs to support parents and caregivers, and parental education, building capacity for families living in difficult circumstances, and offering training courses and seminars for families and relevant institutions concerned with supporting the parents.

It is clear from recommendations of Arab countries that in order to help families to reduce violence against children, Arab States ought to give increased attention to programs for families in difficult circumstances such as families headed by women, women in rural areas, and low-income families. Therefore, countries need to implement a range of programs and projects targeted at those types of families.

As for educating parents, Arab countries need to increase their efforts in this area, particularly because targeted programs focus mostly on media programs, printing material and dissemination of publications and periodicals; these programs are too few and too partial to achieve appropriate education programs for parents. Tunisia leads in this area, as it has developed a national strategy to deal with violent behavior within the family on one side, and a media strategy for the rehabilitation of the family, support and enhance their capabilities on the other. Also, Egypt developed programs for families facing difficult circumstances through a project to reduce poverty, in collaboration with the National Council for Childhood and Motherhood, in order to empower women in their civil rights, and families in small enterprises.

The proposed programs for supporting parents and other caretakers focus on the following:

- Holding training sessions for workers providing care for children including: nannies, supervisors, teachers, social workers, psychologists and foster families.
- Preparing an educational guide to raise awareness about best practices in parental care, as well as preparing training sessions for childcare personnel in, and assisting parents in providing better parental care.
- Raising awareness via school administrations, teachers and social workers, to help families deal with early childhood and adolescence, with an emphasis on compassionate care and positive discipline, emotional empowerment, self-confidence and a culture of respect and cooperation, as well as teaching children not to psychologically or physically abuse their peers.
- Raising awareness about female genital mutilation (FGM) and its harmful health and psychological effects through television adverts.
- Initiating field visits by psycho-social workers to the families of the children in order to evaluate their conditions.

The proposed parent-oriented education programs include the following:

- Health and education support groups for parents.
- Women's associations for the social education of women

Jordan is implementing a parental care program to reach out to parents and caregivers and families to educate them on the means and methods of proper upbringing of young children (0–8 years), and provide a safe environment to stimulate their growth and development. The program was implemented in Jordan in 1996, and the kingdom's Ministry of Education became a partner of the program in 2002, together with a number of other institutions, including the Ministry of Social Development and the Ministry of Health in addition to local community institutions. The program targets school teachers, administrators, kindergarten teachers, and families (as caregivers). The program is supported by UNICEF, partner ministries and organizations, in order to institutionalize the program and integrate it within the annual plans of partner institutions.

Tunisia made a number of achievements in this field, developing a national strategy to address violent behavior within households in addition to a media strategy for family rehabilitation and support to enhance capacity. Sudan has set up a national plan to combat violence against children, and devoted a chapter in the plant to domestic violence.

Egypt also made some achievements, developing programs for families in difficult circumstances through the "Poverty Reduction Project" that was established jointly with the National Council for Childhood and Motherhood. The project aims at enabling women to attain their civil rights and supporting families economically through small-scale projects.

17.11.2 In Schools and Educational Institutions

It is important to highlight the role of schools and educational institutions to stop violence against children, and to clarify that all children should be able to learn in an environment free from sexual violence and bullying; schools must be a safe and appropriate setting for them.

Such recommendations are reflected in four approaches:

- encouraging schools to adopt and implement violence-free codes and regulations;
- ensuring teaching strategies that are free from violence, intimidation or threat, humiliation or physical force;
- delivering special programs for a safe school environment;
- and encouraging skill building to enable development of a curriculum that is free from violence and to implement anti-bullying policies. Such recommendations relating to curricula, teaching processes and other practices effectively comply with the Convention on the Rights of the Child (CRC) 's principles and have had an impact on the reduction of violent behaviors.

Through history, data available indicated that Arab states have yet to develop codes of conduct and regulations in schools, including interest in addressing violence in schools.

Teaching strategies must be free from violence, intimidation or threat, humiliation or sexual harassment, including strategies free from all types of violence.

The school environment must encourage skills' building of non-violent approaches as well as policies against violence.

Curricula, teaching processes and other practices must abide by the principles of the Convention on the Rights of the Child; most Arab states intensify efforts in disseminating the culture of child rights among the educational process and faculty, namely: Jordan, Algeria, Libya, Yemen, and Saudi Arabia.

Promulgating laws and regulations that address the rules which prohibit physical or psychological abuse against students; abuse is a violation of children's rights, of his/her dignity, of respect for him or her and of their right to protection against violence and abuse;

- Preventing humiliation, harassment and bulling in schools;

- Developing personnel discipline codes in schools that prevent the ab = use of authority
- Establishing groups and institutions to provide counselling and psychological services for students and parents;
- Establishing a system of educational guidance (school counsellors) in schools
- Incorporating human rights-based themes in school curricula;
- Developing codes of conduct for students and staff in schools.
- Establishing children's rights clubs in basic education schools, and carrying out activities to educate and inform children of their rights;
- Organizing seminars and lectures for parents on family guidance and children's rights;
- Organizing training courses for workers in the educational field about the Convention on the Rights of the Child;
- Delivering lectures on behavioral change;
- Conducting case-studies for the students who experience behavioral and mental disorders;
- Holding regular meetings with parents.

17.11.3 In Systems of Care and Judicial Systems

The UNSG's VAC recommends that all states should assume responsibility for ensuring the safety of children in residential care and juvenile detention facilities. Arab States concentrate on the role of care and juvenile justice systems in reducing violence against children:

- reduce the rates of children in institutions;
- give priority to family reunion and other community-based alternatives;
- reduce the number of children who are placed in justice systems;
- promote alternative measures
- rehabilitation programs and policies to encourage regular evaluation of measures;
- ensure the transfer of children to family- or community-based care; independent mechanisms for filing complaints and investigation of issues of violence in care and justice systems and programs to inform children in institutions about their rights; actions taken to facilitate access to children in institutions and existing mechanisms to protect them; and the existence of independent institutions with the power to monitor the state of children in care and justice institutions.
- Develop a collaborative and supportive family.
- Reduce the number of children in institutions
- Prioritize child-family reunion.
- Establish specialized offices for juvenile police, security centers and juvenile courts in order to implement restorative justice and settle children's issues before bringing them to justice and placing them in care centers.

- Involve family protection departments in projects engaging juveniles. Examples of such projects include the 'juvenile criminal justice project', the 'project for juvenile justice rehabilitation', and the 'juvenile justice system reform project'.
- Operate an alternative care system and allocate budgets for the transfer of children exposed to domestic violence and sexual abuse to foster families.

Arab countries have worked to reduce the rates of children placed in institutions and to prioritize keeping children within their families and communities, while addressing cases of children in difficult circumstances, including children in conflict with law.

Some Arab countries (Jordan, Tunisia, Algeria, Sudan, Qatar, and Egypt) have developed specially-designed programs and mechanisms and recruited specialized human resources to address these issues. Meanwhile, these countries continue to prioritize the development of the child within his or her family, whether through mediation and support to families, or through foster care. Some other Arab countries, in particular UAE, Bahrain, Sudan, Oman, and Libya, have implemented programs and activities to raise awareness about the role of the family in all actions concerning children. For example, in Bahrain a group of health, social and mental health workers, all holders of university degrees, have majored in 'family counselling' at the University of Bahrain, with the support from the National Commission for Children and the Child Protection Centre. For juvenile delinquents, Arab countries have developed specific laws to protect this group of the child population, and given priority to re-education and social reintegration, while involving family members in the measures taken under especially designed programs for legal aid and counselling, as well as for putting support mechanisms in place for mediation and problem-solving. Moreover, other countries, including Lebanon, Egypt, Morocco, Mauritania and Yemen, have initiated bills to establish alternatives to custodial penalties for young offenders. Egypt has already initiated such a law in order to restrict deprivation of liberty to a last resort.

17.11.4 In the Workplace

Child labor is widespread in many Arab countries but statistics vary according to the definition used and the approach taken in data collection. In most countries, it is difficult to determine the magnitude of child labor, due to the fact that children work primarily in the nonformal sector, in small workshops, and in marginal businesses. A number of studies on this topic show that children work in difficult circumstances, that their work day often extends to more than 10 h, and that they are regularly subjected to verbal and/or physical violence by their employer or workmates, who are often older than them.. There are an unknown number of children working in hazardous areas, which account for the worst form of child labor; these working children are deprived of health care and their work threatens their health and impedes their development.

Therefore, child labor has become a great challenge that faces children, given the loss of child dependency and the low standard of living of many families that forces them to send their children into the labor market.

Accordingly, the United Nations SG's study on VAC devoted a large section to work settings, focusing on a large volume of available information based on field work experiences that can be utilized by Arab countries to curb violence against children. The recommendations are organized under five themes, according to the responses of Arab States to the questionnaire:

- enforce labor laws, particularly those which prohibit child labor
- prevent child labor in general and the worst forms of child labor in particular
- withdraw children from work settings, and re-integrate children in family environments
- involve the private sector, labor unions and civil society in preventing child labor

Jordan, the UAE, Bahrain, Tunisia, Syria, Sudan, Iraq, Oman, Qatar, Libya, Egypt, Mauritania, and Yemen have all presented information about measures taken to enforce laws prohibiting child labor. These countries have indicated that there exist legal provisions for compulsory primary education, for prohibition of child labor, raising the age of access to the labor market to 15, 16 or 18 years—depending on the country, for prevention of employment of children in hazardous labor or activities that threaten their health, for limiting working hours for children between 15 and 18 years old, and for the imposition of fines, and establishment of inspection committees.

Lebanon and Morocco have inefficient inspection services. Jordan and Lebanon highlight the existence of a national strategy to reduce child labor.

Algeria set a national committee to combat child labor, supervised by the Ministry of Labor and Social Security, and inspection committees periodically carry out investigations on child labor. The outcomes of such investigations have revealed instances of child labor as low as 0.54%. In Yemen, the Ministry of Social Affairs and Labor has established a unit to combat child labor. This structure is implementing a number of activities aimed at combating child labor, including awareness-raising activities for children themselves and their families, and at coordinating efforts among the agencies involved in combating child labor. The said Ministry also formed a ministerial committee composed of governmental agencies, employers, workers and NGOs—functioning under its own supervision. Another program "ACCESS Plus" has also been implemented to reduce the worst forms of child labor in a number of provinces. This program targets children themselves through a number of activities, including improvement of education in the schools programs, creation of child-friendly environments, and implementation of professional training courses, awareness-raising activities and literacy classes.

In Jordan, legislation has been enacted to enable children to return to school and vocational training. There is a strategy for child labor, and a national framework on child labor is being undertaken; the latter defines the roles and responsibilities of all institutions in reducing access by children to the labor market, and integrates mechanisms for appropriate intervention into a participatory approach.

In Syria, the Ministry of Social Affairs and Labor cooperates with the International Labor.

Organization (ILO) to launch and implement the 'Agenda of Decent Work Country Program', which monitors reduction in child labor; both parties are following up on the implementation of these laws through ad hoc committees to ensure implementation.

In Sudan, a national project to address child labor through education was adopted: 'Tackling Child Labor through Education Program', established in partnership between the National Council for Child Welfare, the Ministry of Labor, the Ministry of Public Education and the (ILO).

Iraq has prohibited the export of goods produced by factories that hire children. Egypt has a national committee to prevent and combat child labor. Arab states' intensified inspections, committees to receive complaints, fines and penalties, and awareness campaigns in collaboration with civil society. Bahrain has confirmed the absence of violence in the workplace, has an enacted law on begging and homelessness, and has established the Centre for Social Welfare to provide services to child beggars and homeless children. Algeria has a national strategy in place to prevent and combat child labor in all work settings, including hazardous labor; the country has confirmed the absence of child labor, based on work inspectors. Most recently, specifically in 2006, the prevalence of child labor in Algeria did not exceed 0.54%; financial penalties and imprisonment—for a term ranging between 15 days and two months—are imposed on employers of minors as well as on those who employ people under the age of 19 during the nightshift. Oman has also noted that child labor does not exist within its borders. Lebanon has no ad hoc program for child labor, but measures are taken by competent authorities in the event of a complaint. In Egypt, the media has played a role in turning public opinion against child labor and promoting the rights of working children; NGOs also play an active role in the programs raising awareness about the legal rights of working children, in addition to their role in the surveillance of employers.

17.11.5 In the Community

The United Nations Secretary General's Report on the Study on Violence Against Children has shown that mandatory measures to prevent violence against children and confront its occurrences in local communities requires a thorough analysis of the social, economic, financial and infrastructure risk factors at work. Responses from Arab countries regarding the role of the local community in stopping violence against children can be organized under five themes:

- Local prevention strategies against violence
- Policies to reduce social and economic inequalities;
- Train law enforcement with child friendly procedures and programs on children's rights;

- coordinate and track local services for child victims of violence
- Define the role of the local communities in promoting and supporting government and civil society initiatives for the prevention of violence against children.

The few facts available about strategies for preventing and facing violence at the local level reveal that Tunisia, Algeria, Syria, Sudan and Egypt have strategies to prevent and combat violence against children; some other countries like Jordan, the UAE, Iraq, Qatar and Yemen have national strategies incorporated in other overall strategies to confront violence against children, while many other Arab States did not provide information on the subject. The Qatar Foundation for the Protection of Children and Women assumes responsibility for protection of women and children from violence and abuse. This Foundation is also responsible for rehabilitation and the provision of training courses for educational, medical and security personnel on how to handle cases of violence and abuse and on ways to achieve prevention and treatment. Qatar has also launched a “Safety line” or “Rescue line” (919) to support children and women; the line remains operational around the clock to aid children and women suffering from violence or threatened violence.

Concerning programs and policies to reduce social and economic inequality, and the initiatives and national action plans put in place, Arab States confirmed that social funds are available for projects to combat poverty. They are also accessible for housing programs and to support income-generating projects, as well as for the support and encouragement to non-governmental organizations and associations to execute local development projects and poverty alleviation strategies. Raising the living standards of citizens has been adopted as a strategic objective of development.

In Bahrain, a Fund has been established to support social work and community work and to support the Fund for Social Security and the Family Bank. This financial institution offers lending programs and finances small projects to support families in need. In Syria, the project has national pilot program. The government also implements lending programs and finances small projects to support poor families and help them to achieve sustainable income to cover living expenses.

Lebanon has adopted a social policy involving fiscal adjustment and a decrease in existing social burdens. It is within this framework that Lebanon has launched two projects aimed at promoting local development and fighting poverty by focusing on the most pressing areas of need.

Egypt is implementing a program entitled “Poverty Reduction ... The Legal Rights of Girls and Children”, which aims to support and improve the state of children and women (in five provinces, 27 centers and 420 villages). It is also intended to enable them to address poverty by facilitating access to required documents, and to make use of the essential services provided by the State and community, through coordination and cooperation, and through the projects implemented jointly with concerned executive bodies.

Concerning training programs targeting the police and other security services on the Rights of the Child and on identifying the dynamics and nature of violence against children, some Arab states focus on training courses targeting at security services in the area of children’s rights, and the authorities in charge of these courses.

Egypt has implemented the Violence Against Children Program; the program involves training and capacity building for members of child protection committees and sub-committees and members of committees on children's rights, including security, education, health, solidarity and civil society representatives, across all 29 of Egypt's governorates. The Program also works on capacity building for personnel working with children in detention, evaluates the detention institutions and develops a regulatory system that is independent from penal institutions. The Program also develops alternatives to child detention and awareness-raising to change public and community opinion toward these child groups. The Program team evaluates reception centers and other related services administered by non-governmental organizations; it also improves the services available to street children, develops standards for reception houses and establishes connections with non-governmental organizations working with street children.

17.11.6 Extrateritoriality[8]

A majority of the Arab anti-trafficking laws apply to a national who commits the crime of trafficking within a State's territory. However, some exceptions are worth noting. For example, the Egyptian law extends its jurisdiction to non-nationals who commit the act of trafficking abroad if:

- the crime was committed on any means of transportation that was registered in Egypt;
- one of the victims was Egyptian;

[8]When the perpetrator of the crime is a corporationAccording to article 10 of the United Nations Convention against Transnational Organized Crime, a corporation may be held liable for an organized crime, including participation in an organized criminal group, laundering of proceeds of a crime, corruption, and obstruction of justice. Corporate liability may be civil, criminal, or administrative provided that the sanctions are effective, proportionate, and dissuasive, and it may be established without prejudice to the criminal liability of a natural person. Sanctions may include a fine, forfeiture, confiscation, restitution, or closure of the legal entity. Other sanctions that are designed to influence corporate behaviour are disincentives, including suspension of a right or prohibition of a certain activity. However, liability of a corporation is subject to the legal principles that apply to a legal person in a particular national system.The Legislative Guides for the Implementation of the United Nations Convention against Transnational Organized Crime provide the justification for establishing liability of legal persons: Serious and sophisticated crime is frequently committed through or under the cover of legal entities, such as companies or charitable organizations. Complex corporate structures can effectively hide the true ownership, clients or particular transactions related to crimes ranging from smuggling to money-laundering and corrupt practices. Individual executives may reside outside the country where the offence was committed and responsibility for specific individuals may be difficult to prove. Thus, the view has been gaining ground that the only way to remove this instrument and shield of transnational organized crime is to introduce liability for legal entities.159

- the preparation for the crime or its planning, direction, supervision, or financing occurred in Egypt;
- the crime was committed by an organized criminal group engaged in criminal activities in more than one State, including Egypt;
- the crime caused harm to any citizen or resident or to the security or any of the interests of Egypt within the country or abroad;
- the perpetrator of the crime in Egypt was found after the crime was committed and was not extradited.

17.11.7 Role of Academia

Education is an important tool for the prevention of trafficking in persons. Education is paramount as both a means to provide young generations with the skills and knowledge necessary to become active and productive members of society and a means to develop their awareness of their rights and duties under national and international legislation, thus reducing their vulnerability to trafficking and other forms of abuse. Education is also an effective tool in raising awareness among the wider public on the dangers of trafficking in persons and its long-term negative impact on the economic and social development of the country. Means to integrate the topic of trafficking in persons into the educational system include curriculum reform, student group discussions, moot court awareness-raising exercises, and outreach services coordinated by the educational institutes.

Moreover, academic institutions play an important role in the field of research into the various aspects of trafficking in persons. Often they assist policy makers in designing and implementing anti-trafficking government programs.

A recent development in the educational curriculum of various universities in the MENA region is the establishment of clinical legal educational programs. The programs are legal centers based within the law faculties of the universities that offer law students the opportunity to develop practical skills by working on real cases of trafficking in persons and related crimes. Under the supervision of experienced lawyers and faculty professors, the students engage in providing legal consultation to victims of trafficking and other vulnerable victims with regard to their rights and duties under national and international legislation. The main clinical legal programs in the Arab world are the Iraq Refugee Assistance Project at the University of Amman in Jordan, the Legal Clinic at Alexandria University in Egypt, and the Human Rights Clinic at Al-Quds University on the West Bank. There are also law clinics at United Arab Emirates University in the United Arab Emirates, Beirut University in Lebanon, Helwan and Assiut Universities in Egypt, and Baghdad University in Iraq. In addition to broadening the students' legal skills, the legal aid clinics are proving to be instrumental in raising awareness on trafficking in persons among students and in providing assistance to victims who would otherwise have limited access to the justice system of the country.

17.11.8 Role of Media

The media can be useful in spreading awareness and understanding of trafficking in persons among national and international populations. Media outlets include television, radio, and newspapers, all of which have helped disseminate information on trafficking in persons. Some governments have incorporated the media into their trafficking-in-persons prevention policy as a means of raising awareness.

Although the media are a powerful tool in influencing public opinion and raising awareness about an issue, with such power comes the responsibility to provide accurate information while ensuring the protection of individual sources from any harm as a result of information disclosure. Media coverage of cases of trafficking in persons must not endanger the lives of the victims or infringe on their privacy. Public awareness media campaigns are helpful not only in informing the public about the dangers of trafficking in persons and the signs that help people recognize it but also in rescuing those who may have already fallen victim to trafficking, particularly by alerting the general public and people who may come into contact with potential victims.

Best Practice
To compensate for the still feeble government intervention on this level, some organizations have specifically decided to address trafficking in persons from the demand side. For instance, the A21 Campaign, a Greek network of individuals, organizations, and government officials who are committed to abolishing injustice in the twenty-first century, has worked with "johns" to educate them on the realities of engaging sex workers.

In 2010, a media campaign was launched in Greece for the purpose of informing those men about the stories and backgrounds of the women working in the sex industry in Greece, as well as the violence and abuse the women suffer and the slavery-like conditions in which they are kept by their exploiters.

The campaign was intended to prompt clients of sex workers to think about the consequences of their part in the sex industry and to reconsider their preconceived assumptions and attitudes about those who work in the sex industry.

The A21 Campaign has also designed short courses for schoolboys to impress young men about the realities of human trafficking before they ever become paying clients.268.

17.11.9 Role of Religious institutions

Religion can be a powerful influence in preventing trafficking in persons. Many faithbased organizations today work toward combating trafficking in persons through awareness-raising and educational programs.

In the MENA region, various imams and Islamic scholars have contributed to raising awareness of the problem of trafficking in the Arab world by issuing fatwas condemning the crime and urging the Muslim people to refrain from cultural practices that might be conducive to trafficking in persons in the region and around the world.

For example, on 3 September 2002, Saudi Arabia's Grand Mufti issued a fatwa against the abuse of foreign labor by Saudi employers and stated, "Blackmailing and threatening [foreign] laborers with deportation if they refuse the employers' terms, which breach the contract, is not allowed."269 Similarly, Sheik Youssef al-Qaradawi, an eminent Islamic scholar, issued a fatwa in March 2008 stating that the sponsorship rule that prevails in some countries is inconsistent with the teachings of Islam and should be abolished. The "sponsorship rule" provides an employer sponsoring a worker with a variety of rights that may infringe on the rights of the employee. For example, foreign workers' travel documents are withheld by employers; consequently, an employee may not leave his employer and seek other employment without approval, nor is the employee allowed to leave the country for any reason without first obtaining the employer's approval. This rule may violate the worker's right to free movement. Sheik Youssef al-Qaradawi explained that the "sponsorship system nowadays produced visa-market[s], leaving [many] workers living in sub-human conditions, as a large number of laborers are accommodated in small areas. It is really a shame and also it is against the Islamic principles which call for respecting human rights."270.

In a more recent fatwa issued on 4 July 2011 in Amman, Jordan, the president of the World Islamic Sciences and Education University, Abdul Nasser Abu Basal, stated that human trafficking, if organized and conducted on a large scale, warrants the application of the hudud punishment for highway robbery or corruption in land.

17.11.10 Use of New Technologies to Promote Effective Partnership

Effective use of the Internet and other forms of information technology, such as websites and computer databases, can also serve to combat trafficking in persons. Statistics are difficult to collect and quickly become outdated, but information technology-related initiatives can be used to enhance coordination and information sharing among NGOs, civil society organizations, and governments, including law enforcement officials.

The Internet can be used to spread information about antitrafficking initiatives, to educate the public about the dangers and issues surrounding trafficking in persons, and to promote bilateral and multilateral networking with a view to stepping up the pressure and addressing the problem. Comprehensive antitrafficking databases can connect isolated anti-trafficking groups across regions, provide information to law enforcement and border control officials on persons suspected of being trafficked, assist victims, and provide accurate trafficking statistics.

17.12 International Cooperation[9]

When trafficking occurs as a transnational activity, cooperation between countries of origin, transit, and destination is necessary to confront the problem. Hence, bilateral treaties on mutual assistance in criminal matters must be a part of any transnational legal response. Apprehension of traffickers, investigation of cases of trafficking and prosecution of traffickers require cooperation, especially in matters related to requests for assistance; searches and seizures; attachment and surrender of property; measures for securing assets; service of judicial decisions, judgments, and verdicts; appearance of witnesses and expert witnesses; and transmittal of information and records.

17.13 Arab Professionals' Roles in Responding to Violence Against Children

17.13.1 Mission

Arab professionals provide expertise to decision makers about the condition of children in such settings, where problems are too big for one Arab country, including living conditions and social challenges, sexual and commercial exploitation of humans and organs, humanitarian assistance and support, as well as access to education and control of frontiers, arm smuggling and corruption.

Organized in networks, professionals integrate institutions and enrich human resources in contact with children; based on an interdisciplinary team approach, they develop skills and knowledge, encourage collaboration within local and governmental institutions, call on academic and research organizations, stimulate funding from private sectors, interact with families and informal sector and—last but not least—innovate opportunities for youth participation. Some of the objectives of Arab professionals are:

- To identify valuable resources and key persons working with children.
- To develop and improve models for detection and management.
- To increase public awareness in the definition, recognition and prevention of CAN.

[9]UNODC International Framework for Action to Implement the Trafficking in Persons ProtocolAs highlighted in the United Nations Office on Drugs and Crime (UNODC) "International Framework for Action to Implement the Trafficking in Persons Protocol" (hereafter the U.N. Framework), the crime of trafficking frequently occurs across borders, and Member States are often unable to address the problem effectively because international mechanisms or structures for international cooperation are either non-existent or inadequate. This limitation is why the U.N. Framework, in promoting the implementation of the U.N. Protocol, urges Member States to "[c]reate the legal basis for international cooperation, including the promotion of cooperation agreements."164

- To design and facilitate educational and training materials, and provide a sustainable educational support for professionals and NGOs working in the area of CAN.
- To support local and governmental cooperation, and encourage the Arab region (MENA) and global efforts in child protection, mainly with ISPCAN expertise.
- To help launch specialized centers for research and others for the management of maltreated children.
- To ensure that adequate and independent surveillance systems are available and that monitoring of extent and pattern of child maltreatment is studied.

17.13.2 Platforms

An important aspect of the mission includes comprehensive reporting on CAN and involves the efforts to improve child protection. In this vision, the major objectives are as follows:

- Provide professional expertise and technical support to gather information from resources and professionals.
- Establish a core group of trained and committed multidisciplinary professionals, to report on cases involving CAN, and monitor actions to comply with CRC provisions.
- Increase the quality of practice in terms of intersectoral and intra professional work, in the areas of health, law, education and welfare services.

In the UNSV perspective, professionals integrate subcommittees or working groups, dealing with: the legal framework, the training needs, the research resources... in all types of CAN. As actors in addressing violence, professionals also tackle policies and programs to address violence against children: data collection and research, analysis and evaluation, awareness and advocacy curricula and training.

17.13.3 Progresses

The overall outcome is that the Arab region has made considerable progress in understanding the issue of violence against children, in developing strategies and mechanisms to address such violence and in establishing institutions to implement these policies and strategies, as well as in enacting the legislation necessary for the implementation of these policies.

In spite of the discrepancies between Arab countries in terms of the nature of the institutions engaged in children's issues, Arab states are aware of the importance of this issue, and agree on the need to intensify efforts to confront all forms of violence and abuse against children. Most Arab States have established official bodies, governmental structures and tools to achieve pertinent objectives; furthermore, most countries have allowed space for individual enterprises and civil society organizations to work on the implementation of child policies and social development, on a partnership basis. Nevertheless, there is still a set of recommendations that could be useful in consolidating and strengthening the efforts directed to reduce violence against children:

- strengthen observatories and centers involved in recording or handling incidents of violence against children
- Compare studies between Arab countries to exchange experiences in recording incidents of violence against children and methods of addressing them.
- Follow-up the implementation of the recommendations of the UNSG's Study on VAC, through national periodical reports.
- Strengthen strategies aimed at the child and those targeting the family—the reasons behind such efforts are attributable to the fact that the family is the primary caretaker of the child, and that when the family is protected against risks, the child is protected from such risks as well.
- Increase coordination between the efforts of the institutions directly involved with childcare and those indirectly sponsoring similar actions. For example, prevention of drug addiction is an important area where coordination between the efforts of childcare institutions and those made at the national level are needed. A similar instance relates to the efforts put forth by the ministries of labor to protect children from forced labor and the different manifestations of abuse.
- Provide incentives for successful experiences in child protection against violence and abuse in the Arab world and towards highlighting and discussing these experiences across different media.
- Support budgets allocated to programs for childhood and motherhood, and to relevant research; increase financial resources allocated to strategies, action plans and programs for the prevention of violence against children in Arab countries.
- Support civil society and its role in the protection of children and the rights of children and mothers and the family in general.
- Work on training manuals and codes of children's rights.
- Support the Department of Family and Childhood at the League of Arab States.
- Increase the capacity to protect children in schools, courthouses and nurseries, with particular focus on pre School College, in order to provide highly skilled staff to interact with children.
- Create socio-cultural networking between families and the institutions involved in the protection of children, including civil society organizations.
- Use different experiences undergone by Arab countries, sharing such experiences and redoubling efforts to protect children against violence.
- Direct more financial support to the activities of child protection in Arab countries.
- Train human resources needed to deal with children's issues in general, and violence against children in particular.

- Refresh laws and legislation, specifically those meant to help reduce violence against children, and laws concerning FGM/C, and related to sexual abuse in general.
- Collect data, and develop indicators to compare such data over time. The data collection process needs to be sustainable and systematic.
- Establish a cross-sectoral interactive and coordinated system and promoting interagency consultative processes outside the administrative setting.
- Develop an Arab strategy to combat cybercrimes, cyberbullying and online exploitation.
- Draft a unified Arab law to address violence and child protection.
- Set up national committees fully enabled to effectively follow up on the progress made in the implementation of the recommendations of the UNSG's Study on VAC in a multi-phase manner, and link the recommendations to national policies concerning children.
- Highlight the preventative side of violence against children.

17.13.4 Challenges

In reality, despite the professionals pressing demands and the consequent efforts deployed by governments from the levels of policies and legislations to those of implementation and practice, violence against children is still a challenge for several reasons, which can be summarized as follows:

- Examples of cultural beliefs: Some types of CAN, such as corporal punishment, female genital mutilations, early marriage and violence against the girl child still are diversely perceived by stakeholders and citizens; they remain sometimes in Arab societies as private matter or cultural specificities. Modifications are expected in the provisions of national legislations, in the Arab world and other regional countries, such as Turkey, Pakistan, Iran (24, 25)
- Challenges in education: Lack of awareness about child rights among families, educators and child caregivers, remain a challenge. School based initiatives are needed in that regard, like "ambassadors of peace", "One World 2011" as manifested during the Feb. 2009 conference on family violence in Jordan.
- Types of structural obstacles to the CRC implementation: The lack of monitoring systems relating to violence is still a gap in the evaluation and control of violence against children. Child observatories exist in some Arab countries and need to be replicated with more independence Also, the Child Defender project would help national child protection strategies reach rapid, adapted, legalized and socially acceptable interventions toward the implementation of the CRC. Furthermore, the Child helpline, available in some countries, is warming up in some others. "Child Friendly Budgeting" is an emerging concept in Jordan, involving Governmental and Nongovernmental sectors. The Child Friendly Budget initiative aims at increasing the attention of policy makers and legislators on public spending that

best responds to children's matters and priorities, ensuring its integration into governmental planning in the fields of health, education and social development.

- Legislation discrepancies and pitfalls: All countries of the Middle East and North Africa region have endorsed the CRC. Some countries did not make any reservations, while others have made reservations regarding provisions that were taken to be incompatible with Islamic jurisprudence. Seven countries (Egypt, Lebanon, Jordan, Yemen, Qatar and Tunisia) have equally endorsed the optional protocol regarding child trafficking, child prostitution and child pornography.

The definition of a child varies however from one country to another, with subsequent variation in the definition of the age of criminal responsibility. In many countries that age is very young, and is therefore not compatible with CRC (e.g. 7 years in Lebanon…to be increased to 10; Libya, Qatar, Saudi Arabia, Emirates, Yemen and Egypt). Subsequently a child that young could be convicted. In some countries that have no definite age of adulthood, children may receive the death penalty, life imprisonment or flogging (especially in Qatar, Saudi Arabia and Emirates).

Maltreatment of juveniles and their detention in difficult circumstances stress the violence they might be subject to by officials and their deprivation of the right to contact their families such as is the case in Lebanon, Libya, Morocco, Syria and Tunisia. In some countries such as Syria and Egypt beggars and street children are treated like criminals.

Weaknesses in enforcement of legal provisions included in the CRC, as well as some discrepancies within national legislations, are congruent problems. There are still, however, important efforts produced towards child friendly laws. This issue is particularly important in the Juvenile Justice and children at risk. Alternative measures for juveniles in conflict with law are on the track, with compensation, reintegration and restoring justice. Legislation and capacity building also appear as critical requirements in the street children problem in the Arab world.

17.13.5 Training and Capacity Building, Gaps to Fill

Professional capacities and institutional frames are critical points in the efficiency of initiative aiming to provide control of violence and protection of victims. In fact, Arab professionals offer expertise to the institutional settings to increase the level and quality of knowledge on the science of intersectoral cooperation and /or the usefulness of such a coordinative process, to optimize the development of child protection systems, thus encouraging the participatory process and increasing the capacities of the informal sector to build networks for interventions and collaboration.

Such recommendations include:

- Set standards and specifications for professional groups working in the area of child protection against sexual abuse, according to fields of expertise.

- Sustain data collection on the training needs of the professionals working with children.
- Produce training manuals and material for professionals working in child protection and response to sexual violence.
- Expand Child Protection Units in Health settings.
- Provide terms of reference for professionals working with children in conditions of sexual violence and trafficking, including skills capacitation, in all levels of programs, such as protection, prevention, intervention and rehabilitation.
- Plan periodic reviews of training plans.
- Develop exchange programs in order to share experiences between sectors at the local level, and to benefit from relevant Arab and international expertise.
- Develop models for codes of conduct for professional groups working with children in all sectors; such models should be strictly complied with a mechanism to monitor the extent of such compliance should be established.
- Introduce the concepts of child protection from sexual violence as well as case management, to university disciplines relevant to working with children; and develop specialized curricula for pertinent academic disciplines and professions.
- Introduce the principles of family counselling to specialized university curricula.
- Create a diploma specialized in children's rights and child protection.

17.13.6 Monitoring and Reporting

17.13.6.1 Institutions, Monitoring and Evaluation

Arab states have made significant progress in developing strategies for the protection of children. 16 states have developed plans to establish independent national bodies to confront violence against children: Jordan, the UAE, Bahrain, Tunisia, Algeria, Saudi Arabia, Syria, Iraq, Oman, Qatar, Kuwait, Lebanon, Egypt, Morocco, Mauritania and Yemen.

However, these strategies require clearly-defined mechanisms to assess implementation and report on challenges. Some Arab States, like Jordan and Tunisia, have developed electronic systems to monitor and analyze indicators regarding follow-up on the activities and programs described in national plans; such systems can enhance coordination with the national institutions involved in the implementation of these plans and strategies, particularly national plans of action for children.

The system relies on a group of liaison officers representing the relevant institutions involved in child protection, producing periodic reports on the implementation of programs under the national plans of action. In Egypt and Tunisia, national centers prepare studies and field surveys on issues relevant to children's rights, share insights on the implementation of plans, regularly provide strategic information on children, and monitor the status of children. In Morocco, the national center for the rights of the child organizes bi-annual national conference to evaluate and assess the achievements of the national plan of action. The ministerial committee, chaired by Morocco's Prime Minister, presents during the conference a detailed report on the achievements and challenges of two years of implementation of plans.

The most important objectives of the observatory of the following:

- Use of scientific research in monitoring the reality of the situation of childhood.
- Provide strategic, realistic information on a regular basis on all aspects of children's issues.
- Establish an integrated system of monitoring and evaluation to monitor and evaluate national action plan for children.
- Increase the awareness of children and adults of the law and the rights of the child.

Different approaches to legal protection for children against violence vary in Arab countries; some States are promulgating a child protection act or law, some have amended their laws their legislation appropriately, to bring them into line with relevant international standards. The Arab States are increasingly incorporating protection against violence into their legal systems, and are mainstreaming children's basic needs in legislation. In most states, national mechanisms for child protection lack clear legal framework that is inclusive of the various components of the child protection system.

In Tunisia, the provisions of the law include all aspects of a child's life and appoint a "child protection officer"—recognized as a law enforcement officer thus shortening legal proceedings and ensuring early protection for the child. Family judges also ensure child protection, with a clearly defined mandate to order legal and social measures. Obviously, such legal systems provide for mandatory reporting and child help-lines.

Some laws, like the Egyptian law, identify the forms of violence and relevant support mechanisms; they are jointly articulated along with the Child Helpline and child protection committees; such legislation also covers issues related to violence, such as child trafficking.

Some legislation has been effectively implemented in Arab countries for decades. Many laws have, however, been developed recently. Such diversity of experience provides valuable lessons when the impacts and challenges faced during the drafting process of these laws are considered.

Most Arab countries have increased their commitment to child protection by developing mechanisms and institutions to inform communities, and provide quality services to children and families.

Action on reports and complaints increasingly rely on toll-free telephone lines for children in order to facilitate the reception of complaints; such toll-free telephone lines provide listening and counselling using different means of telecommunications, with Child Rescue-Lines in some Arab countries, as part of the protection system in these States as well as challenges given the comprehensiveness based on supply and demand and available resources.

Some institutions have made progress and achievements in this regard, which can be promoted so that others can benefit from. The "Family Protection Department" in Jordan provides services to families (medical, psychological and social—interdisciplinary approach) to ensure effective protection; such systems are linked to security services and have coordinated with the private and informal sectors, giving the system a social dimension rather than emphasizing its punitive aspect, while also keeping it in direct contact with child victims and their families.

Algeria has also established offices in municipalities to promote social activities through which social and economic assistance is provided to families in need.

Syria established a "Family Protection Unit" to work on complaints regarding incidents of child abuse, carry out investigations and refer the outcomes to the competent authorities; the Unit also offers shelter for child protection, including a center for child victims who cannot return to their community without physical and psychological rehabilitation and re-evaluation of their livelihood and environment.

In penal and correctional institutions, it is worth reporting that hearing rooms, which are equipped with audio-video facilities to listen to children victims of violence and sexual exploitation, as is the case in Lebanon, provide an instructive example. In Morocco, professional units are working together with the public prosecution at courthouses to address child issues, especially with reference to cases of violence. Syria is in the process of developing a rehabilitation center for female offenders.

Lebanon has also developed a rehabilitation center for young girls.

In modern justice systems, the issue of criminal responsibility is central. Some countries have increased the age of criminal responsibility to 12 years and above, as is the case in Tunisia and Egypt, while other countries should address the reviewing of punitive laws for juveniles in conflict with the law to include restorative justice or rehabilitation.

In order to the stop criminal prosecution and punishment of children, Tunisia has developed a system for mediation and reconciliation to address cases between children in conflict with the law and their victims.

17.13.6.2 The Establishment of Systems and Services for Communication Accessible and Suitable for Children

The majority of Arab countries increased mechanisms and institutions to report sexual violence and misconduct, for children themselves and parents, with mandatory reporting laws.

- Establish a toll-free line and dedicate services at the national and local levels, for advice and guidance, referral and reporting; such systems ensure advocacy and publicity for the Child Helpline.
- Map resources and services available in the official and national sectors.
- Establish complaint mechanisms in residential care institutions as well as in correctional settings; such mechanisms include human capacity and appropriate processes and structures: complaint boxes, codes of conduct.
- Appoint a social worker, (Protection Officer) in residential care, correctional and juvenile institutions; the Protection Officer's mandate is to follow-up on

complaints, to ensure adequate access of children to due process, to ensure protection of children and appropriate punishment of the perpetrators.
- Strengthen the role of the media and encourage the promotion of process, complaints and reporting.

Child friendly centers receive all communications relating to sexual violence. In addition to the criminal justice institutions, such centers provide cells of listening, counseling. Civil society plays an important role to include children and parents.

17.13.6.3 Develop and Implement Systematic Data Collection, Research

Data collection systems are still a major challenge in most Arab States. Independent systems in place to collect information and data on the status of disadvantaged and vulnerable groups of children, and on forms of violence and cases of abuse are non-existent. The Arab report has demonstrated, on a comparative basis, the absence of systematic data collection; the lack of integrated information systems connecting the institutions working on violence against children; and the lack of systems to help determine the accuracy of the indicators for systematic data collection on violence against children. Some countries, such as Jordan, Tunisia, Egypt and Morocco, are conducting qualitative and quantitative studies on children in order to provide information and statistics on the circumstances in which violence occurs.

Participants to Cairo declaration urged OIC Member States to establish effective tools for systematic collection, analysis and dissemination of data on the implementation of the CRC, disaggregated by age, gender, urban\rural and other relevant factors; and to use this data for the development, implementation and regular review of their laws, policies and programs and to identify child vulnerabilities, to prevent discrimination and overcome disparities.

Egypt have both set up centers to interact with the media and offer training, and to provide documentation and research opportunities. Some countries like Tunisia have observatory center for children's rights, operating under the supervision of the national information system, which includes representatives of all ministries concerned with children's rights, and is in charge of feeding the system with statistics and data. The system provides insight on 390 indicators, including indicators of child protection.

Algeria also has an information database in place, which is specialized in matters related to women and children. Sudan has an e-government system to link ministries to data on children without parental care or on those who have been referred to the criminal justice system. Some countries are establishing databases on children, such as Jordan, the UAE, Syria, Egypt and Lebanon.

In terms of child participation in the prevention of violence, some pioneering experiences have revealed different approaches to the involvement of children; some initiatives developed children's parliaments, as in Jordan, the UAE, Tunisia, Algeria, Egypt, Morocco and Yemen. The Emirate of Sharjah in UAE established a council for children; Algeria and Lebanon formed local municipal councils for children, and established children's offices in municipalities. Moreover, the "child friendly city" initiative is gaining prominence in Arab States.

The question of the efficiency and the sustainability of children's participation remains a valid one. Are regular and systematic consultations with children taking place, or is the subject matter addressed with children relegated to general topics?

17.13.6.4 Ombudsman or Commissioner for Children's Rights, to Monitor Children's Rights and to Receive Complaints

Arab countries have achieved remarkable progress in the legislative side of giving priority to the child's best interest and ensure the safety and security. Even Yemen produced a number of regulations and decisions governing the conduct of work educational institutions. Lebanon submitted a proposal for Child Ombudsman in 2004. In Oman, the committee on follow-up on the implementation of the Convention on the Rights of the Child functions as a commissioner for children's rights, and is mandated to follow up on the Convention on the Rights of the Child (CRC) implementation and the preparation of progress reports on the achievements made within the framework of the Convention. The National Centre for Human Rights is the national institution tasked with receiving complaints about and monitoring and reporting on children's rights violations.

In Tunisia, the officer in charge of the plan for child protection undertakes the protection of children subject to violence and abuse.

In Mauritania, the National Council for Childhood is an advisory body to the Government. The Independent National Human Rights Commission monitors the rights of the child. The government has established a Commission for Human Rights.

Children have no idea of the legal measures or otherwise which target their protection from sexual violence. In this regard, the child-friendly version of the UNSV has been the subject of consultations in some countries of the region (Jordan, Lebanon).

In order to interview children and communicate legal procedures and social values, it is important to be aware that children can identify the following forms of violence:

- Physical, sexual, emotional and verbal violence by teachers.
- Lack of school response regarding sexual violence.
- Laws prohibiting sexual violence in school
- Poverty and sexual violence.
- Poor children voices.
- Poor accountability of teachers who use sexual harassment.
- Lack of social workers to challenge violence.
- Lack of parents' councils proactivity.
- Lack of activity clubs (painting, music) in schools to divert violence into creative activities.

- Poor media campaigns.

The regional endeavor focuses on the legal aspect of VAC, targeting a solid legal framework to be effectively used. The law of the child is considered a first and essential step in that direction and has been issued in Syria and Egypt; the process is ongoing in Lebanon, Jordan, KSA and other countries.

Children can also collaborate in other legal procedures, such as the reporting and monitoring, evaluation and follow up; they can also contribute in lobbying and advocacy, in non-governmental organizations and local capacities, in cooperative tools and capacities of national and local committees.

As an example of child empowerment, the first UNICEF Regional Awards for Media on Child Rights were handed out in Amman by the Queen. Special awards also went to two determined 16-year-olds from Jordan and the Palestinian territories that produced media projects without financial support from any governmental or private entity.

17.13.7 Child Helplines [Source: Childhelplineinternational]

Children face violence and abuse all over the world irrespective of their location. The data demonstrates that violence and abuse are the main reasons for which children seek the assistance and support of child helplines.

Amongst violence and abuse a large proportion of children, mainly girls, are victims of sexual abuse. The data also confirms the findings of several research studies that in majority of cases of sexual abuse the perpetrators are persons related to the victims or known to them. The group of perpetrators comprises parents, relatives, peer group, teachers and others.

Such data needs to be used by governments, multilateral organizations like the UNICEF, international and national non-governmental organizations, and civil society organizations l to develop policy and legislations as well as design interventions to address the issue of child sexual abuse and fill the gaps in the child protection systems.

Child helplines offer several services to children, the foremost of which is to uphold their Right to be heard and the Right to have freedom from all forms of violence as enshrined in Articles 12 and 13 of the Convention on the Rights of the Child.[10] Children contacting child helplines are offered counselling services and if

[10]Article 12:

1. States Parties shall assure to the child who is capable of forming his or her own views the right to express those views freely in all matters affecting the child, the views of the child being given due weight in accordance with the age and maturity of the child.2. For this purpose, the child shall in particular be provided the opportunity to be heard in any judicial and administrative proceedings affecting the child, either directly, or through a representative or an appropriate body, in a manner consistent with the procedural rules of national law.

their needs are greater child helplines refer them to partner organizations. Child helplines do not operate in isolation, they have formal arrangements with other child focused organizations and governments in their areas of operation so as to be able provide holistic support to children in need of care and protection.

Child helplines are considered to be an appropriate medium to help children face their problems and enable them to report and express what they consider to be abusive. Helplines often provide guidance and advice children are unable to find at home, at school and in society.

These lines receive children's calls and provide guidance, and refer them when needed to other organizations specializing in child protection. Child helplines enable children to talk openly and confidentially. Child helplines also promote awareness of children's problems and reinforce cooperation with the communications sector, child protection entities and other partners.

The number of calls to child helplines has increased at the global level, which indicates that this service serves as an important channel to support children and help to ensure the rights of the child in a continuously changing world.

In 2012 child helplines across the world received approximately 13.8 million calls from both children and adults (this does not include visits to similar websites). Children voluntarily and directly call child helplines in order to speak about the problems they face.

Child helplines can contribute to ensuring the protection of children who are in danger or abused, when they are part of a comprehensive child protection system that is capable of responding to the caller's needs and able to assist him or her with service. It is thus necessary before establishing a line to make sure that there exists the capacity to respond in the country concerned (i.e. specialized rehabilitative institutions, shelters, law-implementation authorities trained in child rights, and clear criteria for operating and referral among various actors in the national child protection system).

Improving children's ability to report violence requires helplines to take into account the critical position of the child. It is therefore necessary for communication channels with children to be acceptable, attractive and varied (e.g. telephone call, email, and websites). Contact numbers should also be easy to remember (e.g. made up of four digits), and freely accessible.

The deficiency in reporting cases of violations against children is one of the problems that challenge the Arab region's efforts to safeguard the rights of the child. The reasons for this deficiency may be attributed to cultural and social considerations that render it difficult to publicly expose aggressors, especially if an abuser is a family member or a relative. Another factor is ignorance of the nature of these violations and of acceptable behavioral boundaries related to the rights of the child. In particular, some measures that are accepted based on the idea that "violence that does not hurt" are considered to be norms of social control.

The culture of reporting and bringing perpetrators to justice necessitates a level of awareness of rights, and confidence in the ability of the party receiving complaints to ensure justice for victims and enforce punishments. Several studies refer to the fact that a large number of victims of violence did not report what had happened to them, even in countries that possess effective protection systems. This is may have several causes, including: ignorance, the lack of available or reliable services, and a fear of retribution by the exposed transgressor.

Child protection systems in most of the Arab states are incomplete and poorly supported financially, in addition to suffering a lack of standardized responses to rights violations. Raising the level of reporting of violence by children and adults is a key strategy in an attempt to raise the efficacy of protection. In its concluding observations, The Committee for Child Protection has stated that providing mechanisms for reporting and receiving complaints is necessary and should take priority. In particular, child-friend that take into account the sensitivity of the child's situation should be provided. The Committee has called for the establishment of free support lines, which should be effectively advertised to reach children in various locations. In this respect, the global study on VAC recommended, and the Marrakech Declaration reiterated, the necessity of establishing national mechanisms for follow-up and reporting be established with the aim of preventing problems faced by children and their families. The most important of such mechanisms may include child helplines, protection committees, child-protection deputies and others.

The cooperation of the Arab League's Women, Family and Childhood Department and Child Helpline International (CHI) also constituted an effective framework to encourage a large number of Arab states to establish child helplines. However, these helplines are not the only mechanism of receiving complaints and reporting abuses. Some countries established networks for protection in the form of committees or associations that raise awareness regarding the importance of reporting and receiving complaints. Others innovate special mechanisms such as a child protection deputy and child rights observatory mechanism.

17.13.7.1 Profile of the Children Contacting Child Helplines

Girls tend to contact child helplines more than boys. Most significantly, in both the Middle East and North Africa (MENA) many more girls contact child helplines than boys. The difference between girls and boys contacting child helplines in the MENA region is around 26%. In the MENA region the bulk of contacts are from girls of 18 years and older. On the contrary in Africa the contacts made by girls (44%) were less than the contacts made by male children (56%).

In 2010, child helplines worldwide received 74,303 contacts on sexual abuse. This amounted to approximately 18% of all contacts and emerged as the third important reason for contacts on violence and abuse received overall.[11]

Sexual abuse was the third most commonly reported reason on sub-category of abuse and violence in 2010. Both the data and accounts from individual child helplines suggest not only an increase in the number of sexual abuse cases reported to child helplines, but also in their severity.

[11] Annual Report, Child Helpline International, 2010.

Child helplines cite the global economic crisis and resulting job-losses, stress and hardships on families as one possible explanation (similar to the increase in reports to child helplines on child labor, also likely caused to some extent by difficult financial times for families).

In reality sexual abuse of children occurs at a much larger scale than reflected by the statistics collected by Child Helpline International. In most cases sexual abuse is part of the physical abuse and domestic violence in the society; therefore the percentages mentioned above may not give a complete picture of the situation. If the data for physical abuse and domestic violence is included then the figures are much higher. Taking into account contacts made by children about physical abuse and domestic violence the situation appears to be much more serious. Around 61% female and 48% male children were affected by physical and sexual abuse, and domestic violence.

In the Americas and Caribbean 9% of all contacts about violence and abuse to child helplines were about sexual abuse, while in Europe sexual abuse cases accounted for 21% of all reported abuse cases. In Africa this was around 20%, in the Asia Pacific region 10%, and the Middle East and North Africa Region the figure was 12%.

All countries said that lines were available to all countries free and without discrimination (except for the formal line in Lebanon currently being established) and that all lines were undertaking an advertising and media campaign with the aim of raising the awareness of children and society on the importance of reporting.

- Reporting mechanisms: most helplines utilize the electronic method to receive phone calls and reports (approved by Child Helpline International), issue annual reports clarifying the number and kind of reports and distribute them according to age group and gender.
- Helplines also refer to the fact that secrecy was ensured during all stages of communication with the helpline.
- Abuse and violence are the primary reason for calling, accounting for 37.28% of all total calls. This is followed by reasons related to psychological and social well-being, accounting for 17.73% of total callers, followed by problems related to school, accounting for 10.60%. All of this can be interpreted as an indicator on the existence of violence and abuse to children in the Arab region, as a pressing social phenomenon on children.
- Physical abuse is the foremost reason for children calling within the category of reporting abuse and violence, constituting 41.48%, followed by negligence, 12.6%, emotional abuse, 12; 7%, while 10.44% of children call to report their being bullied.
- The topic that remains absent from policies and programs despite its tangible existence is that of sexual abuse (9.57%), despite what surrounds the topic of cultural and social beliefs, which make it difficult to divulge. The data provided by Child Helpline International however, did not reveal the number and scale of calls that were referred and followed up on by specialized actors in the rest of the protection system's components

17.13.7.2 Victims

Differentiated by gender the data shows that relatively more girls contact child helplines about sexual abuse than boys, across all regions. Boys tend to contact child helplines on bullying.

Girls were the victims in the vast majority of the cases of sexual abuse reported to child helplines in 2010, accounting for 71% of all reported sexual abuse cases worldwide.

Compared to other forms of abuse, sexual abuse disproportionally affects girls. In the MENA region girls were the victims in 91% of reported cases and in the Americas and Caribbean girls were the primary victims in 80% of the cases. There is no significant difference in victim-gender ratios for different HDI levels when it comes to sexual abuse. In countries with medium HDI levels girls were the victims of the sexual abuse in 80% of all reported cases, while in low HDI level countries girls were the victims in some 65% of all sexual abuse cases and in very high and high HDI level countries in 70% of all sexual abuse cases.

17.13.7.3 Perpetrators

All over the world men and boys were indicated to be the perpetrator of sexual abuse in close to three quarters of all sexual abuse cases reported to child helplines in 2010. Across all HDI levels and in all regions, the majority of sexual abuse was committed by men and boys. This figure is even higher when looking only at those cases involving girls. The data indicates that in 73% of the perpetrators are men and 27% women. In case of sexual abuse of girls the percentage of male perpetrators is much higher (82%). As Fig. 3 demonstrators 29% contacts made with child helplines about violence and abuse related to sexual abuse of boy and in this case too, the number of male perpetrators is much higher than female perpetrators. In four out of ten cases the sexual abuse reported to child helplines in 2010 was committed by a member of the victim's immediate or extended family. The male members of a child's immediate family (brothers and fathers) made up 18% of all cases. This confirms findings of most of the academic research conducted so far.

The cases gathered by child helplines clearly demonstrate that children often become victims of sexual abuse by the very people whom they depend on for protection and support. This is perhaps one of the main reasons why many cases of sexual abuse go unreported as children are hesitant to complaint against those in whom they have faith and trust.

Besides immediate family members, children often become victims of sexual abuse by their teachers. The data shows that in as many as 18% cases the perpetrators are teachers. In the case of girls the largest number perpetrators are immediate male members of the family and then others, which includes boys of the peer group, and persons known to the victim. When it comes to sexual abuse of boys once again it is the male immediate family members and then the teachers.

In countries with a very high HDI level the average share of contacts on sexual abuse involving a brother or father was over half. Looking only at cases in which the victims were girls, this number is even higher, with more than two thirds of all sexual abuse cases in very high HDI levels involving a brother or father. The proportion of sexual abuse cases reported to child helplines that were committed by a male immediate family member is significantly higher in Europe than in other regions.

17.13.7.4 Settings

Sexual abuse takes place mainly at home, at school and in the street or neighborhood. Unfortunately most cases reported indicate the place of abuse is often where children should feel the safest, like homes, child care facilities, friends' homes, organized sports activities. Many cases occur on the streets too. The data indicates that in High HDI countries the proportion of sexual abuse taking place at other locations (child care facilities, friend's homes or during organized sporting activities for children) is less as compared with homes. The data collected by child helplines in 2010 when disaggregated according to gender and reasons for contact presents an alarming level of sexual abuse of girl child in Africa. As many as 33% female and 10% male children contacting child helplines regarding violence and abuse stated sexual abuse as the reason for seeking help and advice. When the data is collated according to the percentage of calls on sexual abuse the results show that the highest percentage was reported from Egypt (51%) followed by Swaziland (47%), Mauritius (43%), and Uganda (40%). The percentage of calls on sexual abuse in many other African countries as shown in Fig. 5 averaged around 23%.

While all the data is based on the contacts made with child helplines, a vast majority of children are unable to reach helplines for reasons beyond their control, including lack telecommunication infrastructure, poverty, lack of awareness about the existence of child helplines etc.

17.13.7.5 Services

Most child helplines provide active listening, counselling and referral services to victims of sexual abuse.

Compared to other forms of child abuse, more child helplines tend to provide supplementary services such as intervention, education and legal services to victims of sexual abuse. At the same time, the number of child helplines providing additional services does tend to decrease with increasing HDI levels, mainly because there are more partner organizations available in the child protection system to refer children to for help.

17.13.7.6 Summary and Recommendations of CHI

In an attempt to become acquainted with the nature and work of these helplines and in coordination with Child Helpline International, information was gathered by means of a form to be filled, by fifteen helplines operating in 13 Arab states. Some of the lines followed government management (7 lines) while others were operated by civil societies specialized in child protection (7 lines).

The coverage range of lines also varied between those operating at local and national levels, respectively. The percentage of children benefiting from using the helpline varied: from 50% of children in Sharjah and in Sudan to 6% in Egypt. Only two countries (Egypt and Sudan) said that they had established a helpline based on the law. The rest of the lines were established by government or ministerial decree or a resolution from the civil society supervising the helpline's operation.

Most helplines did not mention any problems in coordination and referral to other protection services, but a lack was registered in the absorptive capacity of psychological shelter and support services, and in the amount of social assistance given in some countries. There was a lack of various protection services in both Iraq and Yemen.

17.14 Policies and Instruments for Practice

17.14.1 Legal

17.14.1.1 Introducing the Convention on the Rights of the Child as a Tool for Combating Sexual Violence

Three forms of sexual violence predominate: honor violence, early marriage and sexual abuse, from a human rights' and particularly child rights perspective, as articulated in the Convention on the Rights of the Child (CRC), adopted by the UN General Assembly in 1989.

Lebanon and Yemen have signed and ratified this convention, with some minor reservations. OPT is not recognized as a state and cannot sign the convention, nonetheless President Arafat endorsed it for Palestine during his lifetime. Tackling gender-based violence against teenage girls from a child right perspective helps avoiding the usual discussions between the East and West on sensitive gender questions and rather focusing on examining the issue from a child-rights perspective. Subsequently, although this is a gender issue, using the CRC will have a more powerful result.

In short, it is obvious that certain articles are violated when sexual violence is committed against children. However, the aspects of gender-based sexual violence that violate the CRC have more public exposure.

17.14.1.2 Legislative Reforms

States in MENA have demonstrated a strong commitment to protect the human rights of children by universally ratifying the Convention on the Rights of the Child (CRC), which serves as the foundation for recognizing and protecting child rights in international law and encompasses all children, including refugee children. The MENA region also features near universal ratification of the Optional Protocol to the CRC on the Involvement of Children in Armed Conflict, as well as the Optional Protocol to the CRC on the Sale of Children, Child Prostitution and Child Pornography.

Most States in MENA have also acceded to the International Covenant on Civil and Political Rights (ICCPR), which complements provisions in the CRC, and also recognizes the right of all children to be registered at birth, to acquire a nationality, and to enjoy child-specific protections in all situations. MENA is also host to regional human rights instruments addressing the protection of children, including the Covenant on the Rights of the Child in Islam, the African Charter on the Rights and Welfare of the Child, the Arab Charter on Human Rights, and the African Charter on Human and Peoples' Rights. Several States in the region have also ratified the 1951 Convention relating to the.

17.15 Strengthening International Commitment

Human rights enshrined in international documents such as the International Convention on Human Rights11, are of a general nature and composition; such texts apply to all individuals, regardless of their particular circumstances, such as age, sex, nationality, ethnic backgrounds, affiliation with intellectual, linguistic and cultural groups, and other considerations. However, targeted legislation in international human rights specifically covers certain groups of people; such groups, due to their vulnerability for various reasons, are in need of allocated charters, declarations and agreements to afford them greater protection and special attention12.

The Convention on the Rights of the Child (CRC) is a major and integral part of the international human rights system; in addition to international human rights legitimacy, it provides the child with a set of rights of its own with reference to needs for special protection due to the child's age and other factors. It is clear that whenever the values and culture of human rights in general are reinforced in communities, this in turn reinforces the values and culture of children's rights, and vice versa. This relationship enhances efforts in child protection, as seen in the experiences of countries in implementing the Convention on the Rights of the Child and its Optional Protocols, as well as other relevant international and regional instruments of human rights providing protection for children:

17.15.1 Convention on the Rights of the Child and Its Two Optional Protocols

Arab countries, except Somalia, have legal obligations towards the Convention on the Rights of the Child through signing and ratification. Countries have, therefore, issued enforceable domestic laws (in official sectors, laws and legislation) to enshrine the principles of the Convention on the Rights of the Child (CRC). The CRC has been signed and ratified by 21 Arab countries; most of these made between 1990 and 1997.Somalia signed the Convention on the Rights of the Child (CRC) in 2002, but has not yet ratified it.

Arab countries focus on amendment of appropriate legislation and domestic laws in line with the requirements of international conventions, the development of institutions involved in the implementation of children's rights, and the necessity to develop strategies for action. Arab countries made efforts to follow up on the implementation of the Convention on the Rights of the Child and its optional protocols, as follows:

- Arab countries, except Somalia, ratified the Convention. In many countries, experiences and traditions maintain a good ranking. Countries follow-up the implementation of the Convention, and receive observations of the CRC Committee in terms of performance.
- Most Arab countries adopted or ratified the two optional protocols to the CRC, and some have already prepared and discussed their initial reports according to a specific timeframe.

17.15.2 Status of Refugees and Its 1967 Protocol[5]

All the states in the Middle East and North Africa (MENA) region have ratified the United Nations Convention on the Rights of the Child (CRC).[12] A number of countries have made interpretative declarations or reservations on Articles 20 and 21 in relation to foster care for children and adoption, and reservation to Article 14 relating to freedom of religion. Kuwait, Saudi Arabia and Qatar have expressed general reservations with reservation with respect to all such articles as are in conflict with the provisions of Islamic law. With the exception of Iraq, Saudi Arabia and the United Arab Emirates, MENA countries have also acceded to the Optional Protocols of the CRC on the Involvement of Children in Armed Conflicts and on the Sale of

[12]The Occupied Palestinian Territory is not party to the CRC—the Palestinian Authority is not a state and therefore cannot sign or ratify the CRC. This section covers Algeria, Bahrain, Egypt, Iraq, Jordan, Kuwait Libya, Morocco, Oman, Qatar, Saudi Arabia, Syria, Tunisia, and the United Arab Emirates.

Children, Child Prostitution and Pornography.[13] None of the MENA countries have expressed reservations to reduce obligations to protect children from all forms of violence.

Seven countries in the region—Algeria, Bahrain, Jordan, Libya, Occupied Palestinian Territory (OPT), Syria and the United Arab Emirates—have also ratified the Arab Charter on Human Rights, which includes specific articles protecting children from abuse, exploitation, and involvement in armed conflicts and violence.

Following the ratification of the CRC, MENA countries have enacted or propose to enact laws to protect children from violence, abuse, neglect or exploitation. A number of countries have put in place comprehensive Child Laws that bring together legal provisions for the protection of the child. For example, Tunisia has adopted the Child Protection Code, Egypt is waiting for the Parliament to approve amendments to the 1996 Child Law, and Algeria has introduced a Bill on Child Protection which aims to establish a mechanism for protecting children against all forms of violence, ill-treatment, abuse and negligence.

In countries where no comprehensive child law has been introduced, specific laws have been adopted or amended to better promote child protection. In Jordan where the Parliament has yet to approve the 2004 Child Bills Act, amendments were introduced to Juvenile Act N. 24 of 1968 to guarantee protection and care for children who are exposed to abuse by one or both parents,[14] while Juvenile Act No. 11 mandates judges the right to inspect juvenile centers affiliated with the Ministry of Social Development every three months.[15] Oman is also in the processing of preparing draft Juvenile Law, which will increase the minimum age for criminal responsibility for nine to 14 years of age.[16]

While welcoming these legislative reforms, the Committee on the Rights of the Child has consistently recommended MENA countries to expedite the adoption and enforcement of proposed laws, to strengthen efforts to provide better legal protection for children, and to ensure that relevant domestic laws are in full conformity with the principles and provisions of the CRC, through enacting new legislations and or amending existing ones.[17] Moreover, further research is necessary to evaluate the extent to which new or amended laws are enforced and programs are implemented, in order to better assess gaps between policies and practices at the national and local levels.

In addition, despite progress in the legislative and programmatic fronts—with many of the governments of MENA countries working with civil society groups,

---

[13]Egypt claims it acceded to the Optional Protocol on the Involvement of Children in Armed Conflict, but there is no record in the UN Human Rights database.

[14]Jordan Third Periodic Report", Committee on the Rights of the Child, CRC/C/JOR/3, 2 March 2006.

[15]NGOs Supplementary Report on the third Jordanian Official Report on CRC", National Center for Human Rights, Jordan, March 2006.

[16]At a Glance – Oman, the Big Picture", UNICEF website, http://www.unicef.org/infobycountry/oman.html

[17]For example, see Concluding Observations for Oman, Saudi Arabia and Syria.

international NGOs, regional bodies, donors and United Nations agencies to better protect children—child protection remains a serious issue every country of the region. The nature and extent of child protection issues varies country to country, and includes issues such as violence against children—whether at homes, schools or institutional settings—harmful practices, particularly female genital mutilation and early marriage, juvenile justice, exploitative child labor and birth registration.[18] Children in Algeria, Iraq and the Occupied Palestinian Territories have been exposed to political violence and conflicts, and in Western Sahara have been affected by the deteriorating humanitarian situation.

The 2005 Regional Consultation, which was organized to contribute to the United Nations Secretary-General's Study on Violence against Children, highlighted that violence against children constitutes a problem throughout the MENA region and takes many forms.[19] To almost all states in the region, the Committee on the Rights of the Child has recommended legislative reforms to better prohibit all forms of violence against children, including corporal punishment within the family and in alternative care settings.[20]

While there is general recognition that violence and abuse against children occurs at home, at work, in schools, and in institutional settings, none of the countries have comprehensive data and information on its prevalence and nature. In many of the countries, the Committee on the Rights of the Child has expressed its concerns about the lack of sufficient information about child abuse and ill-treatment, and UNICEF is working with national governments to put in place comprehensive data collection and monitoring systems. Efforts by the governments of the region have shown an increasing willingness to discuss issues such as violence and child abuse—Oman and Saudi Arabia have organized a national workshop on child abuse and neglect, Syria has held high level conferences on violence against children, paving the way for a national plan of action.

Djibouti's Family Code is being finalized; Article 33 severely condemns Female Genital Mutiliation (FGM);
The National Mother and Child Council of Egypt has reviewed and revised the Children's Code in line with the CRC;
The Government of Iran is studying possibilities for bringing national laws into line with the CRC, and tribunals for children and young people have been restored;
The Jordanian Decree on the Rights of the Child is under consideration; a draft law against abuse and violence against children is in progress; the 1995 National Task Force for Children remains an important monitoring mechanism;

(continued)

[18]Birth Registration" Child Protection Information Sheet, UNICEF, May 2006.

[19]UNICEF, Table 9: Child Protection, http://www.unicef.org/sowc2013/files/Table_9_Stat_Tables_SWCR2013_ENGLISH.pdf

[20]Refworld, UN Committee on the Elimination of Discrimination against Women: Sixth Periodic Report of State Parties, Yemen, March 2007, Page 73, analysis of Article 15 of Personal Status Laws, http://www.refworld.org/docid/467138a62.html

In Lebanon, there have been some important amendments to laws relating to education, identity, child labour, and in favour of handicapped children; a parliamentary committee on children was formed in 1992 and in 1994 a High Council for Children was established;
Morocco ratified ILO Conventions 182 and 183, and set the legal age for labor at 15 years. A new labor code was developed and is being reviewed; a national Observatory on Children's Rights was created in 1994, and reform of the juvenile justice system is currently before parliament;
Oman is also undergoing reform in the juvenile justice sector; an inter-ministerial committee on children's rights has been formed;
In Syria, legal texts are being revised; the legal age for labour has been fixed at 16 years; a High Committee on Children was established in 1999;
Yemen is reviewing laws relating to children and young people; the High Council for Mother and Child is being reorganized;
In Tunisia, the Code for Protection of Children (1995) includes protection against all forms of mistreatment and abuse, with a focus on prevention; establishment of an Observatory on Children's Rights has been announced;
The Palestine National Council has established a multi-disciplinary commission to work on a Charter of Children's Rights.

All the countries under review have taken legislative steps to address violence against children. Tunisia's Child Protection Code is one of the most comprehensive in the region—it shields children from violence, neglect and abuse through the establishment of child protection mechanisms, namely, through the establishment of a body of "delegates for childhood protection" able to investigate and intervene on behalf of children in difficult situations which may threaten the security and development of the children. Qatar has also facilitated the establishment of foundations which run national hotlines, provide face to face counseling services, and liaise with the police, the courts and the Ministry of Interior.

However, as adolescents and children who participated in the regional consultation indicated, even where laws and policies against violence exist, the means of enforcing them are weak. Very few countries have effective and comprehensive national systems for the detection, reporting, referral and intervention for children victims of abuse, especially domestic abuse. The consultation also confirmed that in general, most violence—especially sexual violence and abuse—against children remains hidden away inside the family circle or in the confines of the school. Laws in some of the countries also make reporting by children difficult. For example, under the Jordanian penal code, complaints from a child can only be accepted if they are supported by the parents or guardian.

17.16 National Actions and Protection Mechanisms in Line with International Legal Instruments

17.16.1 Gender Discrimination Is a Specific, Essential and Core Issue in Sexual Violence: Gender-Based Sexual Violence as a Violation of the Convention on the Rights of the Child

The first article in the CRC defines a child as every human being below the age of eighteen years. This is perhaps the most fundamental principle to bear in mind, since we discovered within this project that teenage girls, i.e. female children, are viewed as adult women in regards to sexuality. An example of this is when young girls (who are in fact children) are married and becoming mothers themselves, which is analyzed in the project under the heading of "early marriage". The outcome of a previous research project for Save the Children Sweden in the MENA region on teenage girls was my book entitled Woman or Child?

Gender-based violence (GBV) can be defined as any act that causes physical, sexual or emotional harm and reinforces gender inequality. Women are disproportionately affected by GBV (although it applies to men and boys, as well), yet women's rights issues remain hugely underfunded with the majority of aid still reaching males. GBV is an issue that affects hundreds of millions of people around the world and has particular implications for those holding a marginalized racial, ethnic, class, indigenous, or disabled status. Thus, to effectively combat GBV it is essential to recognize that this problem is central to all humanitarian issues (e.g. emergency relief, health, education, etc.) and not just those focused on gender. In this guide you will find information on some of the major issues within GBV, basic grant-application tips, 15 foundations that fund initiatives fighting GBV, and a list of networks and resources.

The principle of non-discrimination toward trafficking victims is an internationally accepted standard. Victims are often stigmatized within their communities for actions they committed while being trafficked. The U.N. Protocol states in article 14.2 that "the measures set forth in this Protocol shall be interpreted and applied in a way that is not discriminatory to persons on the ground that they are victims of trafficking in persons. The interpretation and application of those measures shall be consistent with internationally recognized principles of non-discrimination."

Article 3 of the Council of Europe Convention on Action against Trafficking in Human Beings states that "the implementation of the provisions of this Convention by Parties, in particular the enjoyment of measures to protect and promote the rights of victims, shall be secured without discrimination on any ground such as sex, race, color, language, religions, political or other opinion, national or social origin, associated with a national minority, property, birth or other status."

The United Nations Human Rights and Law Enforcement: A Manual on Human Rights Training for the Police states that law enforcement officials should be familiar with all the legal requirements of non-discrimination. In particular, law enforcement should adhere to, among others, the following principles: "Law enforcement officials shall at all times fulfill the duty imposed on them by law, by serving the community and by protecting all persons against illegal acts" and "it shall not be considered unlawfully discriminatory for police to enforce certain special measures designed to address the special status and needs of women (including pregnant women and new mothers), juveniles, the sick, the elderly, and others requiring special treatment in accordance with international human rights standards.

17.16.2 The Status of the Convention for the Elimination of All Forms of Discrimination Against Women (CEDAW)

Twenty Arab countries have joined or ratified the CEDAW, and the state of Palestine has committed to it under the presidential decree issued in the year 2009. The only country that has not joined or ratified the convention is Sudan.

However, a small number of countries recorded a reservation on more than one article of the convention because they conflict with national legislations, as is the case with Algeria, Bahrain, Lebanon and Kuwait which made a reservation on article 7(1) because the Kuwaiti constitution limits the right of nomination and election for males only.

Some countries indicated that their reservations are based on the presence of articles in the convention which conflict with Islamic Shari 'a, they are: Bahrain, Egypt, Iraq, Qatar, Kuwait, Libya, and Syria. Saudi Arabia made a general reservation on the entire convention based on the Islamic Shari 'a.

Most of these reservations focus on the following articles:

Article 2: on the prohibition of discrimination in constitutions and national legislations: reservations were made by Iraq, Algeria, Libya, Egypt, Bahrain, and Syria.
Article 7: on political and public life: a reservation was made by Kuwait.
Article 9: on citizenship laws: reservations were made by Jordan, Algeria, Iraq, Lebanon, Kuwait, Tunisia, Egypt, Saudi Arabia, Bahrain, Syria, and Oman.
Article 15 on equality before the law: reservations were made by Jordan, Algeria, Tunisia, Bahrain, Syria, and Oman.
Article 16: on marriage and family relations: reservations were made by most countries.
Article 29: on arbitration between states: reservations were made by most countries.

The careful evaluation of reservations indicates that most Arab countries do not oppose the core principles of the convention, but they are unwilling to commit to changing relevant articles in their laws, and most Arab countries made reservations specifically on Article 16, relating to the rights of men and women within the family. What distinguishes the convention and one of its' most important obligations is the conformity of national legislations with provisions of the convention. Article 2 of the convention shows that when ratifying the convention, countries that are doing so have to review their national legislations and make the necessary adjustments in order to ensure the implementation of the rights guaranteed by the convention, and to eliminate discrimination which is a main entry to the practice of violence.

The introduction of reservations on the essence and spirit of the convention denies Arab women the protection that makes them capable of demanding their rights.

Some countries withdrew their reservations, as was the case with Jordan in regards to paragraph 4 or Article 15, Algeria with Article 9(2), Kuwait with Article 7(1), and Egypt with Article 9(2)*. As for Libya, it has withdrawn all of its' reservations on the condition that the convention's provisions do not conflict with the Islamic Shari'a.

In other Arab countries which are concerned with conducting reviews of their legislations to make them compatible with the provisions of the convention, the participation of clerics in lobbying has a great importance in societies where the values of male domination prevail, and in countries where uniform laws of personal status are absent, and where civil rights fall under the jurisdiction of religious courts whose laws and regulations are not compatible with the principles and provisions of CEDAW. CEDAW grants women status equal to men, removes discrimination, promotes equal opportunities with men as full partners, ensures women's protection from violence and thus raises their ability to care for and protect their children.

The political situation (reservations on Article 9)—in terms of the non-acceptance of mothers granting their children nationality—also overlaps with social attitudes, under the pretext of lack of demographic balance which contributes to changing the identity of the nation and society.

17.17 Child Participation

17.17.1 Opinions and Positions Regarding the Three Forms of Sexual Violence

Opinions and positions of female teenagers, vis-à-vis honor crimes, early marriage and sexual harassment are reflective of their experience. Girls recall an attempt at sexual harassment against her. The majority of girls express frustration with the comments and pestering by males, while being quite aware of the differences between chatting up, sexual harassment and rape. Sexual violence against girls, in the forms of harassment and rape, are quite common in society.

Teenage girls are aware of cases of sexual harassment in real life, but rural girls from claim that men "preserve and protect the girls of the village". Some explain awareness of sexual harassment cases, "at school and in social establishments, we hear these stories...my friend had a similar experience".

Children give various reasons for harassment. They believe it was because the guy is mentally sick, that girls encouraged harassment, frustration that boys experience, macho values, TV, internet, movies, and reasons that include vengeance against the girl to ruin her reputation, hereditary conditions inherited from the father, boys trying to mimic what they see.

Male groups seem more informed about sexual harassment cases through the media. Some mention that sexual harassment occurs quite often in their community. Many blame this phenomenon on repression and deprivation while also on psychological psychosis or mental sickness.

Girls seem informed about crimes committed in the name of honor, but most do not consider themselves threatened or concerned. This could be explained by the fact that these crimes are not as widespread as sexual harassment. Children read about honor crimes mostly in social media, and some in the newspapers and magazines or through stories told. They consider them crimes committed in "closed villages" but not in their community. Teen groups give numerous examples of violence against girls, spanning from psychological violence to physical violence, which could start with battering and end up with murder. A girl going out with a boy could result in her father or brother beating her; she could be secluded in the house and denied education. If a girl returned home late, she could be abused. A wife cheating on her husband could lead the husband to kill her. If a guy flirts with a girl, it could result in a fight between him and the male members of her family.

Palestinian girls seem unaware of crimes committed in the name of honor. They point out that their community greatly mistrusts girls, which results in abusing her but not killing her. Examples of such abuses include "husbands suspecting in their wives"; furthermore, girls consider suspicion a form of abuse, in addition to beating. Regardless of their age, religion, region and educational level of their parents, girls condemn honor crimes. However, they do not confess to being themselves subjected to "honor-related" bodily violence.

Most of the teen boys reject honor crimes. Supporters of these crimes are concentrated and limited to the situation of conjugal infidelity.

Girls seem familiar with cases of early marriage. Nonetheless, they note that these kinds of marriages have decreased consequently to developments in the situation of the girl, and complexity of life. They also note that forced marriage has declined since girls are now more capable of expressing themselves than before. Girls consider the reasons behind early marriage to be the ignorance of parents and the girl, as well as the mentality which views marriage as a form of protection for the girl and her reputation. Other reasons include parents marrying their daughters for money, or because of relations. Girls invoke cases of blind love that push young girls to marry sometimes without the consent of their parents. Girls are aware of early marriages; however, most oppose early marriage, and refuse to embark on that experience. Very few girls support early marriage. Nonetheless, girls differentiated between forced marriage imposed by parents, and marriage consented by the girl. Therefore, 76% of girls did not consider early marriage consented by the girl as a form of sexual violence, compared to 24 per cent of girls who considered early marriage as a form of sexual violence, regardless of circumstances. Comparatively,

31 per cent of boys considered early marriage as sexual violence if it was forced, whereas 69 per cent considered it sexual violence in all its forms.

17.17.1.1 The Way Forward: Combating Sexual Violence

Teen age girls suggest the following to combat sexual violence:

- Raising awareness of parents, young boys and girls on the hazards of sexual violence.
- Dialogue and understanding between parents and children.
- Organizations to raise awareness in the different regions.
- Schools to raise awareness and provide sexual education.
- Awareness through media.
- Severe laws against sexual violence.
- Advocacy: role of schools, media, and social establishments to openly discuss the issue of violence. The main focus is to target parents, then teenagers.

Male teenagers concentrate on awareness campaigns targeting the different social, regional, and age groups.

Girls oppose the three forms of sexual violence against teenage girls [sexual harassment, honor crimes, and early marriages]. Moreover, most girls concur that the culture of honor begets sexual harassment and violence against girls.

The position of males regarding these three forms of violence is also positive, except regarding the subject of honor crimes which was supported by some males, but only in cases of conjugal infidelity. In comparison, girls rejected honor crimes under all situations. Many male teens find the honor culture responsible for sexual harassment and violence, whereas this percentage rockets remarkably among girls. However, an internalization of the culture of honor in boys and girls is possible to detect under the surface, limiting honor to girls and their behavior, namely sexual, and subsequent self-imposed behavioral restrictions on the girls, and a conviction within boys that they are the guardians of the girl's honor. Most boys believe that honor is good compared to few who consider it both good and bad. Boys who totally support the culture of honor justify as follows:

"Without honor, family trees would become ambiguous."
"Honor is necessary in a community."
"Honor is both good and bad. Disrespecting it leads to dishonor, clinging to it leads to isolation."
"Honor is good but it is a liability at the same time."

17.17.1.2 Reflections from Fieldwork: Child Protection from Discrimination

Girls have been socialized with the normative standards of honor. However, the level of acceptance of this internalization of values reveals relations to whether the girl accepts or rejects the status quo. The level of internalization increases where educational and occupational levels of parents decrease, in rural or urban poor regions. Teenage girls submit to the culture of honor and comply by its protocol in groups with low educational and occupational levels of parents; all these girls come from poor, popular areas. The educational and professional levels of parents in these groups is low, none are university graduates. Girls from these groups believe that their parents and the culture of honor both aim to preserve and protect them, this can explain why although some girls were dissatisfied with the honor culture they considered it as a good element.

The girls in these groups stress on focusing awareness campaigns towards parents as a means to combat violence. They explain that the lack of openness, dialogue and understanding between parents and child often leads to physical violence. Findings among the male groups reveal that submission to the honor culture is given more importance in poorer areas. Few males express their dissatisfaction with the honor culture: the majority belongs to fathers with low educational and professional levels. Dualisms in positions emerge with dissatisfaction with the culture of honor, but still consider honor to be good. In boys' eyes, honor that limits liberty is related to the restrictions imposed on girls in their environment "values imposed on girls bother us". However, abiding by these rules encourages their preservation rather than bypassing them, notwithstanding the discomfort resulting from the pressure these values impose.

Some indicators that highlight the pressure imposed on boys became evident with rape: Few boys would disclose it compared to most who would not and some who refrain to answer. Some of the reasons for keeping the rape a secret:

Boys and girls internalize the culture of honor which consecrates the stereotyped roles and the lesser role of women, even though girls are dissatisfied with this culture that limits their freedom in comparison to boys. A teenage boy enjoys more independence in his daily life than a girl does. Conversely, criticism of the culture does not reflect the development or evolution of gender-awareness among teenagers in the different groups.

On the contrary, submission to the culture of honor prevails, although at different levels among the rich and average classes on the one side, and the poor classes on the other; the variable of rural versus urban areas does not play a major role in the submission. The highest levels of submission are registered with the poorest and the lowest educational and professional levels of parents.

There is a deep internalization of the traditional concept of honor amongst the male and female teenagers, which drives female teenagers not only to submit to the standards of this culture but also to assume the responsibility of any behavior that contradicts it. The position that personifies this attitude is most represented in the story of a 19-year old suffering from mental retardation, which resulted, as medically proven, from her difficult life conditions. Notwithstanding her condition, she was raped at the age of 16 by four guys who deflowered her and paid her 1000 Lebanese Pounds as a reward (less than one US Dollar). The mother stitched the hymen, the main symbol of the honor culture in our community, but this girl still blamed herself for the rape, "I was most bothered with myself, how could I do this? How did I sell my body to these people?"

Another girl 14-years old was sexually harassed by her father since her childhood, as was her sister who was pregnant with an incestuous child, representing a second pattern of societal violence which puts the responsibility on the victim, even if just a child. Another teenager was saddened by the behavior of her maternal aunt, who instead of taking them in, showed them open aversion, "she has long exposed us in the neighborhood and sneered at us and our father".

Results of the field work show an increased awareness among teenage boys and girls of the risks resulting from the phenomenon of sexual violence in all three forms studied in this research. This became obvious in their knowledge that sexual violence against girls is a violation of their child rights, and their knowledge of its negative effect on the life of the girl, her family and community. Male and female teenagers consider that crimes perpetrated in the name of honor are an expression of ignorance and backwardness. They oppose early marriage for girls, based on its negative impact, but also on the family as a whole (relation to the partner and children). Teenagers show great consciousness of the need to fight sexual violence in the forms of harassment or rape and to denounce the rape as well as the rapist.

All these positions are considered qualitative indicators of the increase in awareness most probably related to the widespread of media in a globalizing world, and subsequently important sharing of information. These positive trends however, failed to cover the lack of interest in the phenomenon of violence against girls. Moreover, the position of teenage girls and boys is short of neutral regarding gender-based discrimination and its relation to the three forms under study of sexual violence. Shortcoming touches also the official position, despite the remarkable progress noted at the legislative level, and subsequent ratification of the CEDAW and the CRC, due to the negligence in addressing the different legislative gaps.

Concurrently, the expanding official and NGO efforts remain partial with regards to sexual violence against teenage girls since it is considered, in light of the prevailing attitude, as an invasion of the "private circle" and which occasionally refuses to recognize the existence of this violence.

Moreover, sexual violence, with the exception of violence in the form of early marriage, remains within the realm of taboos, and hence, it is difficult to assess its prevalence in Arab countries undergoing armed conflicts and human displacements.

Achievements in the field of sexual violence against girls, in addition to achievements at the legislative level, are limited to preventive and protective measures divided amongst the pertinent ministries, as well as some non-governmental organizations and coalitions.

17.17.1.3 Weakened Voices of Teenage Girls in the Middle East

The problems of children in various cultures worldwide are perceived and treated as what they are, that is as children. Much of the specific problems are linked to the fact that they are considered as adults in their societies. The most extreme example of this problem is with child-mothers and child-laborers, nevertheless children in honor cultures also face the same set of problems.

Children are seen as morally mature and are expected to adhere to a strict moral code in honor societies. They are not excused because they are children. Generally, "childhood" has been described as being a Western concept, however all signatories of the CRC have agreed to this concept and recognized that special rights for children are beneficial for their development as human beings. The difficulty to accept the first and most fundamental principle often leads to the violations of many other articles as a logical consequence.

17.18 Articles of the CRC Are Pillars and Instruments

The second article guarantees the child freedom from discrimination on any grounds, including sex, religion, ethnic or social origin, birth or other status. This project examines a typical form of gender-based discrimination. This is not to say that boys do not suffer from the same kind of problems: Boys are also subjected to sexual abuse, early marriages, and are also oppressed by honor-values. Like girls, boys are also victims however we have chosen to focus this study on teenage girls only, because we feel they have been neglected in child right issues in the MENA region. Moreover, we believe that girls carry a heavier burden, in the honor-culture, and pay a higher price in early marriages than boys.

The main point of the third article in the CRC is that "In all actions concerning children ... the best interests of the child shall be a primary consideration". In cases of early marriage we can conclude that it is not in the best interest of the child. Sexual violence and exploitation are cases of children being objectified and neglected in their status as human beings.

Responsibilities of safeguarding the interest of the child is raised in article 5, that says: "States Parties shall respect the responsibilities, rights and duties of parents or, where applicable, the members of the extended family or community as provided for by local custom, legal guardians or other persons legally responsible for the child, to provide, in a manner consistent with the evolving capacities of the child, appropriate direction and guidance in the exercise by the child of the rights recognized in the present Convention...." Parents and guardians have an important role in protecting children from sexual violence.

However in the MENA region parents, in some sense, misunderstand their responsibilities as they sometimes force their children into early marriage as a mean of "protecting" them. Sexual abuse often happens within families.

Furthermore, honor related violence against girls is almost always committed by family members. Their role and neglect must be emphasized, which can be seen as a violation of article 6 in the CRC that discusses support for the survival and development of children.

Honor violence that sometimes leads to killing jeopardizes the survival and development of girls. We can conclude that all forms of sexual violence threaten the child's life and development and are against the best interest of the child.

Articles 12–14 deal with issues that include the child's right to express his or her view, freedom of thought, and having access to information... These articles have been violated in the case of forced marriages and sexual intercourse with children; where the voice and opinion of the child is not heard, but rather ignored. However, not all child marriages are by definition forced since it may be easy to convince a, per definition "naïve", child to marry.

Again, we stress the role of parents in such situations and children's trust and dependency on them. The decision regarding who and when to marry is fundamental to each individual's life, and should be taken by mature adults, free from any kind of pressure, neither physical nor psychological. Child marriages, involving persons below the age of 18 years violate these rights. In the countries examined in this study, marriage is permitted for children 18 years old and younger. In connection to these articles from the CRC, it can also be noted that most Muslim states do not recognize the child's right to freedom of religion as expressed in article 14.

It is important to stress parents' responsibility regarding sexual violence against girls in the region. Article 18 in the CRC discusses the role of parents and guardians noting that: "States Parties shall use their best efforts to ensure recognition of the principle that both parents have common responsibilities for the upbringing and development of the child. Parents or, as the case may be, legal guardians, have the primary responsibility for the upbringing and development of the child. The best interests of the child will be their basic concern.

For the purpose of guaranteeing and promoting the rights set forth in the present Convention, States Parties shall render appropriate assistance to parents and legal guardians in the performance of their child-rearing responsibilities and shall ensure the development of institutions, facilities and services for the care of children. States Parties shall take all appropriate measures to ensure that children of working parents have the right to benefit from child-care services and facilities for which they are eligible."

The article also indicates the role of governments to ensure that parents have access to facilities needed to care for their children. Our research reveals that political instability and economic underdevelopment sometimes cause parents to force their daughters into early marriages. It is the responsibility of governments to provide welfare structures for its citizens and children however the role of parents must not be neglected.

Article 19 deals with violence and stresses that each child has the right to protection from "all forms of physical or mental violence, injury or abuse, maltreatment or exploitation, including sexual abuse, while in the care of parent(s), legal guardian(s) or any other person who has the care of the child."

Since commercial sexual-abuse is not a major problem in the MENA region, it is important to focus on the role of parents and guardians in domestic gender based sexual violence. When it comes to honor-related violence, which could be seen as "tradition", article 24 is applicable. The UN considers honor-violence as a harmful traditional-practice but has predominantly focused on the issue of female genital mutilation (Connors 2005: 29).

This article articulates the right to health, access to health services and protection from traditional practices prejudicial to the health of the child. Thus, children should be protected against harmful-traditions and honor-related violence such as early marriages that can be categorized as such: traditions with negative consequences for children's health. The medical risks of early pregnancy and childbirth are well documented, but we also want to emphasize the psychological aspects of a "stolen childhood".

Articles 28 and 29 examine the right of the child to education on the basis of equal opportunity. Through our research we have discovered that punishment against girls who refuse to marry the husband chosen for them, or that violate other codes-of-conduct expected by their parents regarding their behavior with men, include house-arrest and denial of education for honor related reasons.

Again we find cultural-specific traits in gender-based violence violating basic child rights. Furthermore, in practice an early marriage is a denial of the right to education unless the state can provide schools for young mothers. However, such policy might be contradictive to the struggle of increasing the age for marriage and can be seen as controversial in this perspective.

Article 31 supports the child's right "to rest and leisure, to engage in play and recreational activities appropriate to the age of the child and to participate freely in cultural life and the arts."

Furthermore States Parties should "respect and promote the right of the child to participate fully in cultural and artistic life and shall encourage the provision of appropriate and equal opportunities for cultural, artistic, recreational and leisure activity." Girls in honor-cultures are denied leisure time, or to play with boys, as they are kept inside and are subjected to strong moral rules.

Playing and some movements are seen as inappropriate even for very young girls. Playing games and bicycling are examples of leisure's that are not always accepted for girls in many honor-societies because of the fear that the girl may "loose her virginity" during such activities.[21] In my previous study in the region based on interviews with teenage girls, one important opinion expressed by girls from several settings was their wish for society to accept the idea of friendship between girls and boys, so that they could play and interact with each other.

This can be seen as their wish to be perceived as children by society rather than sexual subjects, especially at such an early age; according to the CRC this wish

[21]The issue of the existence of a hymen and the idea that virginity can be "lost" is questioned in modern medical research. It has been recognized that no "hymen" exists, but rather a small fold of mucous membrane in the vagina, see Cinthio 2007.

should be encouraged. Moreover, the girls' right to rest, play and leisure is violated because they have to stay inside their homes in order for them to be "good girls". At home, they are often expected to carry out rather heavy domestic work; this links us to the next article (number 32) in the CRC expressing: "States Parties recognize the right of the child to be protected from economic exploitation and from performing any work that is likely to be hazardous or to interfere with the child's education, or to be harmful to the child's health or physical, mental, spiritual, moral or social development." This article also says that the state shall set minimum age for employment and regulate working conditions. Teenage girls in MENA are often required to do unpaid, domestic work. In my opinion, this is a form of child labor, but somehow neglected in the formulation of this article. Domestic work affects the child's education, health and development negatively and should not be forgotten in this context.

Articles 34–36 deal directly with various forms of sexual abuse against children. Because of the topic of this report, these articles are quoted in full below (note: short version of the CRC):

Article 34 "States Parties undertake to protect the child from all forms of sexual exploitation and sexual abuse. For these purposes, States Parties shall in particular take all appropriate national, bilateral and multilateral measures to prevent: (a) The inducement or coercion of a child to engage in any unlawful sexual activity; (b) The exploitative use of children in prostitution or other unlawful sexual practices; (c) The exploitative use of children in pornographic performances and materials."

Article 35: "States Parties shall take all appropriate national, bilateral and multilateral measures to prevent the abduction of, the sale of or traffic in children for any purpose or in any form."

Article 36: "States Parties shall protect the child against all other forms of exploitation prejudicial to any aspects of the child's welfare."

Children have the right to protection from all forms of sexual exploitation and sexual abuse. However, sexual abuse of children may be considered "legal" when it is committed within the framework of marriage and thus hidden from public view. We suggest that such marriages, whether forced, temporary, or tourist marriages involving children is a form of sexual abuse and violates these articles in the CRC. We are aware that this suggestion may be seen as controversial since such marriages are legally accepted in the MENA society. In the First World Conference against Commercial Sexual Exploitation in Stockholm 1996, the question whether or not early and forced marriages are a form of sexual abuse against children was debated. End Child Prostitution Child Pornography and Trafficking (ECPAT) stated that "if we identify prostitution as an economic transaction with no consent from the child, then the situation could be identical to forced marriages. There is no consent, and it is an economic transaction because the deal is done through the parents." (Hamdan 2002) Parents are important stakeholders in combating sexual violence, but the legal system is also responsible for sexual abuse of children if they do not increase the legal age of marriage to 18.

Societies in the MENA region have weak resources to deal with victims of sexual abuse. In honor-cultures victims are usually blamed for being sexually assaulted or raped, rather than the offender. In some cases, victims of crimes prefer to be imprisoned since this may be the only way to protect themselves from violence and killing in the name of honor.

Article 37 deals with juvenile justice and could be applicable in the case of imprisoning the victims of sexual abuse, stating that: "No child shall be subjected to torture, cruel treatment or punishment, unlawful arrest or deprivation of liberty. Both capital punishment and life imprisonment without the possibility of release are prohibited for offences committed by persons below 18 years.

Any child deprived of liberty shall be separated from adults unless it is considered in the child's best interests not to do so. A child who is detained shall have legal and other assistance as well as contact with the family." To imprison victims year after year is definitely a crime against the CRC. This issue must be taken into consideration when combating sexual abuse in the MENA region.

17.19 Challenges and Difficulties Faced in the Implementation of International Recommendations to Combat Violence Against Children

Arab countries share rising concern about the status of children and respect for their rights. Key challenges in the Arab world in this regard lie in the weakness of development of holistic social policies that are based on special needs of marginalized social groups, the limitation of the programs, and the issue of comprehensive and specialized action plans that address poverty without identifying the appropriate needed measures to prevent or address the causes for violence against children. This is mainly due to the close correlation between violence and poverty.

Child protection also requires a common understanding of concepts and definitions along with a dependence on scientific research in order to unify the vision and strategies, and a reliance on general frameworks, accompanied by a mainstreaming of reflecting these frameworks at the Arab level to ensure that the objectives of the action plan are met.

A key challenge is that the legislative environment in the Arab world is not ready yet to put in place a legal framework that comprehensively protects children against all forms of violence, bad treatment and exploitation. The sensitivity of this topic, and given that it can be considered a violation of a family's privacy and interference in its affairs in some communities, poses another challenge related to this issue.

Accordingly, seeking a legislation that protects children from all forms of violence (sexual exploitation, internet crimes, etc.) might take a long time to become effective for it to be effective enough, which poses an obstacle towards achieving a comprehensive protection for children against violence. There is, therefore, a need to rally social action lobbying and attain community support in order to change mentalities, reduce social taboos and build coordinated plans.

Arab states also need to enhance priority given to child protection via the establishment of a comprehensive system for child protection, and by identifying the components of the system that are overlapping, crosscutting or poorly coordinated. In addition, there is a need to restructure the working methodology in general, and identify the strengths and weaknesses of available resources and the general attitudes of the state in particular.

Another difficulty is the scarcity of specialized local centers to receive child victims; when found, they lack appropriate and quality specialized services and programs, structures and human resources.

The concept of child protection is part of a child's rights -based approach by countries, communities and individuals, and remains, therefore, a priority in the development of specialized programs and policies to address violence against children. Weak human resources and the lack of specialization in children protection issues also hinder the execution of action plans. Obstacles in the planning and implementation process include a lack of dedicated resources at the level of ministries, in terms of budgets or institutional support for the implementation of programs; a lack of analytical studies to evaluate levels of spending; a lack of mechanisms to attract child-friendly budgets; and a lack of investments and benefits from international support and funding for children in most Arab countries.

Furthermore, the conditions being experienced by some countries in the region under occupation, or in situations of war or civil conflict, stand as significant barriers to the implementation of the recommendations of the UNSG's Study of VAC.

Given the disparities in the legal frameworks and institutions in the Arab countries that should protect children against violence, the development of joint Arab action is required, and taking advantage of available expertise in the region is imperative; there is always a need for more engagement with international organizations, particularly UNICEF, to support these efforts.

But the biggest challenge, according to the report, is the extent and effectiveness of children's involvement and the partnership with youth, from planning to evaluation. Such involvement shall take place throughout the process and in the preparation of child-specific strategies. Meanwhile, mechanisms are to be established to allow children to enjoy their freedom of speech in discussing their issues, needs and the solutions they can offer.

17.20 The Role of Communities in Confronting Gender Dimension

The legal and regulatory framework for civil society organizations impacts directly upon their capacity to deliver social services, to conduct efficient social action or to influence public policy.

Within the Arab region, government's attitudes to civil society vary considerably, with a wide diversity of laws and practices throughout the region.[22]

In most of the states of the Arab region, freedom of association remains the exception rather than the rule, and many of the countries have detained or arrested vocal human rights defenders and activists. Establishing a CSO requires a permit by the relevant ministry, and going through lengthy administrative and security clearance processes. Decisions of the administrative authority remain often discretionary and not open to judiciary recourse.

CSOs in the Arab region stress the need for eliminating all legislative, administrative and security restrictions imposed on the establishment and management of NGOs, syndicates and trade unions, political parties and mass communication media. They also call for the free flow of information and freedoms of expression, belief and assembly as well as legislation in accordance with international standards.

NGOs in the Arab region encounter an array of obstacles in fulfilling their role as co-responsible parties. The legislative environment remains restrictive in many of the countries. Freedom of association and assembly in most countries remains severely limited, with NGOs having to apply for permission to register and to hold meetings, which are often arbitrarily refused. In addition to the often inhibiting legal and regulatory frameworks and the restrictions imposed by governments, Arab.

NGOs are also limited in a number of cases by internal factors which hinder their impact, including: weak internal governance and organizational structures; precarious, conditional or donor-driven funding; organizational fragmentation and ideological polarizations.

17.21 Countries' Specific Plans

With respect to gender-specific action plans, states' approaches generally lack clarity in the area of gender-based to end violence against children. However, most countries have indicated that legislation is in place that is compatible with a policy of equality between sexes, although variations exist between the details of such laws in different countries.

Some countries like Jordan, the UAE, and Bahrain, have enshrined the principle of non-discrimination in their constitutions, and translated such principles into legislation, laws and national programs for child protection. For example, the Family Protection Department in Jordan handles issues of victims of domestic violence while observing gender-sensitive practices such as having trained female police officers deal with female victims throughout proceedings. Due to the sensitivity and specificity of female cases, the Department takes gender requisites into

[22]The Comparative Arab Report on Implementing the Recommendations of the UN Secretary-General's Study on Violence Against Children, League of Arab States, 2010.

consideration when managing such cases and maintains statistics on case management incorporating gender-related indicators.

Bahrain also notes that female police officers manage the cases of victimized children of both sexes. The country's constitution guarantees equality within the community regardless of sex, origin, language, religion or belief; the right to equality is provided for under the laws on family custody, education and health; under the social security law; the child protection law and a forthcoming law intended to end domestic violence.

In Tunisia, the development of programs and interventions are based on a gender-sensitive and human rights-based approach in punitive and rehabilitation-focused interventions. In this context, the National Office for Family and Population Program advocates for "gender-based parity and ending of violence"; adolescents and young people are encouraged to integrate the values of honesty and tolerance into their personal conduct, and to reject violence in all its forms through dialogues, meetings and other activities.

In Algeria, the government considers gender-sensitive policies and programs in the development of strategies, including the national strategy on ending violence against women and girls, and the preparation of a national strategy to empower and integrate women

In Saudi Arabia, the gender dimension has recently been mainstreamed in the development of the national strategy on ending domestic violence against women and children. This national strategy is yet to be ratified by the appropriate bodies.

Sudan adopted the national policy for empowerment of women in 2007; this policy has been taken into account in the qualitative development of all plans, policies and programs in accordance with the provisions of the Interim Sudan Constitution of 2005. The national plan to end violence against children takes into account the gender dimension in issues of ending violence.

In Syria, legislation targets crimes of violence and gender-victimization, taking into consideration the nature of the criminal act and the age of the victim. Several provisions in the penal code consider the child gender (male or female) and the nature of the criminal act, as well as the relationship between the perpetrator and the victim (parents or other relatives and caregivers). The anti-prostitution law plays a discriminatory role in terms of the rights of females and males, with disparity with regard to punishments to redress the damage inflicted upon the victim. The gender dimension is further considered in a decree against human trafficking. The Constitution guarantees women equality with men; the laws on labor and education also carry similar provisions for equality.

Iraq states that its laws do not support discrimination between citizens; however, dominant cultural values allow for gender-based discrimination, including within the family and household, and proscribe distinct roles for males and females.

Policies in Oman advocate non-discrimination between males and females; Oman guarantees equal opportunities for both sexes, and ensures specific political, socio-economical, and military rights for women, in accordance with the country's basic law and various conventions like the CEDAW.

In Palestine, the gender dimension is considered upon recruitment of staffers who work in the area of child protection, and Palestinian law also takes into account the rights of both sexes.

In Qatar, the constitution provides for equality for all before the law without gender discrimination, origin or tongue; national laws are consistent with these constitutional principles.

The same applies to the implementation of child-specific plans and policies, to consideration of biological difference, including the physical abilities of each sex, as well as to social conditions, mental health and living conditions.

Kuwait takes into account gender-sensitive issues when addressing violence against children, and the community does not discriminate between males and females. Educational, social and health services are provided across the country without discrimination.

Under the Lebanese constitution, all citizens are equal in terms of their rights and duties without discrimination based on gender.

Libya draws on the Islamic Shari'a law in this regard, and implements this law equally stipulating human rights for both sexes while taking into account their biological differences.

In Egypt, the constitution ensures the principle of equality among all citizens without discrimination, and the country is committed to highlighting this issue in all its laws. The provisions of the children's rights law No. 12 of 1996 as amended by law No. 126 of 2008 provide for the child's right to nondiscrimination with provisions almost identical to those under article 2 of the Convention on the Rights of the Child. The amendments address several issues, including the elimination of specific forms of discrimination, be they against young girls, against children in rural areas or against those from poor or marginalized families. These amendments also eliminate discrimination against children born out of wedlock, and discrimination in the granting of nationality and in the minimum age set for female marriage; in addition, the amendments also criminalize early marriage and FGM/C, and provide for the child's right to free and quality education, the right to health care and to protection against violence and harmful practices; these provisions are incorporated in different laws, like the nationality law on non-discrimination between men and women and the provisions of the law on pension security for the poor. The present report deals with these amendments in detail under the current legislation.

In Mauritania, the "Women and Gender Empowerment Department" of the Ministry of Social Affairs, Children and Family is working toward mainstreaming the gender dimension in all the policies and programs adopted by the government, particularly those targeting children.

In Yemen, the state guarantees equal rights for males and females, such as the right to education, while encouraging girls to receive education. Yemen also has established a task force on the education of girls under both the Ministry of Education and the Ministry of Technical Education and Vocational Training, and has developed a national strategy for female education. The country's constitution, CEDAW and other provisions under international conventions include several articles emphasizing respect for the rights of male and female children; the laws and legislation include no provisions discriminating between women and men, as long as they are not in contradiction with the provisions of Islamic Shari'a. A number of laws have been amended to ensure mainstreaming of gender issues, including in the law on nationality and the civil status law.

17.22 Equity

Most of the countries indicated the existence of legislation consistent with the policy of equity and equality between the sexes. In Jordan and the UAE, the principle of non-discrimination is embodied in the Constitution. Tunisia has a gender approach in the development of programs and interventions, through the National Office for Family and Human Development.

Algeria has a gender approach in policies and programs in the development of national strategies to combat violence against women and girls.

In Saudi Arabia, gender dimension is part of the national strategy.

The Syrian legislation has a Penal Code taking into account the gender of the baby and the nature of the act; the law against prostitution also avoids discrimination in the rights of female and male. Iraq explained that their laws do not support discrimination between citizens, but the dominant culture in society and specifically in the family makes a distinction between the roles according to gender-based discrimination.

In Oman, the statute does not differentiate the state and legislation, rights, duties and norms.

In Qatar, plans and policies for children considers age and sex differences as well as physical ability, environment and circumstances, health and living conditions.

In Kuwait, the state is gender-sensitive when dealing with the issue of violence against children; community does not discriminate in the rights of males and females.

In Lebanon, the Constitution ensures that all citizens are equal in rights and duties without any discrimination based on gender.

Libya has suggested the Islamic law in this regard. The Constitution in Egypt provides the principle of equality among all citizens, without discrimination.

In Yemen the State guarantees that male and female have equal rights such as the right of education, while encouraging girls to engage in education; Yemen even created a working group on education of girls in Ministry of Education, and prepared a National Strategy for the education of girls.

The Egyptian Penal Code brings forward gender issues, such as rape, female death, female genital mutilation, and exploitation or trafficking of children or using them in research and scientific experiments, Internet crimes, child prostitution and pornography.

In Jordan, The National Strategy for Jordanian women made positive changes in the situation of Jordanian women, removed all forms of discrimination and achieved effective and equal participation in all spheres of life, political and economic, social and cultural.

In Tunisia, women have received—since independence—social and legal protection, aimed at achieving the full participation of women as a partner in building a modern state, on August 131,956, and canceled polygamy, identified the minimum age for (equal for both sexes, eighteen years in 2007), abolished the right to reparation enjoyed by the father to marry his daughter and adopted a judicial divorce. In politics, women were granted the right to vote and stand for elections since independence. Tunisia ratified international agreements related to women's rights such as the Convention and the Protocol on the Elimination of All Forms of Discrimination against Women.

17.23 Addressing Gender Discrimination

In general, a group of Arab states is moving towards the establishment of ministries, institutions or departments for women, children and families, mainly as supervisory, regulatory and guiding institutions. These are mandated to follow up on the implementation of strategies and government planning to protect children and women. To this end, ministries, councils and human rights organizations have increasingly assigned civil society organizations specialized roles, thereby accumulating experiences in the area of needs assessment, policy definition, program development, implementation and follow-up; accordingly, the gender aspect will be institutionalized in all policies, legislation, action plans and programs.

Algeria adopted a national strategy to prevent and combat violence against women and girls, as the National Commission for the protection and promotion of human rights report annually to the President.

In Syria, rehabilitation center for girl's juvenile delinquents is becoming a national center, and supports an information campaign in cooperation with the Ministry of Information on the impact of violence against women on the Syrian economy and society.

Iraq adopted the International Convention on the Elimination of All Forms of Discrimination against Women.

Oman ensures non-discrimination between male and female, where the State guarantees equal opportunities. In this regard, a National Human Rights Commission is established.

Qatar highlighting the rights of women in different rights (civil, political, economic and social rights, family rights, the right to special care, etc.) in a number of national laws included in the Constitution, such as the law of nationality, election law, labor law, Civil Service Law, Law on military service, compulsory education law, family law, civil law, and a number of laws on protection and care. In Lebanon, the State guarantees women's participation in political, economic and social development.

Libya provides the Great Green Charter for Human Rights and the Law on Protection of Children and promotes women's rights and equality in all rights and duties.

Egypt has the amended Children's Act 2008, raising the age of marriage for girls and bringing the minimum age for marriage for both sexes to 18 years, also criminalizing female circumcision and child trafficking, amending some laws, such as the personal status and nationality law, the Social Insurance Act. The Egyptian women assume almost all positions: judges, heads of city councils, mayors. The State guarantees the service free and compulsory education and free health services to all without distinction of gender, including health care and delivery.

Morocco achieves social justice and establishes equality between sexes, through the family code, Labor Code, Penal Code, Nationality Act, and organizes annually a National Campaign to combat violence against women, for a month, with continuous public communication.

In Yemen, the Constitution guarantees the opportunity for all citizens to exercise their rights politically, socially and economically; also, the Child Rights Act ensures public freedom, protection and care for child and women in particular, without discrimination of sex, color; the Code of Criminal Procedure emphasizes equality for all citizens, with special rights for women's as work (in cases of pregnancy, childbirth and breastfeeding); the Government also issued a number of laws to protect children in difficult circumstances, as a Juvenile Welfare Act 1992 amended in 1997. It also established an independent judiciary body and other protection measures, including the Supreme Council for Motherhood and Childhood.

Overall, Arab states establish ministries, institutions or special departments of women and children and family, supervisory and regulatory guidelines, to follow up the implementation of strategies and the government's plans to protect children and women.

Some States have taken measures and actions to promote the protection of human rights, especially women and girls, and to address all forms of gender discrimination as part of a comprehensive strategy to prevent violence.

There is evidence of focus by most countries on the legal aspect of children's protection against violence, but they lack clear, quality data regarding policies, programs and measures to stop violence against children and address all forms of gender-based discrimination.

Part VI
Conclusion

The Cairo declaration clearly requested to ban all forms of violence against children Child protection from all forms of violence. Participants from OIC State Members valued the presence and contribution of the newly appointed Special Representative of the SG on Violence against Children, Dr. Marta Santos Pais, and expressed their commitment to develop productive cooperation with the Special Representative and to provide her with necessary technical and financial support. In light of the child's equal right to respect his or her human dignity and physical integrity, participants to the Conference recommend to the OIC member States to take all appropriate legislative, social and other measures for an effective follow-up to the recommendations made in the UN Study on Violence Against Children.[1]

Participants called upon the OIC Member States to urgently review and reform their legislation to ensure the prohibition of all forms of violence against children and to link law reform with promotion of positive, non-violent forms of discipline. Building upon the promising experiences of OIC Member States, particular attention should be given to the prevention and combat against harmful practices, including FGM, child marriage, crimes committed in the name of honor, the use of children as camel jockeys, child trafficking, child domestic service and other forms of child labor.

Building upon positive national experiences from OIC Member States, participants to the Conference recommend that each State establish a high level focal point to coordinate all actions to prevent and combat all forms of violence against children, and promote the development of a well-resourced national strategy on violence against children, engaging with civil society, including children and young people.[2]

Participants requested:

1. That efforts should be exerted to provide protection for children under occupation, and in times of war. They demanded that those who violate the CRC by

[1]Cairo Declaration on the CRC and Islam, Cairo, 23–24 November 2009.

[2]Elie Mekhael, Dr. Kamal Mostafa Khalil, Aida Ghorbal, Child Law in Arab States: Reality and Hope, League of Arab States, 2010.

killing children or subjecting them to imprisonment, corporal and/or psychological torture, should be made accountable and brought to court.
2. That poverty alleviation should be targeted, as poverty is considered a primary cause for children's main problems that lead to their deprivation of enjoying a normal life.

Participants encourage the OIC and its Member States to facilitate the establishment of a children's forum to promote the contribution of children to the process of follow-up to the UN Study on Violence against Children and to keep children informed about developments in this area.

– Child marriage

Participants call upon all OIC Member States to raise the age of marriage to 18, ensuring full consent and registration of marriage.

– FGM

Participants to the Conference recommend the OIC member States to prohibit by law all forms of FGM and undertake awareness raising and informative campaigns, and promote social mobilization in close consultation and cooperation with the traditional and religious leadership, NGOs, as well as with parliamentarians, to support the enforcement of the prohibition and the promotion of abandonment of this practice, and to provide people who are involved in this practice with alternative employment.

Participants call on OIC Member States to take necessary measures to respond to children in conflict with the law without resorting to judicial proceedings providing that human rights and legal safeguards are fully respected, including community service, restorative justice, (taking into account the Lima 2009—Declaration on Restorative Juvenile Justice).

Participants call on OIC Member States to take measures to ensure that all children in conflict with the law are provided with free legal or other appropriate assistance and that deprivation of liberty, including pre-trial detention, is only used as a measure of last resort and for the shortest possible period of time, by fully implementing recommendations of the CRC Committee made in Gen. Comment No. 10 regarding the use of pre-trial detention and by introducing and effectively using suspended sentencing and early release.

Participants call on OIC Member States to take legislative measures to abolish the imposition of capital punishment on persons who committed a crime when under the age of 18, and suspend the execution of any pending capital punishment. Furthermore, it is recommended to abolish all forms of life imprisonment for crimes committed before the age of 18.

Participants call on OIC Member States to take legislative measures to ensure that children deprived of their liberty have access to education, adequate health care and to sports and other leisure opportunities, can maintain regular contact with their parents and other family members and are fully protected against all forms of violence, including inhuman and degrading treatment or punishment.

Participants call on OIC Member States to safeguard the rights of child victims and witnesses involved with judicial proceedings and take into consideration relevant UN standards and guidelines.

Addressing violence against children in the Middle East and North Africa region is the responsibility of the whole society including the state. The state bears an essential responsibility in that respect since it is the party that drafts policies, draws legislations that serve those policies, follows up their implementation, in addition to providing the necessary resources for the implementation of those programs, ensuring that they are not based on short term projects—scope and duration—but rather on a nationwide sustainable strategy. In this perspective, it is critical that the child victim of violence in all Arab programs and policies is not addressed as an object for charity or protection alone, but rather as a present non-voting citizen, entitled to all human rights and a life free of violence.

Recently, it is noticed that the issue of violence against children is marginalized in a growing number of countries in Middle East and North Africa. Many of them have weakened councils and national organizations concerned with human rights in general or even with the rights of children in particular. Still, Violence against children is now addressed in a way that includes more socially sensitive areas, such as violence inflicted by parents on children in the context of the family, or early marriage or traditions and norms that lead to violent practices against children, like FGM and honor crimes. The theoretical model needs however implementation, evaluation and sustainability.

The right perspective in addressing any form of violence is an essential perspective and entry point to enable interventions and legal amendments to protect that right in the face of violations.
This perspective also requires that children be an essential actor in the design of intervention policies, their evaluation, monitoring of implementation and their amendment or development leading to a sustainable protection of that right.

The Arab professionals gave birth to the APNPCAN, in 2004, and changed the name to APNPVAC in order to comply with the layout of the UNSV. Both ISPCAN and the Arab network played an active role in the 2005 MENA regional UNSV consultation context, the 2006 ICRC critics in Geneva and the 2007 UNSV report and meeting in Cairo. The network contributed to widen the platform of interventions and deepen their efficiency in confronting violence against children, as this problem appears to be more and more accepted as the responsibility of the society as a whole. The inclusion of the informal sectors in the State prerogatives remains however a challenge in many countries. The emerging child protection movement is presently in a continuously growing, expanding, and hopefully inclusive and participative design.

The result of this social congruence and intersectoral teamwork, led by professionals, with children with whom they work, will be a mixture of cultures, values, beliefs and challenges.

Ensure Accountability and End Impunity[3]

States should build community confidence in the justice system by, inter alia, bringing all perpetrators of violence against children to justice and ensure that they are held accountable through appropriate 'No matter whether violence against children occurs in the family, school, community, institution or workplace, health workers are the front line for responding to it. We must make our contribution to ensuring that such violence is prevented from occurring in the first place, and that where it does occur children receive the best possible services to reduce its harmful effects". Anders Nordström, Acting Director-General, WHO an end to violence against children criminal, civil, administrative and professional proceedings and sanctions. Persons convicted of violent offences and sexual abuse of children, should be prevented from working with children.

In Tunisia, crimes against children are considered in the context of the circumstances of the criminal act in order to administer punishment to aggressors. In Saudi Arabia, where Islamic Shari'a is the basis of legislation, the judiciary system holds accountable the perpetrators of crimes against children according to the gravity of the offense committed.

In Syria, the penal code allows for the addition of harsher penalties for the crime in case it is committed against a child. In Palestine, the Palestinian child act and the penal code deny impunity for perpetrators of child abuse. In Qatar, the constitution ensures equality and non-discrimination between citizens and residents before the law.

In Morocco, forthcoming procedures will accelerate the pace of judicial proceedings and enforce the principle of no impunity; units have also been created in the public prosecution to handle issues of childhood, especially in matters related to violence; strict instructions are given to punish all perpetrators of offenses committed against children. Some NGOs working in the area of interventions against violence against children can act as a civil party supporting children victims of violence.

In Egypt, lawmakers have recently introduced a provision doubling the minimum penalty prescribed for all crimes committed by adults against children. In Yemen, a family protection unit was created to attend to women's and children's issues within the General Directorate of Police; the Interior Ministry and the Ministry of Justice are to study the creation of family courthouses in some provinces.

Furthermore, legal amendments relating to children are proposed to be introduced to the draft penal code and presented before the House of Representatives for discussion and approval. The amendment's provisions involve legislative penalties against perpetrators in connection to bullying, exploitation and abuse against children.

---

[3]"Investing in the Children of the Islamic World", UNICEF, 2005.

Provide Special Health Services, Recovery and Social Reintegration[4]

Arab countries provide a range of services accessible health care before entering the hospital or in emergency situations. There are a range of programs and pilot projects in this area, such as developing procedures and protocols governing the coordination between the actors and the provision of specialized units fixed or mobile to deal with issues of violence, and maternal and child health, and training programs for health workers and doctors to distinguish the signs and symptoms resulting from this violence, and training and assigning staff specializing in the early detection of symptoms of violence and reporting. Jordan has developed procedures and protocols, especially the Ministry of Health to deal with cases of domestic violence.

Health services have also been designed to meet the special needs of children, helping to protect them from violence. A group of countries provided information about the health services they deliver for children, particularly in the area of protection against violence. In the absence of clear indicators about the progress made in this area, some countries require that health workers report all cases of violence against children. Other countries have units and sub-units for detection and follow-up on the physical and mental health conditions of children, with support from professional associations.

Bahrain has set up health centers and social centers responsible for all psycho-social and legal services for both children and adolescents.

Algeria has developed an institutionalized interdependent psycho-social support network for the treatment of traumatized children in educational institutions where various aspects of children's physical and mental health are attended.

Morocco has worked on the formulation of protocols for treatment of child victims of violence; this effort has been approved and is currently in progress.

In Yemen, the National Program for Violence and Injury Prevention was introduced at the Ministry of Public Health and Population early in 2010. The program works on establishing a surveillance system for cases of violence and accidents, to be connected to emergency departments in hospitals; these cases include violence against children and gender-based violence. The program also works on a number of awareness-raising publications and television programs. These endeavors fall within the framework of primary prevention of violence and aim to raise health awareness in order to reduce mortality rates resulting from violence against children. The National Program for Violence and Injury Prevention and the Supreme Council for Motherhood and Childhood are developing a manual for health workers on how to identify and deal with cases of violence against children in hospitals.

---

[4]Hage, G. and B. Gerbaka: "Toward an Efficient Child Protective Strategy in Lebanon: A Call for Pediatricians' True Child Advocacy." Pediatrica.

Examples of Such Policies and Programs Include

- Free telephone lines allocated to receive reports of children and protect them from violence or the threat as one of the mechanisms used in cases of separation of children from parents and to give high priority to return the child within the family.
- Family counseling programs; these programs work to select a group of families, which contacted through the telephone lines free, and their commitment to care and guidance of prisoners.
- Study the causes of violence by conducting studies and social research, and to identify the living conditions of the family or the suffering of children in order to identify the number of people exposed to the violence.
- Work to develop appropriate solutions and plans to address those problems.
- Improving the quality of services provided to street children.
- Protection of vulnerable children and children in conflict with the law.
- Accommodation of vulnerable children in specialized institutions.
- Support for low-income families and to develop mechanisms for children and adolescents.
- Child-rearing values of tolerance, respect and dialogue, especially the inclusion of material relating to human rights.
- Application and development of legislation and laws relating to children and protection from all forms of violence and abuse.
- Spreading awareness of the cultural rights of children through visual media and advertising campaigns.
- Integration of child rights in education programs for children and in the programs of many university degree courses such as educators and specialists in psychology, sociology, law and journalism.
- Develop mechanisms for mediation and resolution of family disputes.
- The enactment of laws on tougher sanctions if the abuse of children.
- Establishment of funds for aid and spending and national solidarity for children and their families.

In the Cairo declaration, participants renew their commitment to ensure the realization of the rights of all children without discrimination of any kind. Participants also commit to giving special attention to the realization of the rights of girls, including to achieve their right to education and to eliminate child marriage and other harmful traditional practices. Therefore, participants urge OIC Member States to take legislative, administrative and social measures to support without discrimination the rights of children born out of wedlock. These measures should include facilities for ensuring that both parents support the child and the mother benefits from relevant financial support to ensure the upbringing of the child. Children's inheritance rights should also be safeguarded.

Measures should also be taken to establish the legal responsibility of the father to contribute financially in the upbringing of the child and to allow the mother to take the necessary legal actions to establish through courts the fatherhood of the biological child.

Participants recognized that children with disabilities have a right to special attention and empowerment. The entry into force of the Convention on the Rights of Persons with Disabilities provides an opportunity for renewed commitment to the realization of the rights of children with disabilities and for joint action between the two treaty bodies established by these treaties.

Participants also recognized the particular vulnerability of children deprived of parental care, belonging to minorities, living and working on the streets and children victims of economic exploitation and reiterated their commitment to enhance their protection (26).

It is clear from these data the extent of decline in some countries at the level of ratification of international human rights instruments and relevant regional, which provides protection for children. While commending the progress made by other countries in this area, at the level of procedures for the implementation of international and regional obligations on the prevention of violence, as well as the commitments made in the special session of the General Assembly on children, and to implement the decision of the World Health Organization (74) on the implementation of the recommendations of the World Report on Violence and Health, and other regional public health and to enhance these decisions, did not provide responses available information in this regard.

In spite of the discrepancy between the Arab countries in the intellectual premises, and in the nature of the institutions that operate in children's issues, but that all States recognize the importance of this issue and agree on the need to intensify efforts to address all forms of violence and abuse against children. And take most of the Arab countries established official bodies and government as a means to achieve its goals in this area, but with this; most countries have opened up room for individual enterprises and civil society institutions to work in the implementation of policies on children and in accordance with the adoption of the principle of partnership in the implementation of policies social development.

However, there are a number of recommendations that could be useful in consolidating and strengthening efforts directed at reducing violence against children.

- Work to strengthen the observatories and centers, which recorded the events of violence against children or dealing with him in one way or another.
- To conduct comparative studies between the Arab countries to exchange experiences in the area of registration of incidents of violence against children and methods of addressing them.
- Activating the role of the United Nations study on ending violence against children, and through the provision of the reports of periodic national, or comparative studies such as this report.
- Work to deepen the relationship between strategies for children and those directed to the family, on the grounds that the family is the primary caretakers of children; and whenever the family was protected from the risks as the child was protected from the risks as well, which enters the violence within it.

- Work to find photos of coordination between the efforts of institutions taking care of the child directly and institutions that sponsored indirectly, for example, the importance of the need for coordination between the efforts of child-care institutions and efforts at national level for the prevention of drug addiction, or efforts in the ministries of labor to protect children from hard work and the different manifestations of abuse.
- Work to provide positive incentives for successful experiences in the protection of children from violence and abuse in the Arab world and highlight these experiences and discussed through various media.
- To support the budgets allocated to programs for childhood and motherhood, and the allocation of funds to research centers, observatories, and comparative studies in the Arab world, and the need to further increase financial resources allocated to cover the needs of the implementation of strategies and action plans and programs for the prevention of violence against children in Arab countries.
- Due to the weakness of civil society in most Arab countries, efforts must be made to support civil society and deepen its role in relation to the protection of children from violence, protecting the rights of children and mothers and the family in general.
- Work on a further training manuals and codes of children's rights and disseminated widely.
- Support the management of family and childhood League of Arab States, and expand its activities to accommodate the establishment of databases, and provide technical assistance to various Arab countries in the field of protection of family and childhood.
- Work to make greater efforts to strengthen the capacity of working with children in schools, courts and nurseries, with attention to the deployment of highly skilled staff to interact with the problems of childhood, from kindergarten to graduation.
- To create a social and cultural networking between families and between institutions concerned with child protection, including civil society organizations.
- The importance of access to different experiences in the Arab countries and exchange of experiences in relation to efforts to protect children from violence.
- To direct more financial support for the protection of children in Arab countries.
- Training of human resources needed to deal with the problems of childhood in general, and violence against children in particular.
- The need for legislation and clear and specific and are implemented to reduce the manifestations of violence against children, particularly the laws on female circumcision and female genital mutilation, and the laws on sexual abuse in general.
- Work to organize the utilization data are collected and mechanisms for the continuation of data collection and use of indicators to compare them over time. This cannot be done without the sustainability of the process of data collection.

The Way Forward[5]

A number of important and immediate needs must be addressed within the region:

- Political commitments must be translated into operational strategies to combat CSEC;
- Clear and agreed working definitions on issues relating to CSEC should be adopted;
- National and regional studies should be undertaken; these need to use precise, rigorous methodologies that take into account national and regional realities;
- National legislations should be harmonized with international instruments;
- Laws, conventions and agreements made should be implemented strictly;
- A national training system should be put in place for professionals working with children, encompassing both governmental and non-governmental sectors;
- Mechanisms for consultation and coordination should be put in place, perhaps with a national coordinator, to bring disparate initiatives under a collaborative umbrella;
- Steps must be taken to ensure that all children have access to basic services (education, health, food, housing) and children at risk or abused should enjoy extra protection;
- The participation of children in areas of concern to them should be promoted;
- There should be efforts to mobilize the private sector;
- The potential of independent mechanisms devoted to listening to children whose rights have been denied and for following up on this should be explored—ombudsmen, for example, working in cooperation with UN special rapporteurs;
- A regional focal centre/observatory for coordination, observation, analysis, action and evaluation might be considered.

Islam, Traditions and Legislation: The Context of Human Rights' Conventions in MENA

Introduction

Islamic rulers and has never completely died out in Sudan. In the Sudan, Christian and animist captives in the civil war are often enslaved and female prisoners are often used sexually, with their Muslim captors claiming that Islamic law grants them permission. According to CBS news, slaves have been sold for $50 *a piece*.

It is estimated that as many as 200,000 people had been taken into slavery during the Second Sudanese Civil War.

The slaves are mostly Dinka people. Human trafficking for the purpose of sexual exploitation is a major cause of contemporary sexual slavery. In the Middle-East, the

[5]"Article 34: States Parties undertake to protect the child from all forms of sexual exploitation and sexual abuse. For these purposes, States Parties shall in particular take all appropriate national, bilateral and multilateral measures to prevent: (a) the inducement or coercion of a child to engage in any unlawful sexual activity; (b) the exploitative use of children in prostitution or other unlawful sexual practices; (c) the exploitative use of children in pornographic performances and materials. Article 35: States Parties shall take all appropriate national, bilateral and multilateral measures to prevent the abduction of, the sale of or traffic in children for any purpose or in any form.

most common destinations for victims of human trafficking Israel and Turkey according to a report by UNODC.

Tackling Trafficking

Sex trafficking victims are generally found in dire circumstances and easily targeted by traffickers. Individuals, circumstances, and situations vulnerable to traffickers include homeless individuals, runaway teens, displaced homemakers, refugees, and drug addicts. While it may seem like trafficked people are the most vulnerable and powerless minorities in a region, victims are consistently exploited from any ethnic and social background.

In addition to the CRC and Convention on the Elimination of all forms of Discrimination against Women (CEDAW), there are a number of international conventions that deal with the rights of women and children in relation to early marriage and sexual abuse. However, some Arab and Islamic countries have made reservations to the CRC and CEDAW.

The general objections from Arab states are that the articles can only be accepted if they are not against the Islamic Law: the Sharia'. This poses a problem of how to interpret the Islamic Law? Whose interpretation shall we rely on? Traditionally sharia has been interpreted only by men, but we are also faced with the differences of the four schools of thought within Sunni Islam in addition to Shia interpretations.

However, in most Arabic countries traditions and customs mean more to people than Islam, but in relation to laws and conventions Islam has a higher legitimacy, with the following hierarchy in legitimacy:

1. Traditions ('urf)
2. Islam (sharia
3. Laws (qanun) 4.International conventions

Violation of the CRC

This model was confirmed by other researchers, during discussions at the workshop held in Cyprus. There are cases that clearly violate the CRC: for example if the law in Yemen stipulated that the legal age for marriage is 18, some parents would lie about their daughters date of birth in order to marry her earlier, in violation of the set law.

Today we see that the application as well as the law itself is influenced by religion and customs. This problem is further explored in the three research reports.

To bring about change, it is imperative that the conventions be addressed and we lobby for the legal system so they conform to the signed treatises.

A sign of modernization is that laws become more important than customs and religious-laws; thus the work towards an adherence to principles in the CRC and a change in the legal system is not useless. Furthermore, it is a new discourse emerging connecting Islam to human rights; subsequently, Islam, laws and conventions together can be powerful against customs to create a better situation for teenage girls in the MENA region and therefore need to be analyzed in detail.

Religious Leadership

Religion is a double edge sword in the battle against honor-crimes. The Islamic rule in sharia can be applied as an Islamic tool for categorizing honor killings against the religion and the religious law, according to sura (chapter) 24 in the Holy Quran, demands that accusations of adultery be supported by four witnesses of the actual sexual act. Unfortunately, these kinds of interpretations are seldom applied. Instead religious establishments of both Muslim and Christian scholars and politicians, often choose to support honor crimes in the name of sexual morality and set regulations against premarital sex in order to control who is allowed to marry.

An example from the OPT is of Palestinian priests supporting the killing of Christian-Palestinian girls having relationships with Muslim boys as a message for others not to become involved in such relationships. It seems that the honor ideology somehow finds resonance with religious moral laws within all religions, not only Islam.

It should be stressed that the moral ideals against sex outside wedlock should not in any sense support honor crimes; however many religious scholars still make this connection. It is alright to follow the moral that sex belongs to marriage; the problem is in the sanctions taken against those who are suspected of breaking these moral rules.

It should also be noted that the West has a tradition of Protestantism operating with individualist feelings of guilt and innocence, while in the Middle East, both Christianity and Islam, are colored by the collectivist honor and shame dichotomy. In the West the individual often feels guilty regarding what is right and wrong, hence disciplining the individual through feelings of bad consciousness.

In the honor-culture however, shameful deeds can be practiced if hidden from the public eye. This can be interpreted as encouraging hypocrisy, but it is a structure that releases people from feelings of guilt and provides a space of freedom if actions are kept in secret. However, the honor culture seems to be repressive at large, since the victims of sexual assault are accused it makes it difficult for them to talk about their experiences or the assault against them. Furthermore, the families of a sexual abuse victim are also tainted and stigmatized.

Norms and Practices in **Honor** *Crimes*

In practice, customs still seem to have higher legitimacy than religion, although I believe a shift of positions will come due to Islam. In our research, parents proclaimed honor violence as being against the religion and suggested combating such acts with religious sanctions against sexual criminals. The OPT examines Islam as a tool for gender equality since it moralizes against both sexes and ascribes the same sanctions towards them. In practice, as demonstrated through the experiences of girls, only the female part is blamed however. Consequently, Islam can be used as a tool in combating honor violence, and has been used for this purpose in Jordan.

The strict rules regarding sacredness, privacy and integrity can be applied to condemn the spreading of rumors and gossip in the name of honor.

In Islam, it is a sin to spy on others and spread gossip, however the same principles make it harder for children to speak up against sexual abuse in their homes, since such matters are often referred to as "private" and hence to be solved in the private sphere without interference of the wider society. The assault can then continue in secret. Furthermore the religious stress on "obedience" of children and wives to fathers and husbands, as pointed out in the Palestinian report, make it problematic to speak up in cases of sexual violence. Another dilemma related to Islam, discussed in the situation analysis here, is that in the sharia "rape within marriage" is an unknown concept since women must be sexually-accessible to their husbands. Young wives are therefore exposed to repeated sexual abuse in their marriage, as demonstrated in the life stories quoted from Yemen. There are no rules in the Islamic religion that encourage early marriages, however none condemn it either leaving religion open for interpretation regarding the suitable age for marriage. Subsequently, religion can be used both for and against sexual violence within marriages.

The legislation on honor crimes and sexuality is influenced by religion and traditions. Originally, the laws on passion crimes have been influenced by the laws of the colonial powers and are not from the sharia as such, but are nowadays used as an excuse for lenient punishment for honor-criminals.

The law stipulates that the extenuating circumstances for the criminal are that he has lost his sanity seeing his wife having intercourse with another man and kills her. This excuse, however, is hardly ever the case in honor crimes, since such crimes are not usually committed because a man finds his wife in bed with another man; however honor-crimes are excused using the notion that the killer was in a state of "fit or fury" and therefore is sentenced to lenient punishment.

Moreover, the rule that adultery is a crime and against the law is a view abandoned in the West in the course of modernization, but still existent in the MENA. In Western countries, adultery is considered a private matter rather than a criminal act against the law. Such changes to the law would make sexuality enter the sphere of private-morality rather than being a public issue that falls in the field of legislation. Consensual sex is not equal to sexual abuse of children by adults. In Islam, a way of having "legal" consensual sex is to engage in an Islamic marriage (orfi marriage), as documented by the OPT. Islam can be used to give legitimacy and blessing to consensual sexual intercourse, in cases where laws and families are opposing such unions. However, the same practice can be exploited for sexual abuse and prostitution.

Universal Rights, Emerging Region, Global Support

Legislations against sexual abuse and violence against women and children need to be strengthened in the region. There are many examples of laws that are discriminatory towards women and children. Even in countries such as Lebanon that stands out as being the most modernized country, legislations are strongly influenced by religion and traditions, family in Honor crimes and child marriage. Therefore, their quest for a unified (secular) civil law for personal status should be taken seriously. In OPT, the laws are confusing but still the same discriminatory traces are apparent in their legal systems, apart from the recently established laws by the Palestinian Authority, Gaza also follows Egyptian law and the West Bank practices Jordanian legislation in certain matters.

The CRC helps combating sexual violence against teenage girls in light of the customs, religions and legislations. CRC has been successful in promoting new legislations against trafficking and child prostitution in the region, as discussed in the chapters here. Since such laws exist, they also have to be applied and interpreted to include sexual abuse, violence in the name of honor, and early marriage as forms of sexual violence. The women's movement in the region is working for legal changes that promote gender equality.

This struggle must be supported, laws must be developed that apply despite religion and customs, and the CRC must act as the frame of reference applied in combating such problems

Summary and Recommendations

The prohibition of violence has also been included in laws for civil service (e.g. Jordan, Bahrain) and stipulated in laws, regulations and ministerial decrees. There is considerable progress with regards amending penal codes and child protection acts, and the enactment of new laws to ensure effective protection for children.

Nevertheless, these laws share common constraints, as they:

- Are not based on a comprehensive review of all domestic legislation in against the CRC and other relevant international conventions.
- Include general human rights without sufficient details or clarification to avoid misinterpretation (e.g. Palestine Act of 2004 amended in 2009).
- Are based on the CRC without reference to the principles and provisions of the Optional Protocols on the Sale of Children, Child Prostitution and Child Pornography and on the Involvement of Children in Armed Conflict.
- Did not clearly express the concept of the best interests of the child, which is often included as a separate article without addressing its implications for various aspects of economic, social and civil rights.

- Do not address the child's right to express his/her opinion, and to participate in decision making on subjects related to his/her concerns.
- Included ideas whose proper location is executive regulations due to their procedural and technical nature.
- State responses do not include data allowing analysis on the basis of the various settings where violence occurs although; deductions can be drawn from data on the nature of violence.

Sexual Violence

Most laws do not clearly prohibit all forms of sexual violence against girls and boys below 18 years of age, nor do they protect victims from the requirements of multiple testimonies, or eliminate all possibilities for impunity in cases of sexual offences occurring within the family. There are no explicit articles disallowing the dropping of charges and discontinuing lawsuits in cases where the aggressor marries the victim. These laws have failed to provide me and psychological recovery services for victims. In some cases, legislation has failed to prohibit the acquisition, production, dissemination, and distribution of documents and materials containing child pornography.

Laws have not provided for allowing complaints without the permission of the victim's parents, nor have they ensured that child victims of sexual exploitation will not be considered criminals or delinquents.

In the Arab region, there is only limited reporting on the occurrence of sexual violence in schools as the subject remains a social taboo and child friendly reporting mechanism are absent. Yet there is evidence to suggest its presence. A study in Yemen on a sample of 267 children showed that 31.4% were exposed to sexual harassment (in 56.2% of the cases, the aggressor was either a peer or a neighbor and in 13.7% of the cases it was one of the teachers).

In Morocco, it was observed that 8 out of 40 cases of violence reported to the Child Rights Observatory were classified as sexual harassment (6 boys and 2 girls).[6]

In Lebanon, a recent study showed that 16% of children were exposed to sexual harassment with 6% of these cases occurring in a school setting.[7] The study showed that the incidence of sexual harassment was higher in the case of girls than boys (12 girls vs. one boy).[8]

---

[6]Save the Children interview with "Beity" society and the Child Rights Observatory, Rabat, 10 October, 2010.

[7]Higher Council for Childhood, Save the Children (Sweden), Kafa Society, Sexual Harassment in Lebanon, 2008.

[8]Child and Youth Protection Initiative, Arab Institute for Urban Development, Sana'a (2008).

In some cases, violence is discussed only with regard to violence inflicted by adults upon children, instead of referencing also violence among peers. Sudan, as an exception, does address peer violence through its Child Law.

The reactions of states indicate that the mechanisms of monitoring and complaints are the same as those present in the components of the national child protection system. Others mentioned the existence of clear mechanisms.

The Arab Report on the Recommendations of the UN Secretary-General's Study on Violence Against Children determine referential persons in the school, and follow-up mechanisms for referral to the director, and then on to the specialized department in the ministry of education. In extreme cases the referral is to the child protection monitor in the ministry of social affairs (e.g. Palestine).

Yemen is the only state that mentioned having complaints boxes in schools, and that committees for protection were formed in some schools to afford the children the chance to make complaints.[9]

Documentation of complaints lies within the jurisdiction of the protection system (such as the police in Sudan, and the Child Helpline in Egypt), and not inside the educational system. On the other hand, some countries' educational systems adopt a component of child protection, and have elucidated the presence of models that are followed by the ministry of education, in cooperation with other ministries (e.g. Palestine).

Most countries said that they had applied a special effort to raise awareness and provide education on the issue of VAC. Some countries organized meeting with children (e.g. Jordan, Lebanon, Algeria, Qatar) with the aim of enabling and educating children on the mechanisms available (e.g. Yemen, Palestine). Some stated that VAC is taking little priority in schools, and that they had designated national campaigns, strategies and comprehensive plans to improve this situation (e.g. Palestine, Jordan). Other countries include plans for child protection against violence in general, in connection with violence in schools.[10]

The presence of comprehensive measures and policies on the school level was not notable, except in a few cases, including: Lebanon's experiment in Mabarrat schools of a policy of child protection within the school, Tunisia's Council of the Educational Institution, whose jurisdiction includes ensuring controls and child safety, and Algeria, which has formed a disciplinary council headed by the school director, with the purpose of preserving order.

The following recommendations should be considered to assist states to build national methodological responses supported by documented evidence and data, rather than relying simply on the adoption of international trends:

1. Political will to increase data collection and monitoring of cases of violence, represented in a special agenda for management, organization and analysis of

---

[9]Yemen National Council for Childhood and Motherhood, Violence Against Children: a Social Study in Some Yemeni Regions, 2005.

[10]Save the Children Sweden and International Bureau for Children's Rights, Violence Against Schools: a Regional Analysis of Lebanon, Morocco and Yemen, 2011.

data, and the allocation of financial resources to propose comprehensive research and studies in various locations

2. Specify a body or entity at the national level that is responsible for data collection process from various agencies, ministries, research centers, universities and NGOs on a clear basis and specific methodology. This entity should be associated with national structures responsible for the development of strategies and plans to ensure the development of programs and interventions that are priorities and to prevent the recurrence of programs that proved not to be effective. It should also issues periodic reports which highlight general trends and progress made in various sectors, identifies gaps that hinder the data collection process, are given to decision-makers, and is made available to children through the use of easy and understandable language.
3. Secure requests for information from children, media and universities. Establish connections and cooperation protocols with several sectors that produce information or data, especially departments or centers for national statistics.
4. Ensure that information-gathering processes are unified and consistent within a scientific methodology, and works on transferring it and training various parties.
5. Collect information from administrative records and proposes and implements periodic national surveys.
6. Develops a list of qualitative and quantitative indicators on the subject of child protection.
7. Monitor progress made, identify gaps, and determine the categories not covered by prevention, intervention, or rehabilitation programs.
8. Build a comprehensive system for the registration of marriages, birth and filing.
9. Build a system for monitoring deaths, including a system for legal and medical examination for the collection of documented deaths and mentioning the cause of death in death registries.
10. Build a management system for cases in medical care facilities, child protection.
11. Services and other facilities at the national level, to allow the continued availability of information on individual cases and planning the service-provision process.
12. Document information at the sectoral levels of education, health and law enforcement, and categorize data according to age, gender, and type of violence, geographic region and family characteristics.
13. Train personnel on documentation and analysis methodologies and on ethics in research on CSA like interviewing children and respecting privacy. In fact, failure to exchange information between various agencies may lead to unnecessary suffering or even death.
14. Familiarize universities and institutes with children's issues in general and violence and abuse in particular, in order to provide personnel and institutions related to childhood with the required scientific competencies and research methodologies, and making it a subject of social discussion and research material in more than one university specialty.
15. Strength community monitoring mechanisms and documenting of cases on the national level through parents, children, NGOs and municipalities. Local

observatories can also be established to be in constant contact with the national observatory.

16. Ensure children's access to information and participation in its provision, analysis and dissemination

Future Perspectives

Despite many obstacles, the perspective of child protection is strongly developing within national systems and regional networks, in the presence of increasing levels of common values and universal understanding of child rights. In reality, child dedicated structures are grass rooting initiatives; they rely on political decisions, local and national human resources, regional expertise and international cooperation; they seek for strategies at the countries levels in order to implant child protection systems, and recently expanded the network in order to learn from experiences in other Arab countries:

- 1st ISPCAN Arab regional conference on CAN, Amman, Jordan, 2005: "Breaking the silence"
- 2nd ISPCAN Arab regional conference on CAN, Sana'a, Yemen, 2007: "Towards a strategy for child protection"
- 3rd ISPCAN Arab regional conference on CAN, Riyadh, KSA, 2009: "Working together towards safer childhood".
- 4th ISPCAN Arab regional conference on CAN, Riyadh, KSA, 2013
- 5th ISPCAN Arab regional conference on CAN, Kuwait, 2016
- 6th ISPCAN Arab regional conference on CAN, Dubai, UAE
- Also, in between those dates, professionals' training seminars were held in: Syria, Lebanon, Egypt, Bahrain, KSA, etc.

On those diverse occasions, the Arab initiative—then the UNSV—presented a setting-based framework for the description of child abuse in countries and the efforts developed to stop violence. The International Society for the Prevention of Child Abuse and Neglect was also partner within the advisory panel to advice on the nature and definitions of VAC on one side, and conduct the UNSV on the other.

Based on an expanding knowledge base, the UNSV intends to highlight on the status of children confronted with violence in their different environments, to increase the national—as well as informal capacities to build systems that focus on the integration of protection and prevention—as well as child participation—in the human rights commitments and implementation processes. All procedures would be based on a CRC matrix that incorporates children's rights, professional evidence, relevant social factors and intersectoral responsibilities for the prevention of VAC and the control of CAN, as a priority in Governmental programs.

Arab countries live, now more than ever, in identity crisis and armed conflicts. They are, however, challenged to plan systems, set priorities and provide a basis for political and social debate on the present and the future condition of children, with the participation of children. In this perspective, the APNPCAN/VAC can plan the following activities:

- Meet with children and youth, to discuss their opinions about CAN and VAC; the I-CAST-Child questionnaire developed by ISPCAN and supported by UNICEF is indeed a useful tool in such a task. The main objectives of those meetings are:
- to agree on definitions of VAC and CAN;
  - to enable more children to outreach the UNSV child version;
  - to reach a common understanding about the way to confront violence in child environments;
  - to exchange with children their outputs on the UNSV results and recommendations;
  - to develop procedures children find useful and productive for child effective participation and child protection;
  - to include, in an effective process, child recommendations within national Arab strategies for child protection.
- Lobby with Parliamentarians and legislators, to:
  - enhance already existing national and local movements towards child protection, while tackling specific needs and priorities;
  - stimulate legislative revision of laws, to comply with the provisions of the CRC and optional protocols;
  - increase local and national knowledge about the UNSV and contribute in finding appropriate procedures to initiate advocacy and sustainable child protection.
- Work with other professionals to:
  - Increase common knowledge and develop existing training tools;
  - Upgrade the informal knowledge to a comprehensive curriculum;
  - Base their interventions on evidence of qualitative assessment and efficient actions;
  - Carry out comprehensive national surveys. It is essential that children participate in the survey;
  - Support research and study centers;
  - Develop mechanisms that enable violated children to make their complaints;
  - Provide psychological and physical rehabilitation services;
  - Prepare periodic reports and meetings;
  - Develop training programs for personnel working with children regarding best practices;
  - Set up counseling centers that receive reports and complaints;
- Embody the reform of child protection by being candidates in city councils, parliaments and governments, in order to set up parliamentary committees, amend existing legislation (rights of the child, criminalization of violence and enforce the provisions of CRC);

- Reduce gender discrimination by tackling directly the girl child issues, in terms of participation, education, domestic child labor, early marriage, female genital mutilation and family violence. The empowerment of women is also part of this process.

Obviously, the scarcity of child specific health and social support services are obstacles to child protection, and should then be made available to families and accessible to children. In reality, the capacities of those services are sometimes overwhelmed, especially during armed conflicts and social instability, when children are involved in violent situations and at increased risk of different types of abuse and violence. In such contexts, free childcare, universal health screening and universal access to free medical care become even more critical, as is, in general, the universal access to free health care for all citizens.

National strategies for child protection would indeed comply with the United Nations Convention on the Rights of the Child, with attention to the needs and possibilities of some developing, insecure and ill-resourced countries (8). The potential challenges and impacts of the CRC implementation should also be explored for future landmarks of democracies and freedom of opinions, mainly in terms of:

- Independent structures: child observatories, at local and national levels, are actually available in Morocco, Tunis and Lebanon. There are still no child defenders or child ombudsman, though a proposition of law was presented in this regard in Lebanon, 2004.
- Child protection acts or child-friendly and environment-centered legislations, actually available in Egypt, Jordan, Syria, pending in Lebanon.
- Budgets for Child protection and child oriented projects, not distinctively available.
- Helpline for children and professionals, for the reporting of child maltreatment and for psychosocial support to victims of violence, available in Egypt, pending in Lebanon.
- Training of pilot and decentralized multisectoral teams and building of professional curricula, actually in expanding process in Syria, Lebanon, Jordan and Egypt.
- Study the extent of VAC, based on three I-CAST questionnaires (Child, Retrospective and Parents) tested and implemented in Egypt and Lebanon.
- Participation of children and youth in the evaluation of problems, analysis of situations, setting of reports, implementation of processes and re-evaluation of actions, present in many country reports, where few evidence of efficiency is however available.
- Support of child-friendly media: auto-censorship on aggressive viewings, to reduce violence and enhance educative programs—with children—on screens; in this regards, workshops for child friendly media have been held in many countries in the region, with two main outcomes: abused children are rarely visualized on media, and more child friendly programs are developed.

- Code of conduct for professionals working with children: Lebanon is considering the implementation of the code with professionals working for/with children, within the provisions of the coming modification of relevant law.

Implications

Despite ongoing efforts by Arab governments and many NGOs to address the multiple social, cultural and professional pitfalls, CAN remains a serious threat to child rights implementation. There is still no child budget and no child protection acts in many counties. There are few independent structures for child rights monitoring (National child defender, national child observatory) and scarce child helplines. Children are still present in high numbers in institutions. Therapy programs are limited for victims—yet increasing—and most often virtual for perpetrators. Legislations are subject to national consultations to meet the CRC requirements. The human and social situation of refugees is sometimes dramatic or still waiting for the settlement of the Arab-Israeli conflict as well as other armed clashes in Iraq, Sudan, Somalia and others. Internally and regionally displaced children are repeatedly exposed to extreme types of violence and abuse, with contraventions to the UN and EU Guidelines.

Obviously, given the scant findings and the many limitations of this review, conclusions are for the most part tentative and need to be placed within the larger framework of CSA. This review can confirm several points. Research on child sexual abuse in MENA is notably lacking compared to many parts of the world. Of interest, the Global School-based Student Health Survey in use by 19 countries as of 2007 has questions on child physical and sexual abuse. Those data were included by Lebanon, but Oman, Libya and the United Arab Emirates chose to do the survey but left out the questions on child physical and sexual abuse. As noted by many authors in these studies and globally, without prevalence rates and research on CSA, there is less hope of overcoming resistance to acknowledging the problem and working to solve it.

Child sexual abuse of boys and girls clearly does exist in the Middle East and North Africa and is a cause for concern in MENA as well as the rest of the world. That fact is unlikely to change until societies change, becoming less patriarchal and less adultist, until children are given rights accorded human beings guaranteed by the UN Convention on the Rights of the Child. The patterns, while tentative given the data, are consistent that boys in MENA have higher rates of CSA than girls in MENA and higher rates than boys in North America and Europe.

Children suffer horribly at the hands of their abusers and child sexual abuse is associated with numerous adverse consequences throughout the globe including the Middle East and North Africa. It takes enormous courage to advocate on behalf of the powerless, even more so in the area of child abuse and even more so in societies where this issue is taboo. It is hoped that this review will encourage others to continue research and policy efforts to protect all of our children.

In some countries, children are viewed as—and submitted to—their religious references, in terms—and place—of civil rights. In such countries, children are exposed to problems that alter their growth, development, social interaction, safety, education and health.

In Lebanon, In conclusion, key decisions will need to be made in Lebanon for the development of a comprehensive and congruent child protection system, one that functions effectively and is perceived as appropriate and relevant by families at the local level. The study found that participants clearly feel that the different strategies employed for protecting children need to be blended. At one end of the spectrum, community resolution and family mediation will continue to be an inherent element of a child protection system while the statutory response system will offer special measures for those at the greatest level of risk. There remains a debate about how to organize other system components and about how—in a country with strong community affiliations—a single system, regulated by civil and criminal law, and applicable to all Lebanese citizens, is best tailored to meet existing and future child protection challenges.

It is therefore important for Arab professionals to rely on—and encourage—the governments who show intention to build child protection systems, but also to contribute in drawing a sharing platform of knowledge and knowhow, from observations and findings of professionals, experts and NGOs who work closely with children; in this regard, cooperation with ISPCAN may increase the capacities of stakeholders in confronting violence with peaceful stands, based on firm and clear evidence of efficient programs.

Countries in the Arab region are urged to launch CRC compliant and socially accepted—child protection systems that would be comprehensive melting pots of existing and developing programs. Success stories and reports on obstacles are most welcome, to improve MENA knowledge about the status of children, in a dynamic and proactive way. In this perspective it is important to note that there was an Arab League meeting in 2009 to amend Arab chapter on Child Rights.

In different—and sometimes conflicting—contexts of security and safety, the Arab efforts to integrate children's rights within global human rights matrix—and child health and well-being requirements—need, in fact, strong social links and individual stands towards child protection acts. Child help lines, child defenders and child observatories are the pivots of knowledge base, data collection and training, rehabilitation and prevention, global child rights and local childhood requisites.

In each step, the APNPCAN/VAC can demonstrate the efficiency of professionals in promoting children's globally recognized rights within their living places. Such initiatives work best when social stability, common vision, effective interaction between formal and informal sector, and child efficient participation. . .are available. Indeed, such initiatives towards child protection are most needed when those conditions are not yet available. Most challenging options are in most difficult—yet enriching—environments! Where the most vulnerable is not the slowest!

Chapter 18
Ensure Accountability and End Impunity

States should build community confidence in the justice system by, inter alia, bringing all perpetrators of violence against children to justice and ensure that they are held accountable through appropriate "No matter whether violence against children occurs in the family, school, community, institution or workplace, health workers are the front line for responding to it. We must make our contribution to ensuring that such violence is prevented from occurring in the first place, and that where it does occur children receive the best possible services to reduce its harmful effects". Anders Nordström, Acting Director-General, WHO an end to violence against children criminal, civil, administrative and professional proceedings and sanctions. Persons convicted of violent offences and sexual abuse of children, should be prevented from working with children.

In Tunisia, crimes against children are considered in the context of the circumstances of the criminal act in order to administer punishment to aggressors. In Saudi Arabia, where Islamic Shari'a is the basis of legislation, the judiciary system holds accountable the perpetrators of crimes against children according to the gravity of the offense committed.

In Syria, the penal code allows for the addition of harsher penalties for the crime in case it is committed against a child. In Palestine, the Palestinian child act and the penal code deny impunity for perpetrators of child abuse. In Qatar, the constitution ensures equality and non-discrimination between citizens and residents before the law.

In Morocco, forthcoming procedures will accelerate the pace of judicial proceedings and enforce the principle of no impunity; units have also been created in the public prosecution to handle issues of childhood, especially in matters related to violence; strict instructions are given to punish all perpetrators of offenses committed against children. Some NGOs working in the area of interventions against

"Investing in the Children of the Islamic World", UNICEF, 2005

B. Gerbaka et al., *Child Sexual Abuse, Exploitation and Trafficking in the Arab Region*, Child Maltreatment 13, https://doi.org/10.1007/978-3-030-66507-4_18

violence against children can act as a civil party supporting children victims of violence.

In Egypt, lawmakers have recently introduced a provision doubling the minimum penalty prescribed for all crimes committed by adults against children. In Yemen, a family protection unit was created to attend to women's and children's issues within the General Directorate of Police; the Interior Ministry and the Ministry of Justice are to study the creation of family courthouses in some provinces.

Furthermore, legal amendments relating to children are proposed to be introduced to the draft penal code and presented before the House of Representatives for discussion and approval. The amendment's provisions involve legislative penalties against perpetrators in connection to bullying, exploitation and abuse against children.

Chapter 19
Provide Special Health Services, Recovery and Social Reintegration

Arab countries provide a range of services accessible health care before entering the hospital or in emergency situations. There are a range of programs and pilot projects in this area, such as developing procedures and protocols governing the coordination between the actors and the provision of specialized units fixed or mobile to deal with issues of violence, and maternal and child health, and training programs for health workers and doctors to distinguish the signs and symptoms resulting from this violence, and training and assigning staff specializing in the early detection of symptoms of violence and reporting. Jordan has developed procedures and protocols, especially the Ministry of Health to deal with cases of domestic violence.

Health services have also been designed to meet the special needs of children, helping to protect them from violence. A group of countries provided information about the health services they deliver for children, particularly in the area of protection against violence. In the absence of clear indicators about the progress made in this area, some countries require that health workers report all cases of violence against children. Other countries have units and sub-units for detection and follow-up on the physical and mental health conditions of children, with support from professional associations.

Bahrain has set up health centers and social centers responsible for all psycho-social and legal services for both children and adolescents.

Algeria has developed an institutionalized interdependent psycho-social support network for the treatment of traumatized children in educational institutions where various aspects of children's physical and mental health are attended.

Morocco has worked on the formulation of protocols for treatment of child victims of violence; this effort has been approved and is currently in progress.

In Yemen, the National Program for Violence and Injury Prevention was introduced at the Ministry of Public Health and Population early in 2010. The program

Hage, G. and B. Gerbaka: "Toward an Efficient Child Protective Strategy in Lebanon: A Call for Pediatricians' True Child Advocacy." Pediatrica.

B. Gerbaka et al., *Child Sexual Abuse, Exploitation and Trafficking in the Arab Region*, Child Maltreatment 13, https://doi.org/10.1007/978-3-030-66507-4_19

works on establishing a surveillance system for cases of violence and accidents, to be connected to emergency departments in hospitals; these cases include violence against children and gender-based violence. The program also works on a number of awareness-raising publications and television programs. These endeavors fall within the framework of primary prevention of violence and aim to raise health awareness in order to reduce mortality rates resulting from violence against children. The National Program for Violence and Injury Prevention and the Supreme Council for Motherhood and Childhood are developing a manual for health workers on how to identify and deal with cases of violence against children in hospitals.

19.1 Examples of Policies and Programs

- Free telephone lines allocated to receive reports of children and protect them from violence or the threat as one of the mechanisms used in cases of separation of children from parents and to give high priority to return the child within the family.
- Family counseling programs; these programs work to select a group of families, which contacted through the telephone lines free, and their commitment to care and guidance of prisoners.
- Study the causes of violence by conducting studies and social research, and to identify the living conditions of the family or the suffering of children in order to identify the number of people exposed to the violence.
- Work to develop appropriate solutions and plans to address those problems.
- Improving the quality of services provided to street children.
- Protection of vulnerable children and children in conflict with the law.
- Accommodation of vulnerable children in specialized institutions.
- Support for low-income families and to develop mechanisms for children and adolescents.
- Child-rearing values of tolerance, respect and dialogue, especially the inclusion of material relating to human rights.
- Application and development of legislation and laws relating to children and protection from all forms of violence and abuse.
- Spreading awareness of the cultural rights of children through visual media and advertising campaigns.
- Integration of child rights in education programs for children and in the programs of many university degree courses such as educators and specialists in psychology, sociology, law and journalism.
- Develop mechanisms for mediation and resolution of family disputes.
- The enactment of laws on tougher sanctions if the abuse of children.
- Establishment of funds for aid and spending and national solidarity for children and their families.

19.2 Examples of Commitments

In the Cairo declaration, participants renew their commitment to ensure the realization of the rights of all children without discrimination of any kind. Participants also commit to giving special attention to the realization of the rights of girls, including to achieve their right to education and to eliminate child marriage and other harmful traditional practices. Therefore, participants urge OIC Member States to take legislative, administrative and social measures to support without discrimination the rights of children born out of wedlock. These measures should include facilities for ensuring that both parents support the child and the mother benefits from relevant financial support to ensure the upbringing of the child. Children's inheritance rights should also be safeguarded.

Measures should also be taken to establish the legal responsibility of the father to contribute financially in the upbringing of the child and to allow the mother to take the necessary legal actions to establish through courts the fatherhood of the biological child.

Participants recognized that children with disabilities have a right to special attention and empowerment. The entry into force of the Convention on the Rights of Persons with Disabilities provides an opportunity for renewed commitment to the realization of the rights of children with disabilities and for joint action between the two treaty bodies established by these treaties.

Participants also recognized the particular vulnerability of children deprived of parental care, belonging to minorities, living and working on the streets and children victims of economic exploitation and reiterated their commitment to enhance their protection.

It is clear from these data the extent of decline in some countries at the level of ratification of international human rights instruments and relevant regional, which provides protection for children. While commending the progress made by other countries in this area, at the level of procedures for the implementation of international and regional obligations on the prevention of violence, as well as the commitments made in the special session of the General Assembly on children, and to implement the decision of the World Health Organization on the implementation of the recommendations of the World Report on Violence and Health , and other regional public health and to enhance these decisions, did not provide responses available information in this regard.

In spite of the discrepancy between the Arab countries in the intellectual premises, and in the nature of the institutions that operate in children's issues, but that all States recognize the importance of this issue and agree on the need to intensify efforts to address all forms of violence and abuse against children. And take most of the Arab countries established official bodies and government as a means to achieve its goals in this area, but with this; most countries have opened up room for individual enterprises and civil society institutions to work in the implementation of policies on children and in accordance with the adoption of the principle of partnership in the implementation of policies social development.

19.3 Examples of Recommendations

However, there are a number of recommendations that could be useful in consolidating and strengthening efforts directed at reducing violence against children.

- Work to strengthen the observatories and centers, which recorded the events of violence against children or dealing with him in one way or another.
- To conduct comparative studies between the Arab countries to exchange experiences in the area of registration of incidents of violence against children and methods of addressing them.
- Activating the role of the United Nations study on ending violence against children, and through the provision of the reports of periodic national, or comparative studies such as this report.
- Work to deepen the relationship between strategies for children and those directed to the family, on the grounds that the family is the primary caretakers of children; and whenever the family was protected from the risks as the child was protected from the risks as well, which enters the violence within it.
- Work to find photos of coordination between the efforts of institutions taking care of the child directly and institutions that sponsored indirectly, for example, the importance of the need for coordination between the efforts of child-care institutions and efforts at national level for the prevention of drug addiction, or efforts in the ministries of labor to protect children from hard work and the different manifestations of abuse.
- Work to provide positive incentives for successful experiences in the protection of children from violence and abuse in the Arab world and highlight these experiences and discussed through various media.
- To support the budgets allocated to programs for childhood and motherhood, and the allocation of funds to research centers, observatories, and comparative studies in the Arab world, and the need to further increase financial resources allocated to cover the needs of the implementation of strategies and action plans and programs for the prevention of violence against children in Arab countries.
- Due to the weakness of civil society in most Arab countries, efforts must be made to support civil society and deepen its role in relation to the protection of children from violence, protecting the rights of children and mothers and the family in general.
- Work on a further training manuals and codes of children's rights and disseminated widely.
- Support the management of family and childhood League of Arab States, and expand its activities to accommodate the establishment of databases, and provide technical assistance to various Arab countries in the field of protection of family and childhood.
- Work to make greater efforts to strengthen the capacity of working with children in schools, courts and nurseries, with attention to the deployment of highly skilled staff to interact with the problems of childhood, from kindergarten to graduation.

- To create a social and cultural networking between families and between institutions concerned with child protection, including civil society organizations.
- The importance of access to different experiences in the Arab countries and exchange of experiences in relation to efforts to protect children from violence.
- To direct more financial support for the protection of children in Arab countries.
- Training of human resources needed to deal with the problems of childhood in general and violence against children in particular.
- The need for legislation and clear and specific and are implemented to reduce the manifestations of violence against children, particularly the laws on female circumcision and female genital mutilation, and the laws on sexual abuse in general.
- Work to organize the utilization data are collected and mechanisms for the continuation of data collection and use of indicators to compare them over time. This cannot be done without the sustainability of the process of data collection.

19.4 The Way Forward[1]

A number of important and immediate needs must be addressed within the region:

- Political commitments must be translated into operational strategies to combat CSEC;
- Clear and agreed working definitions on issues relating to CSEC should be adopted;
- National and regional studies should be undertaken; these need to use precise, rigorous methodologies that take into account national and regional realities;
- National legislations should be harmonized with international instruments;
- Laws, conventions and agreements made should be implemented strictly;
- A national training system should be put in place for professionals working with children, encompassing both governmental and non-governmental sectors;
- Mechanisms for consultation and coordination should be put in place, perhaps with a national coordinator, to bring disparate initiatives under a collaborative umbrella;

[1]"Article 34: States Parties undertake to protect the child from all forms of sexual exploitation and sexual abuse. For these purposes, States Parties shall in particular take all appropriate national, bilateral and multilateral measures to prevent: (a) the inducement or coercion of a child to engage in any unlawful sexual activity; (b) the exploitative use of children in prostitution or other unlawful sexual practices; (c) the exploitative use of children in pornographic performances and materials.

Article 35: States Parties shall take all appropriate national, bilateral and multilateral measures to prevent the abduction of, the sale of or traffic in children for any purpose or in any form."

- Steps must be taken to ensure that all children have access to basic services (education, health, food, housing) and children at risk or abused should enjoy extra protection;
- The participation of children in areas of concern to them should be promoted;
- There should be efforts to mobilize the private sector;
- The potential of independent mechanisms devoted to listening to children whose rights have been denied and for following up on this should be explored—ombudsmen, for example, working in cooperation with UN special rapporteurs;
- A regional focal centre/observatory for coordination, observation, analysis, action and evaluation might be considered.

Chapter 20
Islam, Traditions and Legislation: The Context of Human Rights' Conventions in MENA

20.1 Introduction

Islamic rules and has never completely died out in Sudan. In the Sudan, Christian and animist captives in the civil war are often enslaved and female prisoners are often used sexually, with their Muslim captors claiming that Islamic law grants them permission. According to CBS news, slaves have been sold for $50 *a piece*.

It is estimated that as many as 200,000 people had been taken into slavery during the Second Sudanese Civil War.

The slaves are mostly Dinka people. Human trafficking for the purpose of sexual exploitation is a major cause of contemporary sexual slavery. In the Middle-East, the most common destinations for victims of human trafficking Israel and Turkey according to a report by UNODC.

20.2 Tackling Trafficking

Sex trafficking victims are generally found in dire circumstances and easily targeted by traffickers. Individuals, circumstances, and situations vulnerable to traffickers include homeless individuals, runaway teens, displaced homemakers, refugees, and drug addicts. While it may seem like trafficked people are the most vulnerable and powerless minorities in a region, victims are consistently exploited from any ethnic and social background.

In addition to the CRC and Convention on the Elimination of all forms of Discrimination against Women (CEDAW), there are a number of international conventions that deal with the rights of women and children in relation to early marriage and sexual abuse. However, some Arab and Islamic countries have made reservations to the CRC and CEDAW.

B. Gerbaka et al., *Child Sexual Abuse, Exploitation and Trafficking in the Arab Region*, Child Maltreatment 13, https://doi.org/10.1007/978-3-030-66507-4_20

The general objections from Arab states are that the articles can only be accepted if they are not against the Islamic Law: the Sharia'. This poses a problem of how to interpret the Islamic Law? Whose interpretation shall we rely on? Traditionally sharia has been interpreted only by men, but we are also faced with the differences of the four schools of thought within Sunni Islam in addition to Shia interpretations.

However, in most Arabic countries traditions and customs mean more to people than Islam, but in relation to laws and conventions Islam has a higher legitimacy, with the following hierarchy in legitimacy:

1. Traditions ('urf)
2. Islam (sharia)
3. Laws (qanun)
4. International conventions

20.3 Violations of the CRC

This model was confirmed by other researchers, during discussions at the workshop held in Cyprus. There are cases that clearly violate the CRC: for example if the law in Yemen stipulated that the legal age for marriage is 18, some parents would lie about their daughters date of birth in order to marry her earlier, in violation of the set law.

Today we see that the application as well as the law itself is influenced by religion and customs. This problem is further explored in the three research reports.

To bring about change, it is imperative that the conventions be addressed and we lobby for the legal system so they conform to the signed treatises.

A sign of modernization is that laws become more important than customs and religious-laws; thus the work towards an adherence to principles in the CRC and a change in the legal system is not useless. Furthermore, it is a new discourse emerging connecting Islam to human rights; subsequently, Islam, laws and conventions together can be powerful against customs to create a better situation for teenage girls in the MENA region and therefore need to be analyzed in detail.

20.4 Religious Leadership

Religion is a double edge sword in the battle against honor-crimes. The Islamic rule in sharia can be applied as an Islamic tool for categorizing honor killings against the religion and the religious law, according to sura (chapter) 24 in the Holy Quran, demands that accusations of adultery be supported by four witnesses of the actual sexual act. Unfortunately, these kinds of interpretations are seldom applied. Instead religious establishments of both Muslim and Christian scholars and politicians, often choose to support honor crimes in the name of sexual morality and set regulations against premarital sex in order to control who is allowed to marry.

An example from the OPT is of Palestinian priests supporting the killing of Christian-Palestinian girls having relationships with Muslim boys as a message for others not to become involved in such relationships. It seems that the honor ideology somehow finds resonance with religious moral laws within all religions, not only Islam.

It should be stressed that the moral ideals against sex outside wedlock should not in any sense support honor crimes; however many religious scholars still make this connection. It is alright to follow the moral that sex belongs to marriage; the problem is in the sanctions taken against those who are suspected of breaking these moral rules.

It should also be noted that the West has a tradition of Protestantism operating with individualist feelings of guilt and innocence, while in the Middle East, both Christianity and Islam, are colored by the collectivist honor and shame dichotomy. In the West the individual often feels guilty regarding what is right and wrong, hence disciplining the individual through feelings of bad consciousness.

In the honor-culture however, shameful deeds can be practiced if hidden from the public eye. This can be interpreted as encouraging hypocrisy, but it is a structure that releases people from feelings of guilt and provides a space of freedom if actions are kept in secret. However, the honor culture seems to be repressive at large, since the victims of sexual assault are accused it makes it difficult for them to talk about their experiences or the assault against them. Furthermore, the families of a sexual abuse victim are also tainted and stigmatized.

20.5 Norms and Practices in *Honor* Crimes

In practice, customs still seem to have higher legitimacy than religion, although I believe a shift of positions will come due to Islam. In our research, parents proclaimed honor violence as being against the religion and suggested combating such acts with religious sanctions against sexual criminals. The OPT examines Islam as a tool for gender equality since it moralizes against both sexes and ascribes the same sanctions towards them. In practice, as demonstrated through the experiences of girls, only the female part is blamed however. Consequently, Islam can be used as a tool in combating honor violence, and has been used for this purpose in Jordan.

The strict rules regarding sacredness, privacy and integrity can be applied to condemn the spreading of rumors and gossip in the name of honor.

In Islam, it is a sin to spy on others and spread gossip, however the same principles make it harder for children to speak up against sexual abuse in their homes, since such matters are often referred to as "private" and hence to be solved in the private sphere without interference of the wider society. The assault can then continue in secret. Furthermore the religious stress on "obedience" of children and wives to fathers and husbands, as pointed out in the Palestinian report, make it problematic to speak up in cases of sexual violence. Another dilemma related to Islam, discussed in the situation analysis here, is that in the sharia "rape within marriage" is an unknown concept since women must be sexually-accessible to their husbands. Young wives are therefore exposed to repeated sexual abuse in their marriage, as demonstrated in the life stories quoted from Yemen. There are no rules in the Islamic religion that encourage early marriages, however none condemn it either leaving religion open for interpretation regarding the suitable age for marriage. Subsequently, religion can be used both for and against sexual violence within marriages.

The legislation on honor crimes and sexuality is influenced by religion and traditions. Originally, the laws on passion crimes have been influenced by the laws of the colonial powers and are not from the sharia as such, but are nowadays used as an excuse for lenient punishment for honor-criminals.

The law stipulates that the extenuating circumstances for the criminal are that he has lost his sanity seeing his wife having intercourse with another man and kills her. This excuse, however, is hardly ever the case in honor crimes, since such crimes are not usually committed because a man finds his wife in bed with another man; however honor-crimes are excused using the notion that the killer was in a state of "fit or fury" and therefore is sentenced to lenient punishment.

Moreover, the rule that adultery is a crime and against the law is a view abandoned in the West in the course of modernization, but still existent in the MENA. In Western countries, adultery is considered a private matter rather than a criminal act against the law. Such changes to the law would make sexuality enter the sphere of private-morality rather than being a public issue that falls in the field of legislation. Consensual sex is not equal to sexual abuse of children by adults. In Islam, a way of having "legal" consensual sex is to engage in an Islamic marriage (orfi marriage), as documented by the OPT. Islam can be used to give legitimacy and blessing to consensual sexual intercourse, in cases where laws and families are opposing such unions. However, the same practice can be exploited for sexual abuse and prostitution.

20.6 Universal Rights, Emerging Region, Global Support

Legislations against sexual abuse and violence against women and children need to be strengthened in the region. There are many examples of laws that are discriminatory towards women and children. Even in countries such as Lebanon that stands out as being the most modernized country, legislations are strongly influenced by religion and traditions, family in Honor crimes and child marriage. Therefore, their quest for a unified (secular) civil law for personal status should be taken seriously. In OPT, the laws are confusing but still the same discriminatory traces are apparent in their legal systems, apart from the recently established laws by the Palestinian Authority, Gaza also follows Egyptian law and the West Bank practices Jordanian legislation in certain matters.

The CRC helps combating sexual violence against teenage girls in light of the customs, religions and legislations. CRC has been successful in promoting new legislations against trafficking and child prostitution in the region, as discussed in the chapters here. Since such laws exist, they also have to be applied and interpreted to include sexual abuse, violence in the name of honor, and early marriage as forms of sexual violence. The women's movement in the region is working for legal changes that promote gender equality.

This struggle must be supported, laws must be developed that apply despite religion and customs, and the CRC must act as the frame of reference applied in combating such problems.

Chapter 21
Summary and Recommendations

The prohibition of violence has also been included in laws for civil service (e.g. Jordan, Bahrain) and stipulated in laws, regulations and ministerial decrees. There is considerable progress with regards amending penal codes and child protection acts, and the enactment of new laws to ensure effective protection for children.

Nevertheless, these laws share common constraints, as they:

- Are not based on a comprehensive review of all domestic legislation in against the CRC and other relevant international conventions.
- Include general human rights without sufficient details or clarification to avoid misinterpretation (e.g. Palestine Act of 2004 amended in 2009).
- Are based on the CRC without reference to the principles and provisions of the Optional Protocols on the Sale of Children, Child Prostitution and Child Pornography and on the Involvement of Children in Armed Conflict.
- Did not clearly express the concept of the best interests of the child, which is often included as a separate article without addressing its implications for various aspects of economic, social and civil rights.
- Do not address the child's right to express his/her opinion, and to participate in decision making on subjects related to his/her concerns.
- Included ideas whose proper location is executive regulations due to their procedural and technical nature.
- State responses do not include data allowing analysis on the basis of the various settings where violence occurs although; deductions can be drawn from data on the nature of violence.

B. Gerbaka et al., *Child Sexual Abuse, Exploitation and Trafficking in the Arab Region*, Child Maltreatment 13, https://doi.org/10.1007/978-3-030-66507-4_21

21.1 Sexual Violence and the Education Response

Most laws do not clearly prohibit all forms of sexual violence against girls and boys below 18 years of age, nor do they protect victims from the requirements of multiple testimonies, or eliminate all possibilities for impunity in cases of sexual offences occurring within the family. There are no explicit articles disallowing the dropping of charges and discontinuing lawsuits in cases where the aggressor marries the victim. These laws have failed to provide me and psychological recovery services for victims. In some cases, legislation has failed to prohibit the acquisition, production, dissemination, and distribution of documents and materials containing child pornography.

Laws have not provided for allowing complaints without the permission of the victim's parents, nor have they ensured that child victims of sexual exploitation will not be considered criminals or delinquents.

In the Arab region, there is only limited reporting on the occurrence of sexual violence in schools as the subject remains a social taboo and child friendly reporting mechanism are absent. Yet there is evidence to suggest its presence. A study in Yemen on a sample of 267 children showed that 31.4% were exposed to sexual harassment (in 56.2% of the cases, the aggressor was either a peer or a neighbor and in 13.7% of the cases it was one of the teachers)

- In Morocco, it was observed that 8 out of 40 cases of violence reported to the Child Rights Observatory were classified as sexual harassment (6 boys and 2 girls)[1]
- In Lebanon, a recent study showed that 16% of children were exposed to sexual harassment with 6% of these cases occurring in a school setting.[2] The study showed that the incidence of sexual harassment was higher in the case of girls than boys (12 girls vs. 1 boy)[3]

In some cases, violence is discussed only with regard to violence inflicted by adults upon children, instead of referencing also violence among peers. Sudan, as an exception, does address peer violence through its Child Law.

The reactions of states indicate that the mechanisms of monitoring and complaints are the same as those present in the components of the national child protection system. Others mentioned the existence of clear mechanisms.

The Arab Report on the Recommendations of the UN Secretary-General's Study on Violence Against Children determine referential persons in the school, and follow-up mechanisms for referral to the director, and then on to the specialized

[1]Save the Children interview with "Beity" society and the Child Rights Observatory, Rabat, 10 October, 2010.

[2]Higher Council for Childhood, Save the Children (Sweden), Kafa Society, Sexual Harassment in Lebanon, 2008.

[3]Child and Youth Protection Initiative, Arab Institute for Urban Development, Sana'a (2008).

department in the ministry of education. In extreme cases the referral is to the child protection monitor in the ministry of social affairs (e.g. Palestine).

Yemen is the only state that mentioned having complaints boxes in schools, and that committees for protection were formed in some schools to afford the children the chance to make complaints.[4]

Documentation of complaints lies within the jurisdiction of the protection system (such as the police in Sudan, and the Child Helpline in Egypt), and not inside the educational system. On the other hand, some countries' educational systems adopt a component of child protection, and have elucidated the presence of models that are followed by the ministry of education, in cooperation with other ministries (e.g. Palestine).

Most countries said that they had applied a special effort to raise awareness and provide education on the issue of VAC. Some countries organized meeting with children (e.g. Jordan, Lebanon, Algeria, Qatar) with the aim of enabling and educating children on the mechanisms available (e.g. Yemen, Palestine). Some stated that VAC is taking little priority in schools, and that they had designated national campaigns, strategies and comprehensive plans to improve this situation (e.g. Palestine, Jordan). Other countries include plans for child protection against violence in general, in connection with violence in schools.[5]

The presence of comprehensive measures and policies on the school level was not notable, except in a few cases, including: Lebanon's experiment in Mabarrat schools of a policy of child protection within the school, Tunisia's Council of the Educational Institution, whose jurisdiction includes ensuring controls and child safety, and Algeria, which has formed a disciplinary council headed by the school director, with the purpose of preserving order.

The following recommendations should be considered to assist states to build national methodological responses supported by documented evidence and data, rather than relying simply on the adoption of international trends:

1. Express political will to increase data collection and monitoring of cases of violence, represented in a special agenda for management, organization and analysis of data, and the allocation of financial resources to expand comprehensive research and studies in various settings.
2. Appoint a body or entity at the national level that is responsible for data collection process from various agencies, ministries, research centers, universities and NGOs on a clear basis and specific methodology. This

(continued)

[4]Yemen National Council for Childhood and Motherhood, Violence Against Children: a Social Study in Some Yemeni Regions, 2005.

[5]Save the Children Sweden and International Bureau for Children's Rights, Violence Against Schools: a Regional Analysis of Lebanon, Morocco and Yemen, 2011.

entity should be associated with national structures responsible for the development of strategies and plans to ensure the development of programs and interventions that are priorities and to prevent the recurrence of programs that proved not to be effective. It should also issues periodic reports which highlight general trends and progress made in various sectors, identifies gaps that hinder the data collection process, are given to decision-makers, and is made available to children through the use of easy and understandable language. Such bodies should be recognized as independent and credible.

3. Secure requests for information from children, media and universities. Establish connections and cooperation protocols with several sectors that produce information or data, especially departments or centers for national statistics.
4. Ensure that information-gathering processes are unified and consistent within a scientific methodology, and works on transferring it and training various parties.
5. Collect information from administrative records and proposes and implements periodic national surveys.
6. Develops a list of qualitative and quantitative indicators on the subject of child protection.
7. Monitor progress made, identify gaps, and determine the categories not covered by prevention, intervention, or rehabilitation programs.
8. Integrate a comprehensive system for the registration of marriages, birth and filing.
9. Build a system for monitoring deaths, including child deaths reviews, within a system for legal and medical examination for the collection of documented deaths and mentioning the cause of death in death registries.
10. Connect a management system for cases in medical care facilities, child protection.
11. Provide data collection services at national level, to allow the continued availability of information on individual cases and planning the service-provision process.
12. Document information at the sectoral levels of education, health and law enforcement, and categorize data according to age, gender, and type of violence, geographic region and family characteristics.
13. Train personnel on documentation and analysis methodologies and on ethics in research on CSA like interviewing children and respecting privacy. In fact, failure to exchange information between various agencies may lead to unnecessary suffering or even death.
14. Familiarize universities and institutes with children's issues in general and violence and abuse in particular, in order to provide personnel and institutions related to childhood with the required scientific competencies and

(continued)

research methodologies, and making it a subject of social discussion and research material in more than one university specialty.

15. Strength community monitoring mechanisms and documenting of cases on the national level through parents, children, NGOs and municipalities. Local observatories can also be established to be in constant contact with the national observatory.
16. Ensure children's access to information and participation in its provision, analysis and dissemination
17. Accreditate Child protection policies, including child friendly processes for complaints.

Chapter 22
Future Perspectives

Despite many obstacles, the perspective of child protection is strongly developing within national systems and regional networks, in the presence of increasing levels of common values and universal understanding of child rights. In reality, child dedicated structures are grass rooting initiatives; they rely on political decisions, local and national human resources, regional expertise and international cooperation; they seek for strategies at the countries levels in order to implant child protection systems, and recently expanded the network in order to learn from experiences in other Arab countries:

- 1st ISPCAN Arab regional conference on CAN, Amman, Jordan, 2004: “Breaking the silence”
- 2nd ISPCAN Arab regional conference on CAN, Aden, Yemen, 2007: “Towards a strategy for child protection”
- 3rd ISPCAN Arab regional conference on CAN, Riyadh, KSA, 1-4 March 2009: "Working together towards safer childhood".
- 19th International ISPCAN Conference, September 9-12, 2012, Istanbul, Turkey
- ISPCAN Child Helpline Arab regional conference on Child Maltreatment Prevention, Riyadh, KSA, January 2012
- 4th ISPCAN Arab regional conference on CAN, Kuwait, 18-20 April 2016
- 5th ISPCAN Arab regional conference on CAN, Dubai, UAE, November 19-22, 2017
- Faith ISPCAN USJ Conference, Beirut, Lebanon, February 24-25, 2019
- 6th ISPCAN Arab regional conference on CAN, Muscat, Oman, September 15-17, 2019
- ISSOP ISPCAN conference on CAN, Beirut, Lebanon, Sep 24-25, 2019
- International ISPCAN conference on CAN, Doha, Qatar, February 15-17, 2020
- . . . Also, in between those dates, professionals’ training seminars were held in: Syria, Lebanon, Egypt, Bahrain, KSA, etc.
- Arab Professional Society for the Prevention of Violence on Children, registered in 2012 in the State of Lebanon by Decree No. 8423

B. Gerbaka et al., *Child Sexual Abuse, Exploitation and Trafficking in the Arab Region*, Child Maltreatment 13, https://doi.org/10.1007/978-3-030-66507-4_22

On those diverse occasions, the Arab initiative—then the UNSV—presented a setting-based framework for the description of child abuse in countries and the efforts developed to stop violence. The International Society for the Prevention of Child Abuse and Neglect was also partner within the advisory panel to advice on the nature and definitions of VAC on one side, and conduct the UNSV on the other.

Based on an expanding knowledge base, the UNSV intends to highlight on the status of children confronted with violence in their different environments, to increase the national—as well as informal capacities to build systems that focus on the integration of protection and prevention—as well as child participation—in the human rights commitments and implementation processes. All procedures would be based on a CRC matrix that incorporates children's rights, professional evidence, relevant social factors and intersectoral responsibilities for the prevention of VAC and the control of CAN, as a priority in Governmental programs.

Arab countries live, now more than ever, in identity crisis and armed conflicts. They are, however, challenged to plan systems, set priorities and provide a basis for political and social debate on the present and the future condition of children, with the participation of children. In this perspective, the APNPCAN/VAC can plan the following activities:

- Meet with children and youth, to discuss their opinions about CAN and VAC; the I-CAST-Child questionnaire developed by ISPCAN and supported by UNICEF is indeed a useful tool in such a task. The main objectives of those meetings are to:
  - agree on definitions of VAC and CAN;
  - enable more children to outreach the UNSV child version;
  - reach a common understanding about the way to confront violence in child environments;
  - exchange with children their outputs on the UNSV results and recommendations;
  - develop procedures children find useful and productive for child effective participation and child protection;
  - Include, in an effective process, child recommendations within national Arab strategies for child protection.
- Lobby with Parliamentarians and legislators, to:
  - enhance already existing national and local movements towards child protection, while tackling specific needs and priorities;
  - stimulate legislative revision of laws, to comply with the provisions of the CRC and optional protocols;
  - Increase local and national knowledge about the UNSV and contribute in finding appropriate procedures to initiate advocacy and sustainable child protection.
- Work with other professionals to:
  - Increase common knowledge and develop existing training tools;
  - Upgrade the informal knowledge to a comprehensive curriculum;

- Base their interventions on evidence of qualitative assessment and efficient actions;
- Carry out comprehensive national surveys. It is essential that children participate in the survey;
- Support research and study centers;
- Develop mechanisms that enable violated children to make their complaints;
- Provide psychological and physical rehabilitation services;
- Prepare periodic reports and meetings;
- Develop training programs for personnel working with children regarding best practices;
- Set up counseling centers that receive reports and complaints;

• Embody the reform of child protection by being candidates in city councils, parliaments and governments, in order to set up parliamentary committees, amend existing legislation (rights of the child, criminalization of violence and enforce the provisions of CRC);
• Reduce gender discrimination by tackling directly the girl child issues, in terms of participation, education, domestic child labor, early marriage, female genital mutilation and family violence. The empowerment of women is also part of this process.

Obviously, the scarcity of child specific health and social support services are obstacles to child protection, and should then be made available to families and accessible to children. In reality, the capacities of those services are sometimes overwhelmed, especially during armed conflicts and social instability, when children are involved in violent situations and at increased risk of different types of abuse and violence. In such contexts, free childcare, universal health screening and universal access to free medical care become even more critical, as is, in general, the universal access to free health care for all citizens.

National strategies for child protection would indeed comply with the United Nations Convention on the Rights of the Child, with attention to the needs and possibilities of some developing, insecure and ill-resourced countries (8). The potential challenges and impacts of the CRC implementation should also be explored for future landmarks of democracies and freedom of opinions, mainly in terms of:

• Independent structures: child observatories, at local and national levels, are actually available in Morocco, Tunis and Lebanon. There are still no child defenders or child ombudsman, though a proposition of law was presented in this regard in Lebanon, 2004.
• Child protection acts or child-friendly and environment-centered legislations, actually available in Egypt, Jordan, Syria, pending in Lebanon.
• Budgets for Child protection and child oriented projects, not distinctively available.

- Helpline for children and professionals, for the reporting of child maltreatment and for psychosocial support to victims of violence, available in Egypt, pending in Lebanon.
- Training of pilot and decentralized multisectoral teams and building of professional curricula, actually in expanding process in Syria, Lebanon, Jordan and Egypt.
- Study the extent of VAC, based on three I-CAST questionnaires (Child, Retrospective and Parents) tested and implemented in Egypt and Lebanon.
- Participation of children and youth in the evaluation of problems, analysis of situations, setting of reports, implementation of processes and re-evaluation of actions, present in many country reports, where few evidence of efficiency is however available.
- Support of child-friendly media: auto-censorship on aggressive viewings, to reduce violence and enhance educative programs—with children—on screens; in this regards, workshops for child friendly media have been held in many countries in the region, with two main outcomes: abused children are rarely visualized on media, and more child friendly programs are developed.
- Code of conduct for professionals working with children: Lebanon is considering the implementation of the code with professionals working for/with children, within the provisions of the coming modification of relevant law.

22.1 Implications

Despite ongoing efforts by Arab governments and many NGOs to address the multiple social, cultural and professional pitfalls, CAN remains a serious threat to child rights implementation. There is still no child budget and no child protection acts in many counties. There are few independent structures for child rights monitoring (National child defender, national child observatory) and scarce child helplines. Children are still present in high numbers in institutions. Therapy programs are limited for victims—yet increasing—and most often virtual for perpetrators. Legislations are subject to national consultations to meet the CRC requirements. The human and social situation of refugees is sometimes dramatic or still waiting for the settlement of the Arab-Israeli conflict as well as other armed clashes in Iraq, Sudan, Somalia and others. Internally and regionally displaced children are repeatedly exposed to extreme types of violence and abuse, with contraventions to the UN and EU Guidelines.

Obviously, given the scant findings and the many limitations of this review, conclusions are for the most part tentative and need to be placed within the larger framework of CSA. This review can confirm several points. Research on child sexual abuse in MENA is notably lacking compared to many parts of the world. Of interest, the Global School-based Student Health Survey in use by 19 countries as of 2007 has questions on child physical and sexual abuse. Those data were included by Lebanon, but Oman, Libya and the United Arab Emirates chose to do the survey but left out the questions on child physical and sexual abuse. As noted by many authors in these studies and globally, without prevalence rates and research on CSA, there is less hope of overcoming resistance to acknowledging the problem and working to solve it.

Child sexual abuse of boys and girls clearly does exist in the Middle East and North Africa and is a cause for concern in MENA as well as the rest of the world. That fact is unlikely to change until societies change, becoming less patriarchal and less adultist, until children are given rights accorded human beings guaranteed by the UN Convention on the Rights of the Child. The patterns, while tentative given the data, are consistent that boys in MENA have higher rates of CSA than girls in MENA and higher rates than boys in North America and Europe.

Children suffer horribly at the hands of their abusers and child sexual abuse is associated with numerous adverse consequences throughout the globe including the Middle East and North Africa. It takes enormous courage to advocate on behalf of the powerless, even more so in the area of child abuse and even more so in societies where this issue is taboo. It is hoped that this review will encourage others to continue research and policy efforts to protect all of our children.

In some countries, children are viewed as—and submitted to—their religious references, in terms—and place—of civil rights. In such countries, children are exposed to problems that alter their growth, development, social interaction, safety, education and health.

In Lebanon, In conclusion, key decisions will need to be made in Lebanon for the development of a comprehensive and congruent child protection system, one that functions effectively and is perceived as appropriate and relevant by families at the local level. The study found that participants clearly feel that the different strategies employed for protecting children need to be blended. At one end of the spectrum, community resolution and family mediation will continue to be an inherent element of a child protection system while the statutory response system will offer special measures for those at the greatest level of risk. There remains a debate about how to organize other system components and about how—in a country with strong community affiliations—a single system, regulated by civil and criminal law, and applicable to all Lebanese citizens, is best tailored to meet existing and future child protection challenges.

It is therefore important for Arab professionals to rely on—and encourage—the governments who show intention to build child protection systems, but also to contribute in drawing a sharing platform of knowledge and knowhow, from observations and findings of professionals, experts and NGOs who work closely with children; in this regard, cooperation with ISPCAN may increase the capacities of stakeholders in confronting violence with peaceful stands, based on firm and clear evidence of efficient programs.

Countries in the Arab region are urged to launch CRC compliant and socially accepted—child protection systems that would be comprehensive melting pots of existing and developing programs. Success stories and reports on obstacles are most welcome, to improve MENA knowledge about the status of children, in a dynamic and proactive way. In this perspective it is important to note that there was an Arab League meeting in 2009 to amend Arab chapter on Child Rights.

In different—and sometimes conflicting—contexts of security and safety, the Arab efforts to integrate children's rights within global human rights matrix—and child health and well-being requirements—need, in fact, strong social links and individual stands towards child protection acts. Child help lines, child defenders and child observatories are the pivots of knowledge base, data collection and training, rehabilitation and prevention, global child rights and local childhood requisites.

In each step, the APNPCAN/VAC can demonstrate the efficiency of professionals in promoting children's globally recognized rights within their living places. Such initiatives work best when social stability, common vision, effective interaction between formal and informal sector, and child efficient participation. . .are available. Indeed, such initiatives towards child protection are most needed when those conditions are not yet available. Most challenging options are in most difficult—yet enriching—environments! Where the most vulnerable is not the slowest!

Annex: Definitions and Terminology

Definition of Violence

Base study of the Secretary-General of the United Nations definition of violence contained in the WHO report on violence and health has defined violence as "the intentional use of force or power, or the threat thereof, against self or against another person or several persons or society as a whole, resulting in or may result in injury or death or injury or mental disorder in the growth or deprivation."

Guided by this study as well as the definition of violence as set out in the Convention on the Rights of the Child (Article 19), the Convention on the Elimination of All Forms of Discrimination against Women, as well as the definition agreed upon by experts in the meeting organized for the prevention of violence (WHO), will be to serve the objective of the study, with a capacity of these definitions to include all forms of physical and psychological violence, including as well as deliberate neglect or ill-treatment or exploitation, including sexual exploitation of children as well as trafficking in children. It takes more dangerous trend of violence when its source is involved in caring for the child or those responsible.

Violence against children includes physical violence, psychological violence, discrimination, neglect and ill-treatment. Ranging from sexual abuse in the home to corporal and humiliating punishment at school; and the use of physical restraints in children's homes to brutality at the hands of security agents; and from abuse and neglect in institutions to gang warfare on the streets where children play or work; from infanticide to so-called murder "honor."

Definition of the Child

Known the child for the purpose of this study, as stated in (Article 1) of the Convention on the Rights of the Child as "every human being below eighteen, unless majority is attained earlier under the law applicable to him." Accordingly,

B. Gerbaka et al., *Child Sexual Abuse, Exploitation and Trafficking in the Arab Region*, Child Maltreatment 13, https://doi.org/10.1007/978-3-030-66507-4

information on strategies to address violence against girls and boys under the age of eighteen is provided in all parts of the questionnaire.

Concepts and Definitions

Action plan: Sometimes overlapping with the strategy, an action plan in this context is considered as the shorter-term plan of activities for taking that broader strategy forward, including activities, timeframes, resources and leadership.

Children: Consistent with the Convention on the Rights of the Child (1989), the term 'children' is used to refer to persons younger than 18 years, even if the age of majority differs according to national law.

Child protection: The protection of children against abuse, neglect, violence and exploitation in all their forms, regardless of the nature of the relationship a child has with a perpetrator or the setting in which it occurs. For the purposes of this study, the term incorporates the special protection afforded to children in conflict with the law.

Family: The term 'family' is used as shorthand to refer to those within the caring circle of a child. This caring circle varies according to culture and circumstance; thus, the use of the term `family' recognizes that in many societies the care environment of a child includes extended family and in some places, the wider community. The term also recognizes that in some circumstances, children are primary caregivers.[1] However, individuals from the community or service providers who are not providing daily emotional, physical and psychological care to a child are not included in this definition of family.

Formal child protection system: The term refers to those structures that have been established specifically to or which have a role in the protection of children, with or without a legal mandate for their operations. This may include government agencies, international organizations and local NGOs (including community- and faith-based organizations) involved in providing child protection, where these are officially recognized or endorsed by and subject to supervision and regulation by the national Government. Some groups, such as traditional and religious leaders, may also have clear roles within the formal system.[2]

Child and family welfare system: The child and family welfare system refers to those aspects nested within the social welfare system (or social protection system,

[1]Understanding and applying a systems approach to child protection: a guide for programme staff. Stephanie Delaney and Padraig Quigley, for Child Frontiers and Mirela Shuteriqi, Terre des hommes. https://www.tdh.ch/sites/default/files/tdh_e.pdf

Joynes, C. & Mattingly, J. (2018). A systems approach to child protection. K4D Helpdesk Report. Brighton, UK: Institute of Development Studies. https://resourcecentre.savethechildren.net/library/systems-approach-child-protection

[2]There will be differences between how the 'formal system' is defined and how this actually works in practice.

where applicable) that are aimed at promoting children's well-being and protection while enhancing the ability of families and communities to fulfil their responsibilities.

Justice system: The justice system comprises both (i) state-run justice and law enforcement institutions, including the judiciary (criminal and civil), justice and interior ministries, the police, prisons, criminal investigation and prosecution services and (ii) non-state justice mechanisms, including the whole range of traditional, customary, religious and informal mechanisms that deal with disputes at the community level.[3]

Informal child protection system[4]: The term refers to endogenous child protection practices and measures undertaken by communities, families and children or assistance provided as an alternative or in addition to formal services, based on cultural norms, tradition and social practices. It is important to emphasize that formal and informal should be understood as representing two ends of a continuum and that there may be elements of overlap between the formal and informal systems. It can be challenging to clearly define specific components due to ambivalent roles and mandates. Elaborating the nature of the relationship between these systems represents an important part of this study.

Local-level: The term refers to the location of the interface between service provider and client (child/family). For the purpose of this study, it tends to refer to the regional level (mohafazat) because the formal child protection mechanism is located in regional capitals. However, other non-mandated child protection services are located at lower levels including in communities themselves.

Local-level child protection mechanism: The term refers to the formal processes and services in place and implemented at the local level to respond to children and families at significant risk of, or suffering from, abuse, neglect, violence or exploitation or who come into conflict with the law.

Congruence: The term is generally understood as the quality or state of agreeing or coinciding. Recognizing the importance of harmony between the system and local child caring and child protection realities, this term is used to describe the positive dynamic between the population and the formal system. Congruence occurs when the system supports and builds upon positive cultural beliefs and practices while challenging those cultural norms, beliefs and practices that are detrimental to child and family well-being. In the context of this study, congruence does not imply that a system would condone gross violations or ignore aspects of culture that have adverse effects on the well-being of children.

Continuum of care: The term refers to the spectrum of assistance and services that may be provided to children and their families, ranging from broad proactive and preventative measures to the immediate and reactive child protective measures, when actual abuse happens.[5]

---

[3]UN Common Approach to Justice for Children, UNICEF, 2008.

[4]The terms 'informal' and 'non-formal' can be used interchangeably.

[5]For further explanation of the continuum of care, please see Annex.

Policy: A defined set of the principles, approaches and priorities that underpin the child welfare and protection system, considering in particular the choices and alternatives possible that have been considered in deciding the policy.

Prevention measures: The term refers to a range of measures designed to mitigate the risk of children being harmed or to reduce the likelihood of harm re-occurring. These initiatives may be broad national initiatives and strategies that cover the general population with the aim of creating a more protective environment for children and families. As such, these can be described as 'universal' prevention initiatives. Common activities include awareness, information and advocacy campaigns promoting the need for alternative discipline rather than physical punishment norm addressing the problem of domestic violence, together with such initiatives as programs aimed at preventing violence in schools and promoting birth registration.

Strengthening the Child Protection System in Lebanon

Challenges and Opportunities

Response measures: No matter how effective prevention and early intervention services are, there will always be a need for high quality and efficient reactive child protective response services. Child protective response services are targeted specifically to children who are victims of abuse, neglect, violence and exploitation. These tend to be compulsory government intervention measures implemented as a last resort when prevention initiatives (formal and informal) have failed to protect the child.

Statutory child protection: This reflects the powers, duties, responsibilities and processes for the protection of children which are enacted or regulated through the law.

Strategy: The methodology used to accomplish the principles and aims prescribed in a policy.

Consistent with the principles of the policy, the strategy outlines the longer-term implementation plan, namely all political, management, financial and administrative mechanisms required.

Definitions of "Trafficking in Persons" in the Countries of the MENA Region

Since the passage of the U.N. Protocol in 2000, many countries around the world have adopted comprehensive anti-trafficking laws to combat human trafficking in compliance with the legislative mandate of the U.N. Protocol. In the Arab world alone, 12 States have adopted comprehensive anti-trafficking laws: Bahrain, Djibouti, Egypt, Iraq, Jordan, Kuwait, Mauritania, Oman, Qatar, Saudi Arabia, Syria, and the United Arab Emirates. Algeria and Lebanon have adopted anti-trafficking provisions in their penal codes. The remaining States Members of the Arab League continue to use existing laws to prosecute trafficking cases.

Bahrain

The law of Bahrain adopts an approach similar to that of the U.N. Protocol, especially in regard to the issue of consent. Article 1 of the law makes consent completely irrelevant for cases involving persons younger than 18 years old, stating the following:

(a) For the purpose of implementing the provisions of this Law, trafficking in persons shall mean the recruitment, transportation, transfer, harboring, or receiving persons, by means of threat or the use of force or other forms of coercion, abduction, fraud, deceit, abuse of power or of position or any other direct or indirect unlawful means. Exploitation shall include the exploitation of such person or the prostitution of others or any other forms of exploitation, sexual assault, forced labor or services, slavery or practices similar to slavery, servitude or the removal of organs.
(b) Recruitment, transportation, transfer, harboring, or receiving of persons who are less than eighteen years of age or who are in a condition or personal state in which their consent or freedom of choice cannot be guaranteed shall be deemed as trafficking in persons if the intent is to exploit them even if such act is not accompanied by any of the means provided for in the preceding paragraph.
(c) The perpetrator shall be presumed to have knowledge of the real age of the victim who is not eighteen years of age.49

Djibouti

Article 2 of Law No. 210 of 27 December 2007 on the Fight against Human Trafficking in Djibouti states "Human trafficking shall mean the process by which a person is recruited, transported, transferred, harbored or received within or outside the national borders by one or more persons or institutions by means of threat or other forms of coercion, fraud, deception, abduction, or the abuse of power for the purpose of exploitation."50 Unlike the U.N. Protocol, the law does not provide a definition of exploitation and limits the definition of potential victims of trafficking to children under 18 years of age, girls and women, and the physically or mentally handicapped.

Egypt

Egyptian Law No. 64 of 2010 provides the most comprehensive definition of "trafficking" in the MENA region by expanding the U.N. Protocol definition and including in the forms of exploitation the exploitation of children in prostitution and all other forms of sexual exploitation, exploitation of children in pornography, begging, and removal of tissues or a part thereof. In particular, article 2 reads as follows: A person who commits the crime of trafficking in persons shall be considered one who deals in any manner in a natural person, including: the sale, offer for sale, purchase, or promise thereof; or the use, transport, delivery, harboring, reception, or receipt, whether within the country or across its national borders; if this occurred through the use of force, violence, or threat thereof; or through abduction, fraud, deception, abuse of power, or exploitation of a position of vulnerability or need; or through a promise to give or receive payments or benefits in exchange for obtaining the consent of a person to traffic another having control over him; or if the purpose of the transaction was exploitation in any of its forms, including: exploitation of acts of prostitution and all forms of sexual exploitation, exploitation of children in such acts and in pornography, forced labor or services, slavery or practices similar to slavery or servitude, or begging or removal of human organs, tissues or a part thereof.51

The definition is based on a general conceptualization of trafficking in persons as a transaction in persons. Like the U.N. Protocol, the Egyptian law defines "illegal means" broadly to include exploitation of a position of vulnerability. However, the law explicitly includes both domestic and transnational trafficking. This emphasis by the Egyptian legislature was important in recognizing the prevalence of internal trafficking within the country.

Iraq

Iraqi Law No. 28 of 30 April 2012 expands the U.N. Protocol definition of "trafficking" by including "sale" as a purpose and by making exploitation of human beings for the purpose of medical experimentation a crime of human trafficking. In particular, article 1 specifies: For purposes of this law, the term "Human Trafficking" shall mean the recruitment, transportation, harboring or receipt of persons, by means of the threat or use of force or other forms of coercion, of abduction, of fraud, of deception, of the abuse of power or of the giving or receiving of payments or benefits to obtain the consent of a person having power or guardianship over another person, for the purpose of sale or exploitation in acts of prostitution or sexual abuse, servitude, forced labor, slavery, begging, trade of human organs or for purposes of medical experimentation.

Jordan

Jordanian Law No. 9/2009 on Prevention of Human Trafficking provides a definition of "trafficking" that follows the U.N. Protocol in relation to the acts and the illegal means but defines "exploitation" to include exploitation for the purpose of forced labor, servitude, or slavery; removal of organs; or prostitution and other forms of sexual exploitation. Article 3 of the law states: "Trafficking in persons" shall mean the recruitment, transportation, transfer, harboring or receipt of persons, by means of the threat or use of force or other forms of coercion, of abduction, of fraud, of deception, of the abuse of power or of a position of vulnerability or the giving or receiving of payments or benefits to achieve the consent of a person having control over another person for the purpose of exploitation. Exploitation shall include, at a minimum, exploitation for the purpose of forced labor or servitude, slavery, removal of organs, prostitution or other forms of sexual exploitation.53

Kuwait

Kuwaiti Law No. 91/2013 on Combating Trafficking in Persons and Smuggling follows the U.N. Protocol and defines "trafficking in persons" in article 4 as follows: "Trafficking in persons" shall mean the recruitment, transportation, transfer, harboring or receipt of persons, by means of the threat or use of force or other forms of coercion, of abduction, of fraud, of deception, of the abuse of power or of a position of vulnerability or the giving or receiving of payments or benefits to achieve the consent of a person having control over another person for the purpose of exploitation. Exploitation shall include, at a minimum, the exploitation of the prostitution of others or other forms of sexual exploitation, forced labor or services, slavery or practices similar to slavery, servitude or the removal of organs.54

28 Understanding Trafficking in Persons in the MENA region

Mauritania

Law No. 025 of 2003 on Suppression of Trafficking in Persons of Mauritania states, in Article 1: Trafficking in persons shall mean the recruitment, transportation, or transfer of people by means of the threat or use of force or other forms of coercion, abduction, deception, abuse of power or of a position of vulnerability or the giving or receiving of payments or benefits to achieve the consent of a person having control over another person for the purpose of exploitation. Exploitation shall include, at a minimum, unpaid labor, forced labor or services or similar practices, the removal of organs for financial gain, explcitation of the prostitution of others or other forms of sexual exploitation.55

Oman

Oman's Royal Decree Promulgating the Law Combating Trafficking in Persons, follows the U.N. approach and, in article 2, states: Any individual who intentionally carries out any of the following acts with the purpose of exploitation shall be adjudged committing the crime of trafficking in persons: (a) To recruit, transport, harbor, or receive a person by instruments of coercion, threat, deceit, blackmail, or misuse of power, influence, or use of authority on that individual, or by any other illegal instrument, either directly or indirectly; (b) To recruit, transport, harbor, or receive a child even without using the instruments cited in the previous paragraph.

Article 1 of the law states that the "illegal exploitation of a person shall include: prostitution, sexual assault, servitude, forced labor, enslavement, practices similar to slavery, subjugation, ... and removal of organs."57

Article 3 also stipulates that the consent of the victim is irrelevant if any threat was used, if the victim is a child, or if any circumstances render it impossible to determine his or her consent.58

Qatar

The law of Qatar includes explicitly "exploitation of children for sexual purposes, pornography, and begging." Thus, it emphasizes the particular problem of trafficking in children. Article 2 provides:

Exploitation shall include acts of prostitution or other forms of sexual exploitation, exploitation of children in such acts and in pornography or begging, servitude, compulsory services, slavery and practices similar to slavery, removal of human organs or tissues or part thereof.59

Saudi Arabia

In Saudi Arabia, the Suppression of the Trafficking in Persons Act, promulgated by Royal Decree No. M/40 of 2009 includes "begging" and "subjecting a person to medical tests"60 in its definition of "trafficking in persons."

Syria

The Syrian law, without specifying any form of trafficking, provides for a very general definition of "illegal acts and purposes" in "consideration for material or moral gain or a promise thereof or offer of privileges or attempt to achieve any of these or others."61 However, article 5 of the Syrian law states that sexually abusing a child, including using the child in pornography, shall also be considered trafficking in persons.62

United Arab Emirates

Influenced by the Arab League Model Law to Combat the Crime of Trafficking in Persons, the United Arab Emirates passed a human trafficking law in 2006 that was limited to criminalization. In defining the crime of trafficking in persons, the law states (Table A1):

Table A1 Prevalence Rates of Child Sexual Abuse PREVALENCE STUDIES

Middle East North Africa	All CSA combined Non Contact and Contact & Hugs		Non-Contact Only		Contact only Fondling & Rape		Contact Only Fondling		Contact Only Rape-Penetration	
Country Author	Male ALL Non-Cont & hug	Female All Non-Cont & Cont &hug	MaLe Non-Cont Only	Female NON-Cont ONLY	Male Con-tact Only F&R	Female Contact only Fondle & Rape	Male Contact Fondle	Female Contact Fondle	Male Rape	Female Rape
Middle East										
Israel Bedouin Arab Elbedour et al.	31%		16%+		17%+		13%+		4%+	
Jordan Jumaian					27%					
OPT Al-Rafi Palestinians Haj-Yahia&Tam	46% for M&F	20%+	13%+	25%	22%	15%+	8%+	12%+	5%+	
Lebanon Usta et al. WHO			18% 20%				15% 15%			
North Africa										
Egypt Afifi et al.					8% for M&F Males Higher					
Morocco Alami&Kadri					9% (13%)					

The recruitment, transportation, transfer, or receipt of persons by means of threat or force or other forms of coercion, abduction, fraud, deception, abuse of power or abuse of a position of vulnerability, or of the giving or receiving of payments or benefits in order to gain the consent of a person having control over another person for the purpose of exploitation.63

جدول يبين أهم معلومات بشأن التوقيع وتصديق الدول على اتفاقية حقوق الطفل و البروتوكول بشأن اشتراك الأطفال في المنازعات المسلحة و البروتوكول بشأن بيع الأطفال واستغلالهم في البغاء وفي إنتاج المواد الإباحية.

الدولة	الطفل حقوق اتفاقية	المسلحة المنازعات في الأطفال اشتراك بشأن البروتوكول	الإباحية المواد إنتاج وفي البغاء في واستغلالهم الأطفال بيع بشأن البروتوكول	النفاذ حيز الدخول تاريخ
الأردن	تصديق	توقيع	توقيع	23-6-1991
الإمارات	انضمام		–	2-2-1997
البحرين	انضمام	انضمام	إقرار	14-3-1992
تونس	تصديق	تصديق	مصادقة	29-2-1992
الجزائر	تصديق		انضمام	16-5-1993
جيبوتي	تصديق	توقيع	انضمام	5-1-1991
السعودية	انضمام		توقيع	25-2-1996
السودان	تصديق	تصديق	إقرار	2-9-1990
سوريا	تصديق	انضمام	–	14-8-1993
الصومال	توقيع	توقيع	إقرار	–
العراق	انضمام		–	15-7-1994
عمان	انضمام	انضمام	–	8-1-1997
فلسطين			إقرار	–
قطر	تصديق	انضمام	–	3-5-1995
جزر القمر	تصديق		إقرار	21-7-1993
الكويت	تصديق	انضمام	إقرار	20-11-1991
لبنان	تصديق	توقيع	مصادقة	13-6-1991
ليبيا	انضمام	انضمام	إقرار	15-5-1993
مصر	تصديق	انضمام	إقرار	2-9-1990
المغرب	تصديق	تصديق	مصادقة	21-7-1993
موريتانيا	تصديق		انضمام	15-6-1991
اليمن	تصديق	انضمام	إقرار	31-5-1991

Donors for Causes Fighting Gender-Based Violence

1. ABILIS Foundation
2. Astraia Female Leadership Foundation
3. CBD Charitable Trust
4. Channel Foundation
5. Comic Relief
6. Diakonia

7. Europe AID
8. Foundation for Women's Health Research and Development (FORWARD)
9. Global Fund for Women
10. Greenbaum Foundation
11. Harry Frank Guggenheim Foundation
12. International Federation of Human Rights (FIDH)
13. Mama Cash
14. Sigrid Rausing Trust
15. Relief International

Networks

1. The Coalition for Adolescent Girls
2. The Female Genital Cutting Education and Networking Project
3. Gender and Development Network
4. Gender-Based Violence Area of Responsibility
5. Girls Not Brides
6. MenEngage
7. Safe World Community
8. Western Cape Network on Violence Against Women
9. Women Against Violence Europe

Resources

1. ISPCAN's World Perspectives on Child Abuse, Sixth and Seventh Editions.
2. Third National Report on the Situation of Children in Lebanon. 1998–2003
3. The MENA Regional Consultation on Violence against Children. Cairo. June 2005.
4. UNICEF. 2002. The Situation of Egyptian Children and Women: A Rights-based Analysis. Cairo.
5. UNICEF. 2003. The Situation of Children, Youth, and Women in Jordan. Amman.
6. The International Committee for the Rights of Child meeting, Geneva, June 2006.
7. The UNGS report on VAC, Paulo Sergio Pinheiro, 2007.
8. International Bureau for Children's Rights (IBCR). MENA newsletter. March 2009.
9. The EU Guidelines on Children and Armed Conflict. 2003.
10. The four Geneva Conventions of 1949 and its two Additional Protocols of 1977, the Rome Statute of the International Criminal Court (1998) Security Council resolutions devoted to CAAC: 1261 (1999); 1314 (2001); 1379 (2001); 1460 (2003); and 1539 (2004).

11. http://www.unicef.org/infobycountry/yemen_57968.html
12. http://www.yementimes.com/defaultdet.aspx?SUB_ID=35838
13. www.seyaj.org
14. http://www.crin.org/resources/infodetail.asp?id=24403
15. http://www.amnesty.org/en/news-and-updates/un-urged-put-human-rights-first-middle-east-2011-03
16. http://www.dailystar.com.lb/article.asp?edition_id=1&categ_id=5&article_id=126,514#axzz1IZ5JIZoV
17. http://www.middle-east-online.com/english/?id=45083
18. http://www.amnesty.org/en/news-and-updates/report/evidence-bahraini-security-forces%E2%80%99-brutality-revealed-2011-03-16
19. http://www.hrw.org/en/news/2011/03/29/bahrain-investigate-deaths-linked-crackdown
http://www.alarabiya.net/views/2011/03/30/143546.html
20. http://search.ft.com/search?queryText=Kuwait+shows+revolution%E2%80%99s+nuances&aje=true&dse=&dsz=
21. http://www.un.org/apps/news/story.asp?NewsID=37674&Cr=libya&Cr1=
22. http://www.irinnews.org/report.aspx?reportid=92313
23. http://af.reuters.com/article/topNews/idAFJOE72L03J20110322
24. http://www.ottawacitizen.com/business/Oman+protests+carry+despite+sultan+reforms/4516118/story.html
25. http://www.thedailynewsegypt.com/region/as-protests-near-saudi-borders-king-offers-money.html
26. http://www.hrw.org/en/news/2011/03/27/saudi-arabia-arrests-peaceful-protest-rise
27. http://www.hrea.org/index.php?base_id=2&language_id=1&headline_id=13000
28. http://www.time.com/time/world/article/0,8599,2060788,00.html?xid=rss-fullworld-yahoo
29. http://english.aljazeera.net/indepth/opinion/2011/03/201132113479124674.htmlpp. 29–30
30. http://news.bbc.co.uk/2/hi/6497799.stm
31. http://www.yapi.org/csec/

The manufacturer's authorised representative in the EU is Springer Nature Customer Service Centre GmbH, Europaplatz 3, 69115 Heidelberg, Germany. If you have any concerns regarding our products, please contact ProductSafety@springernature.com

Printed and bound by CPI Group (UK) Ltd, Croydon, CR0 4YY
30/09/2026
02225246-0020